Cancer of the Liver, Esophagus, and Nasopharynx

Edited by Gustav Wagner and You-Hui Zhang

With 46 Figures and several Tables

Springer-Verlag Berlin Heidelberg NewYork
London Paris Tokyo

Professor Dr. med. Gustav Wagner

Deutsches Krebsforschungszentrum
Im Neuenheimer Feld 280
D-6900 Heidelberg 1, FRG

Professor Zhang You-Hui

Director, Cancer Institute and Hospital
Chinese Academy of Medical Sciences
Pan Jia Yao
Zuo Anmen Wai
Beijing, P. R. China

Sponsored by the Federal Ministry for Science and Technology, Bonn, and Behringwerke A. G., Marburg

ISBN-13:978-3-540-16967-3 e-ISBN-13:978-3-642-71510-5
DOI: 10.1007/978-3-642-71510-5

Library of Congress Cataloging in Publication Data.
Cancer of the liver, esophagus, and nasopharynx.
Proceedings of the Chinese-German Symposium on Cancer of the Liver, the Esophagus, and the Nasopharynx, held in Heidelberg, July 3-5, 1985, and sponsored by the German Cancer Research Center.
Includes index. 1. Liver-Cancer-Congresses. 2. Esophagus-Cancer-Congresses. 3. Nasopharynx-Cancer-Congresses. 4. Cancer-China-Congresses. I. Wagner, Gustav. II. Zhang, You-Hui.
III. Chinese-German Symposium on Cancer of the Liver, the Esophagus, and the Nasopharynx (1985: Heidelberg, Germany)
IV. Deutsches Krebsforschungszentrum Heidelberg. [DNLM: 1. Esophageal Neoplasms-congresses. 2. Liver Neoplasms-congresses. 3. Nasopharyngeal Neoplasms-congresses. WI 735 C215 1985]
RC280.L5C36 1986 616.99'436 86-26029
ISBN-13:978-3-540-16967-3 (U.S.)

2119/3020-543210

List of Contributors

Bannasch, P.

Institut für Experimentelle Pathologie, Deutsches Krebsforschungszentrum,
D-6900 Heidelberg, FRG

Bornkamm, G. W.

Institut für Virologie, Zentrum für Hygiene der Universität,
D-7800 Freiburg, FRG

Chen Ai-Mei

Cancer Institute, Sun Yat-Sen University of Medical Sciences,
Guangzhou, PRC

Chen Han

Changhai Hospital of the Second Military Medical College,
Shanghai, PRC

Chui Shao-Xing

Cancer Institute, Chinese Academy od Medical Sciences,
Beijing, PRC

De Thé, G.

Laboratoire d'épidémiologie et immunologie des tumeurs, Faculté de médecine Alexis Carrel
F-69372 Lyon, Cédex 08, France

Dhom, G.

Pathologisches Institut des Saarlandes,
D-6650 Homburg/Saar, FRG

Dong Zhi-Wei

Beijing Institute of Cancer Research, Dept. of Biochemistry and Molecular Biology,
Beijing, PRC

Ebbers, J.

Hals-, Nasen- und Ohrenklinik der Universität,
D-4000 Düsseldorf, FRG

Fang Ru-Kang

Huatung Teschers University,
Shanghai, PRC

Feng Luo
Cancer Institute, Chinese Academy of Medical Sciences,
Beijing, PRC

Freytag von Loringhoven, A.
Herwarthstraße 25
D-5300 Bonn, FRG

de Villiers, E.-M.
Deutsches Krebsforschungszentrum,
D-6900 Heidelberg, FRG

Gao Ru-Nie
Shanghai Cancer Institute, Dept. of Epidemiology,
Shanghai 200032, PRC

Gu Biu-Chang
Shanghai Medical Laboratory,
Shanghai, PRC

Gu Jian-Ren
Dept. of Biochemistry and Molecular Biology, Shanghai Cancer Institute,
Shanghai, 200032, PRC

Gu Xiang-Zhi
Cancer Institute and Hospital, Chinese Academy of Medical Sciences,
Beijing, PRC

He Li-Ji
Cancer Hospital, Yangcheng County, Shanxi Province,
Taiyuan, PRC

Hecker, E.
Biochemisches Institut am Deutschen Krebsforschungszentrum,
D-6900 Heidelberg, FRG

Hong Jing-Xing
Shanghai Cancer Institute, Dept. of Immunology and Cell Biology,
Shanghai 200032, PRC

Hu Li-Fu
Shanghai Cancer Institute, Dept. of Biochemistry and Molecular Biology,
Shanghai 200032, PRC

Huang Guo-Chun
Cancer Institute and Hospital, Chinese Academy of Medical Sciences,
Beijing, PRC

Huang Yu-Long
Chongming County Center Hospital
Chongming Island, PRC

Jiang Ji-Wen
Dept. of Hygiene Chemistry, Hunan Medical College,
Changsha, PRC

Li Chen-Chuan
Tumor Hospital and Cancer Institute, Sun Yat-Sen University of Medical Sciences,
Guangzhou, PRC

Li Guang-Weng
Vice President, Chinese Anti-Cancer Association,
Tianjin, PRC

Li Jun-Yao
Cancer Institute, Chinese Academy of Medical Sciences, Dept. of Epidemiology,
Beijing, PRC

Li Zhen-Pu
Beijing Institute of Cancer Research, Dept. of Biochemistry and Molecular Biology,
Beijing, PRC

Liang Hao-Cai
Wuhan Medical College, Unit of Cancer Epidemiology,
Wuhan 430033, PRC

Liang Yi-Ren
Cancer Institute, Sun Yat-Sen University of Medical Sciences,
Guangzhou, PRC

Liu Yu-Gu
Wuhan Medical College, Dept. of Environmental Toxicology,
Wuhan 430033, PRC

Lu Jiang-Bang
Dept. of Epidemiology, Henan Cancer Institute,
Zheng Zhou, PRC

Lu Shih-Hsin
Cancer Institute, Chinese Academy of Medical Sciences,
Beijing, PRC

Montesano, R.
International Agency for Research on Cancer,
F-69372 Lyon, France

Muñoz, N.
International Agency for Research of Cancer,
F-69372 Lyon, France

Pan Jie-Ping
Shanghai Municipal Anti-epidemic Station,
Shanghai, PRC

Preußmann, R.

Institut für Toxikologie und Chemotherapie, Deutsches Krebsforschungszentrum,
D-6900 Heidelberg, FRG

Rabes, H.M.

Pathologisches Institut der Universität,
8000 München, FRG

Rajewsky, M.F.

Institut für Zellbiologie, Universität Essen,
D-4300 Essen, FRG

Rimkus, K.

Pathologisches Institut des Saarlandes,
D-6650 Homburg/Saar, FRG

Saffhill, R.

Paterson Laboratories, Christie Hospital and Holt Radium Institute,
Manchester M20 9BX, UK

Shanmugaratnam, K.

University Department of Pathology, General Hospital,
Singapore 0316

Tang Zhao-You

Shanghai First Medical College, Zhong Shan Hospital, Liver Cancer Research Unit,
Shanghai 200031, PRC

Tu Ji-Tao

Shanghai Cancer Institute, Dept. of Epidemiology,
Shanghai 200032, PRC

Umbenhauer, D.

Dept. of Biochemistry, Vanderbilt University School of Medicine,
Nashville, TN 37232, USA

Vosteen, K.H.

Hals-, Nasen- und Ohrenklinik der Universität,
D-4000 Düsseldorf, FRG

Wagner, G.

Institut für Dokumentation, Information und Statistik des Deutschen
Krebsforschungszentrums,
D-6900 Heidelberg, FRG

Wahrendorf, J.

International Agency for Research on Cancer,
F-69372 Lyon, France

Wan Da-Feng

Shanghai Cancer Institute, Dept. of Biochemistry and Molecular Biology,
Shanghai 200032, PRC

Wan Wen-Hui

Beijing Institute of Cancer Research, Dept. of Biochemistry and Molecular Biology,
Beijing, PRC

Wang Ru-Kuan

At present Deutsches Krebsforschungszentrum, Institut für Dokumentation,
Information und Statistik,
D-6900 Heidelberg, FRG

Wei Shu-Min

Beijing Institute of Cancer Research, Dept. of Biochemistry and Molecular Biology,
Beijing, PRC

Wolf, H.

Max von Pettenkofer Institut der Ludwig-Maximilians-Universität, Molekulare und
Tumorbiologie,
D-8000 München, FRG

Wu Bo-Wen

Changhai Hospital of the Second Military Medical College,
Shanghai, PRC

Wu Meng-Chao

Changhai Hospital of the Second Military Medical College, Dept. of Hepatobiliary Surgery,
Shanghai, PRC

Wu Peng-Nian

Dept. of Epidemiology, Hunan Medical College,
Changsha, PRC

Xu Guang-Xiong

Shanghai Cancer Institute, Dept. of Epidemiology,
Shanghai 200032, PRC

Xu Guan-Nan

Changhai Hospital of the Second Military Medical College,
Shanghai, PRC

Xu Xiu-Lai

Beijing Institute of Cancer Research, Dept. of Biochemistry and Molecular Biology,
Beijing, PRC

Yang Bing-Hui

Shanghai First Medical College, Zhong Shan Hospital, Liver Cancer Research Unit,
Shanghai 200031, PRC

Yang Jia-Mei

Changhai Hospital of the Secondary Military Medical College,
Shanghai, PRC

Yao Kai-Tai

Cancer Research Laboratory, Hunan Medical College,
Changsha, PRC

Yao Xiao-Ping

Changhai Hospital of the Second Military Medical College,
Shanghai, PRC

Yu He

Shanghai Cancer Institute, Dept. of Epidemiology,
Shanghai 200032, PRC

Yu Song-Ling

Wuhan Medical College, Unit of Cancer Epidemiology,
Wuhan 430033, PRC

Yu Ye-Qiu

Shanghai First Medical College, Zhong Shan Hospital, Liver Cancer Research Unit,
Shanghai 200031, PRC

Zeng Yi

National Centre for Preventive Medicine, Institute of Virology,
Beijing 100052, PRC

Zerban, Heide

Institut für Experimentelle Pathologie am Deutschen Krebsforschungszentrum,
D-6900 Heidelberg, FRG

Zhang Dan-Hua

Chongming County Anti-epidemic Station,
Chongming Island, PRC

Zhang Ming-Shu

Cancer Institute, Chinese Academy of Medical Sciences,
Beijing, PRC

Zhang Yiao-Hua

Changhai Hospital of the Second Military Medical College,
Shanghai, PRC

Zhang You-Hui

Cancer Institute, Chinese Academy of Medical Sciences,
Beijing, PRC

Zhou Xiao-Han

Shanghai First Municipal Hospital,
Shanghai, PRC

zur Hausen, H.

Deutsches Krebsforschungszentrum,
D-6900 Heidelberg, FRG

Preface

To stimulate greater German-Chinese cooperation in the field of oncology, the German Cancer Research Center (DKFZ) carried through a "Chinese-German Symposium on Cancer of the Liver, the Esophagus, and the Nasopharynx" in Heidelberg from 3 to 5 July 1985. These three forms of cancer were chosen as they are extremely rare in Europe but some of the most frequently found forms in China. Almost half of the roughly 260000 cases of primary liver cancer occurring annually worldwide are Chinese; of the roughly 300000 esophagus cancers occurring annually, more than half are Chinese; nasopharyngeal cancer is roughly 100 times more frequent among Chinese people than in Caucasians.

Under these circumstances, it is not surprising that the Chinese guest speakers of the Heidelberg symposium - selected specialists in the three subsections of oncology mentioned - were able to report about extensive experiences with patient populations of a size hardly imaginable in Europe. The great clinical experience of the Chinese guests was supplemented by special contributions of European experts. Thus, this volume permits a topical survey of the state of the art in these three cancers, with subsections of epidemiology, pathology, and clinical treatment.

The editors wish to thank the Federal Ministry of Research and Technology (BMFT) for their encouragement and direct help in preparing and carrying through the symposium, the Management Board of the DKFZ for their generous assistance and Springer-Verlag for the publication and excellent production of this volume.

Heidelberg, Peking, October 1986

Gustav Wagner
Zhang You-Hui

Contents

III Cancer of the Esophagus

IV Cancer of the Nasopharynx

I Opening Presentation

Selenium as a Possible Chemopreventive Agent Against Cancer

Zhang You-Hui

Evidence has indicated that selenium as a trace element supplemented to a normal diet decreases tumor incidence in animals exposed to chemical carcinogens and in animals with a high tendency to develop spontaneous tumors. A striking example is that observed by Schrauzer and Ishmael [1] in which the incidence of mammary tumors afflicting 80% of aged C3H mice can be reduced to 10% by the long-term feeding of subtoxic levels of sodium selenite. This protective effect of selenium has naturally led people to think that selenium deficiency, on the other hand, would render the hosts susceptible to carcinogenic insults.

Epidemiological studies have indicated that this is indeed the case. According to recently published data from Yu and her associates [2], the blood selenium levels in man in 24 different regions in 8 provinces of China showed a close negative correlation to the age-adjusted mortality of cancers of all sites. This correlation was particularly marked for the three major types of cancers in China, i.e., cancer of the esophagus, stomach, and liver, which account for more than 60% of all cancer deaths. When the areas surveyed were divided into three categories according to the blood Se level of their inhabitants, significantly lower cancer death rates were observed in high-Se areas as compared with those in areas with medium and low Se levels (Fig. 1). In Qi-dong, a county with an exceptionally high mortality rate for primary liver cancer (PLC), an inverse correlation was observed between the blood Se level and the mortality rate when the analysis was made on the commune level

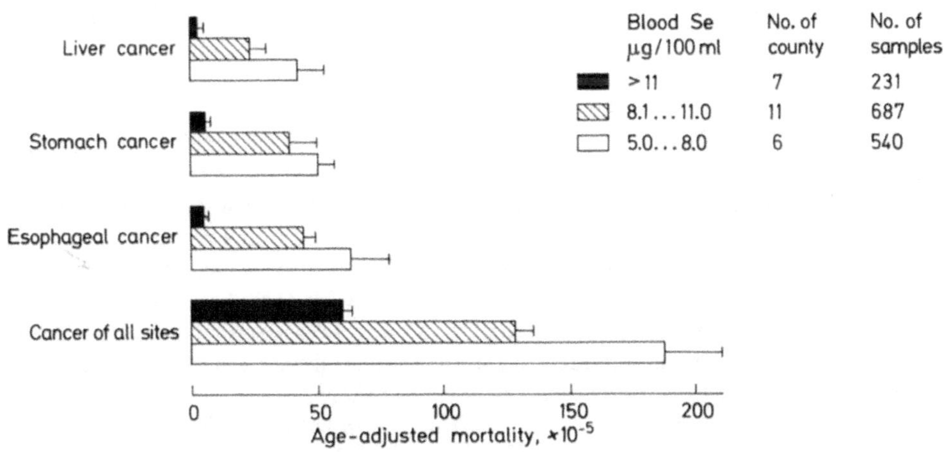

Fig. 1. Mortality of different cancers according to blood selenium levels

Cancer of the Liver, Esophagus, and Nasopharynx
Edited by G. Wagner and Zhang You-Hui

Table 1. Regional variation in the incidence of liver cancer and its relationship to selenium level [2]

Commune	Age-adjusted mortality rate ($\times 10^{-5}$)	Blood Se level (μg/100 ml)
San-jia	30.2	13.5
Dong-yuan	43.7	6.8
Wei-dong	51.9	4.4

Table 2. Correlation between mortality of liver cancer and selenium content in barley [2]

Age-adjusted mortality rate ($\times 10^{-5}$)	No. of communes	Se content (ppb)
>50	18	23.2 ± 5.1 (85)[a]
40–49	17	24.5 ± 8.0 (84)
30–40	5	29.8 ± 8.2 (25)
<20	3	63.1 ± 11.5 (15)

[a] No. of samples analyzed in parenthesis

(Table 1). The higher the mortality rate for PLC, the lower the blood Se level, and vice versa. When the Se content in barley was determined, such an inverse correlation was also noted (Table 2).

The possible mechanisms of Se as a cancer-protecting agent were studied from an immunological viewpoint. In the Lewis lung cancer (LLC) model in B6 mice, it was found that LLC was very weak in immunogenicity since spleen cells both from tumor-bearing mice and from mice with tumor resected could not be induced in a secondary mixed lymphocyte tumor cell culture (MLTC) to become cytotoxic to LLC in an in vitro isotope ([^{125}I]UdR) release assay. Nevertheless, if the mice were given 2 ppm sodium selenite in the drinking water after tumor resection, the spleen cells not only showed high natural cytotoxicity but were induced in MLTC to become highly cytotoxic to LLC (Fig. 2).

Owing to the difficulty of inducing cytotoxic T-lymphocytes (CTLs) in primary MLTC, a mixed lymphocyte culture (MLC) was adopted to explore how Se affects CTL induction. In MLC, spleen cells from B6 mice (H-2^b) were stimulated with mitomycin C-treated spleen cells from Balb/c mice (H-2^d) in a responder to stimulator (R/S) ratio of 10 to 1. The activity of the allospecific CTLs generated in MLC was tested using [^{125}I]UdR-prelabeled target cells with H-2^d haplotype, NS-1 and P815. The allospecific CTLs so induced led to 45%–47% specific lysis of target cells. When sodium selenite at a concentration of 100 ng/ml was added to the MLC, the percentage specific lysis increased to 61%–64% (Table 3).

Thus, Se significantly enhances CTL induction in MLC, but it was not known if this is a result of an activation of the accessory cell function of the adherent cell population. Spleen cells were then depleted of adherent cells by nylon-wool column filtration. When the nylon-wool nonadherent spleen cells were stimulated with

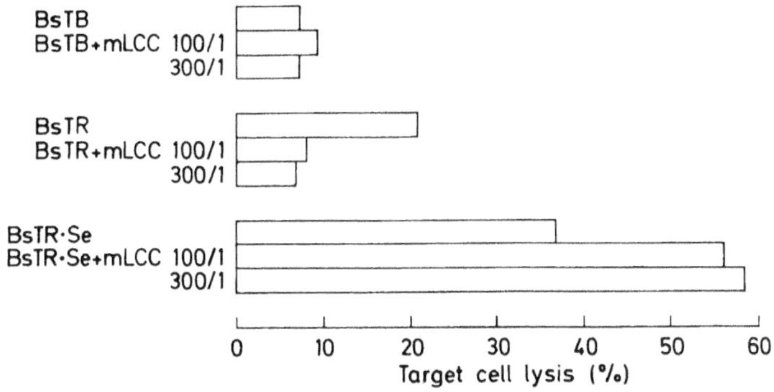

Fig. 2. Effect of selenium on the generation of cytotoxic T cells against LLC in MLTC. BsTB, spleen cells of B6 mice with transplanted LCC; BsTR, spleen cells of B6 mice with transplanted LCC resected; BsTR Se, spleen cells of B6 mice with LCC resected and with supplemented Na_2SO_3 (2 ppm) in drinking water. In vitro cytotoxicity assayed by the release of isotope from [125 I] UdR-labeled LCC

Table 3. Effect of selenium on the generation of allospecific cytotoxic T cells in MLC[a]

Cells cultured	% Cell lysis			
	NS-1		P815	
	100/1	30/1	100/1	30/1
Bs	11.8	-7.6	20	6.3
Bs + Se (100 ng/ml)	–	–	25.8	6.1
Bs + mCs (10/1)[b]	47.9	9.5	45.1	11.7
Bs + mCs (10/1) + Se (100 ng/ml)	61.8	28.0	64.3	32.7

[a] B6 (H-2^b) spleen cells (Bs) cocultured with mitomycin-treated Balb/c (H-2^d) spleen cells (mCs)
[b] Responder to stimulator ratio

mitomycin C-treated allogeneic spleen cells, no CTLs were generated. CTLs reappeared, however, if the MLC was reconstituted with splenic adherent cells from normal B6 mice. This result indicates that the induction of allospecific CTLs in MLC necessitates the participation of splenic adherent cells in the responder cell population as accessory cells. If splenic adherent cells from B6 mice fed with sodium selenite were used for the reconstitution, the cytolytic activity of CTLs was further enhanced (Table 4). Nonetheless, splenic adherent cells from normal B6 mice treated in vitro with phorbol myristic acetate (PMA) failed to restore CTL induction when nonadherent spleen cells were allostimulated. These data are in favor of the view that the accessory cell function can be modulated and Se and PMA have just the opposite effect.

Now there is consensus that the mechanism of action of accessory cells is to present antigen to T-lymphocytes. Therefore, the effect of Se on antigen presentation by splenic adherent cells was also studied. The experimental system used was the lymphoproliferative response of trinitrochlorobenzene (TNCB)-primed T cells stimulated in vitro with TNP-conjugated splenic adherent cells. When adequate

Table 4. Effect of selenium in vitro on the accessory cell function of splenic adherent cells in MLC[a]

Cells cultured	% Cell lysis	
	100:1	30:1
NABs + mCs (10/1)	10	7
NABs + mCs + AdBs (20/1)	45	25
NABs + mCs + AdSeBs[b] (20/1)	59	40
NABs + mCs + AdPMABs[c] (20/1)	-6	4.5

[a] Nonadherent spleen cells from B6 mice (NABs) were obtained by glass adherence and passing through a nylon-wool column twice. Adherent spleen cells (AdBs) were collected from spleen cells adhered to glass surface
[b] Splenic adherent cells were obtained from B6 mice with supplemented Na_2SO_3 (1 ppm) in the drinking water for 11 days
[c] Splenic adherent cells were treated with phorbol myristate acetate (100 ng/ml) for 2 h

Table 5. Effect of selenium in vitro on antigen presentation by splenic adherent cells[a]

Responder to stimulator	T-cell proliferation[b]				
	0	5	50	100	500 (ng/ml)
4/1	1	2.06	2.09	1.29	1.18
4/2	1	1.45	1.83	–	1.10

[a] TNP-primed T-cell-enriched lymph node cells were stimulated with TNP-conjugated splenic adherent cells in vitro
[b] Measured by [^{3}H]TdR incorporation, taking those untreated with selenium as unity

Table 6. Effect of selenium in vitro on antigen presentation by splenic adherent cells[a]

Responder to stimulator	T-cell proliferation			
	0	500	1000	5000 (ng/ml)
4/1	1	3.11	3.02	1.99
4/2	1	2.39	3.15	1.28

[a] TNP-primed T cell-enriched lymph node cells were stimulated in vitro with TNP-conjugated splenic adherent cells. Splenic adherent cells were treated in vitro with different doses of Na_2SO_3 for 2 h and then washed

amounts of Se were added to the in vitro system, an increase in T-cell proliferation was observed. When sodium selenite was present throughout the 3-day culture period at concentrations of 5–50 ng/ml, lymphocyte proliferation was doubled (Table 5). If the splenic adherent cells were pretreated with sodium selenite for 2 h and then thoroughly washed, a more marked increase in T-cell proliferation occurred. The incorporation of [^{3}H]TdR was three times as high as that of the untreated control (Table 6).

Table 7. Effect of selenium on IL-1 secretion by P388D$_1$ cells

P388D$_1$ cells	Thymocyte proliferation (cpm ± SD)[a]		
	No Con A	Con A	P
Not treated	200 ± 30	4765 ± 485	
Treated with LPS	207 ± 29	13744 ± 1204	< 0.05
Treated with LPS and Se	192 ± 27	22233 ± 1702	

[a] The mitogenic activity of culture supernatant of P388D$_1$ cells was assessed by thymocyte proliferation assay

Inasmuch as antigen presentation is a complex, multistep process, at this moment we have had only data concerning the effect on interleukin 1 (IL-1) secretion. A mouse macrophage cell line, P388D1, was used to examine its ability to produce IL-1 when treated in vitro with bacterial lipopolysaccharide (LPS). Mouse thymocyte proliferation assay was used to measure IL-1 activity in the culture supernatant. It was found that, when P388D1 cells were pretreated with Se, LPS induced more marked IL-1 secretion (Table 7). This is circumstantial evidence indicating that the augmentation of the antigen-presenting activity of Se might at least in part be mediated by an increase in IL-1 secretion.

We know that macrophages behave as antigen-presenting cells which actively participate in the induction of cell-mediated immunity, but they can also suppress T-cell-mediated immunity. This has been considered as a normal feedback mechanism in the down regulation of the T-cell response. However, excessive suppression by macrophages, as seen in tumor-bearing animals and in cancer patients, would diminish or repeal an effective T-cell-mediated response. We have been trying to modulate the macrophage-mediated suppression and have found that Se can abrogate the suppressive effect of macrophage in concanavalin A-induced lymphoproliferative assay (Table 8). When peritoneal exudate macrophages from normal mice were added to the culture, significant suppression of lymphocyte proliferation occurred. If, on the other hand, macrophages were from mice orally treated with sodium selenite, only moderate suppression was seen, even when the spleen cell to macrophage ratio was high (4:1). At a ratio of 8:1, the suppression by macrophages from Se-treated mice completely disappeared, whereas macrophages from untreated mice could induce 83.5% inhibition. It is interesting to see that, while Se-treated macrophages lost their suppressive activity to lymphocyte proliferation, their cytostatic and cytolytic effect on tumor cells was augmented. Peritoneal macrophages of Se-treated mice were found to have higher than normal reactivity to the macrophage-activating factor (MAF). When the macrophages were separated into different subpopulations by discontinuous gradient centrifugation on Percoll, the increased response to MAF was observed mainly in the low-density subset.

All above-mentioned experimental data provide convincing evidence indicating that the anticancer acitivity of Se has a profound immunological basis. Se is a very promising agent for the immunoprophylaxis of human cancer regardless of whether or not Se deficiency is present. But Se should be first used in low-Se regions with a

Table 8. Abrogation by selenium of macrophage-mediated suppression of Con A-induced T-cell proliferation[a]

Cells cultured		Cpm (mean ± SD)	Inhibition (%)
Bs		430 ± 102	
Bs + Con A (4 μg/ml)		11906 ± 1203	
Bs + Con A + BpEc			
Bs/BpEc	4/1	361 ± 84	97
	8/1	1923 ± 132	83.8
	16/1	4008 ± 111	66.3
Bs/SeBpEc	4/1	6774 ± 1090	43.1
	8/1	12027 ± 2222	-1.0
	16/1	11945 ± 2351	-0.3
SeBs		379 ± 70	
SeBs + Con A (4 μg/ml)		14258 ± 2010	

[a] Macrophages were collected from peritoneal exudate cells (PEC) from untreated mice or from mice supplemented with sodium selenite in drinking water (2 ppm)

Table 9. Selenium content of cereals [2]

Selenium given[a] (g/ha)	Selenium content (ppb)	
	Maize	Barley
0	11.3	20.6
0.5	46.3	–
1.0	65.8	132.7

[a] Sodium selenite in 20 kg water sprayed onto the leaves

high cancer rate as a simple measure of cancer control. Se supplementation can be achieved by increasing the Se content in the staple food. Sodium selenite solution sprayed onto the leaves of maize and barley increased their Se content six fold (Table 9). Prospective studies of the effect of Se supplementation on the incidence of PLC are being planned.

References

1. Schrauzer GN, Ishmael D: Effects of selenium and arsenic on the genesis of spontaneous mammary tumors in inbred C3H mice. Ann Clin Lab Sci 4 (1974) 441-447
2. Yu SY, Chu YJ, Gong XL et al.: Biol Trace Element Res 7 (1985) 21-29

II Cancer of the Liver

Epidemiology of Primary Liver Carcinoma

G. Wagner

For several reasons it is difficult to make exact statements about the epidemiology of primary liver cancer:

1. Differential diagnosis of the various liver tumors is rather difficult
2. There are no corresponding data from many countries
3. The coding of the various subgroups of category 155 of the International Classification of Diseases (ICD) differs from country to country, as Aoki [2] was able to show with the aid of the WHO databank
4. Comparisons of present with past epidemiology are difficult or even impossible because, up to the 8th Revision of the ICD, malignant tumors of the liver and the gallbladder or bile duct were combined under a common code number. Only since 1968 (8th Revision of the ICD) have malignomas of the liver (ICD No. 155) been differentiated from those of the gallbladder (ICD No. 156).

However, notwithstanding these limitations, there can be no doubt that the incidence rates of primary liver cancer fluctuate considerably throughout the world. While this tumor form is relatively rare in western industrial countries, liver cancer is one of the most frequent forms of cancer in parts of Africa, southeast Asia, and China. If we take the age-standardized incidence rates of men from *Cancer Incidence in Five Continents,* vol. IV [18] as a standard of comparison, we obtain the rank order presented in Table 1 for the most recent comparative worldwide figures for the period 1973-1977, with Hong Kong at the top (incidence rate = 34.4 per 100000), followed by Shanghai (31.7), Singapore Chinese (32.2), and Senegal (25.6).

In the early 1970s the figures from the former Rhodesian Cancer Registry of Bulawayo (today Zimbabwe) were still the highest worldwide, with rates of 64.6 per 100000 men and 25.4 per 100000 women. Unfortunately, the data from this registry are no longer represented in the latest volume of *Cancer Incidence in Five Continents,* which appeared in 1982. However, it is to be assumed that the high incidence rate in this area of central Africa will not have changed considerably.

According to estimates by Parkin et al. [11], 259000 cases of liver cancer were recorded in 1975 (182000 in men and 77000 in women); of these, 110000 cases (42.5%) were recorded for the People's Republic of China, 81000 men and 29000 women (44% and 37.7%, respectively, of all registered cases of primary liver cancer worldwide). Liver cancer takes eighth place worldwide (seventh place in men, ninth place in women) among all forms of cancer.

Table 1 differentiates between countries with an age-standardized incidence rate over 10.0 per 100000 and those with rates below 10.0 per 100000. The considerable difference in frequency between Asian and African countries on the one hand and the United States and Europe on the other hand is clearly shown. Rumania (registry

Cancer of the Liver, Esophagus, and Nasopharynx
Edited by G. Wagner and Zhang You-Hui

Table 1. Primary liver cancer – age-standardized incidence rates (world population) 1975. (Data from *Cancer Incidence in Five Continents*, vol. IV [18])

Male				Female			
> 10.0/100000		< 10.0/100000		> 5.0/100000		< 5.0/100000	
Hong Kong	34.4	Switzerland (Geneva)	9.7	Shanghai	9.1	Poland (Warsaw)	4.9
Singapore (Chinese)	32.2	Poland (Warsaw)	8.3	Senegal	9.0	Italy (Varese)	2.7
Shanghai	31.7	Italy (Varese)	6.9	Hong Kong	8.9	FRG (Hamburg)	1.6
Senegal	25.6	FRG (Hamburg)	3.6	Rúmania (Cluj)	7.9	Denmark	1.6
United States (Bay Area-Chinese)	18.1	Denmark	2.9	Singapore (Chinese)	7.1	FRG (Saarland)	1.5
United States (Los Angeles-Chinese)	12.0	FRG (Saarland)	2.4	Spain (Zaragoza)	5.1	Switzerland (Geneva)	1.3
Japan (Nagasaki)	11.9	United States (Los Angeles-White)	1.8			United States (Los Angeles-White)	0.8
Rúmania (Cluj)	11.8	U.K. (Birmingham)	1.4			U.K. (Birmingham)	0.4

in Cluj), with 11.8 per 100000 shows the highest European rate, while the lowest values are reported from England (registry in Birmingham, 1.4 per 100000).

In women, Shanghai with an incidence rate of 9.1 per 100000 and Senegal with 9.0 per 100000 are top worldwide; the lowest incidence (0.4 per 100000) is again reported from Birmingham.

As can be seen, the incidence rates in men are higher throughout; the sex ratio men: women fluctuates between 1.5:1 and 7.5:1. In both sexes the relationship between the highest and lowest incidence rates is roughly 25:1.

Since the diagnosis of a primary liver cancer is almost always made relatively late (about half the tumors have already metastasized at the time of diagnosis) and the survival times often only amount to months, mortality largely corresponds to incidence. The 5-year survival rate in the United States at the end of the 1960s was about 5%.

Within China several regions with high death rates from liver cancer can be recognized; in particular the region around Shanghai and in the south the region of Nanning show high rates according to the maps from the Chinese Cancer Atlas.

The regional comparison of death rates in the Federal Republic of Germany [4] shows a similar pattern for men and women. There is a tendency toward higher death rates in the Saarland, in Rhineland Palatinate, and in parts of Northrhine Westphalia as well as in the city states Hamburg, Bremen, and Berlin. However, the differences are not big enough to allow etiological conclusions to be drawn.

Temporal comparisons of the incidence or mortality of liver cancer are hardly possible, the reasons being classification difficulties and improvements in diagnostic methods. Moreover, up to a short time ago, secondary neoplasms located in the liver were also coded under ICD category 155 (liver carcinoma). Finally, up to the 7th Revision of the ICD, carcinomas of the liver and the gallbladder had been combined under No. 155. It is only since the 8th Revision that the ICD has differen-

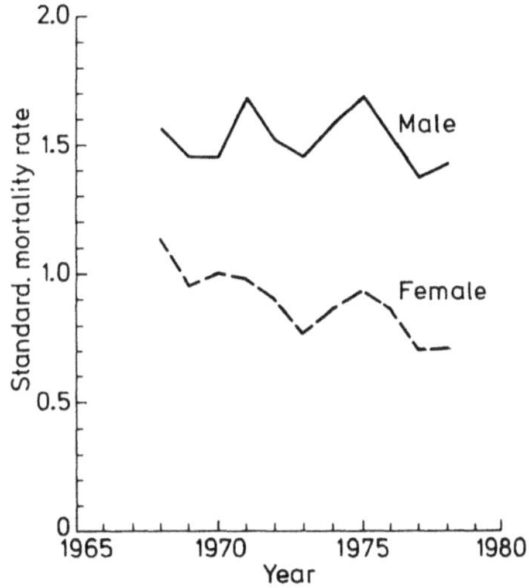

Fig. 1. Temporal trend of the age-adjusted mortality rates for men and women

tiated between No. 155 (liver cancer) and No. 156 (cancer of the gallbladder and bile duct).

It is, therefore, only since 1968 that, with the introduction of the 8th Revision of the ICD, trend analyses have become possible. Since then, however, primary liver tumors have not shown a noticeable decrease. The slight decrease in age-standardized mortality rates in the Federal Republic of Germany from 1968 to 1978 (Fig. 1) should be considered as a result of improved diagnostics and therapy.

In California the death rates from primary liver cancer in the white population from 1958 to 1969 remained about stationary (1.1/100000 and 1.05/100000 respectively); in the nonwhite population they rose from 1.2 to 1.6/100000. The reason for this is seen in an increased immigration of Chinese [8].

While in the countries with a low frequency of liver cancer the peak incidence lies in the higher *age groups,* the countries with a high frequency, particularly in Africa, show the highest incidence rates in the age range 35-45 years.

Primary liver cancer and liver cirrhosis occur at about the same age and with no obvious connection between each other, while in western countries cirrhosis is considered as a precursor lesion and mostly precedes cancer by several years.

Practically nothing is known about the part played by genetic factors in the development of primary liver cancer, although in all places where comparisons are possible Asian races show higher incidence and mortality rates than Caucasians (Table 2).

Etiology

The most essential etiological factors which have been discussed are alcohol, aflatoxins, and the hepatitis B virus. The *consumption of alcohol* and liver cirrhosis are closely related. Furthermore, it is not contested that cirrhosis patients are at a higher

Table 2. Age-standardized incidence rates in different groups in selected locations. (*Data from Cancer Incidence in Five Continents*, vol. IV [18])

Location and *Population groups*	Males	Females
Singapore		
Indian	14.0	4.8
Malay	17.1	3.1
Chinese	32.2	7.1
Hawai		
White	2.7	1.4
Chinese	7.8	3.1
Hawaiian	10.3	7.2
San Francisco Bay Area		
White	2.9	1.1
Black	3.9	1.8
Chinese	18.1	3.6
Los Angeles		
White	1.8	0.8
Black	3.8	0.9
Chinese	12.0	3.8
Atlanta		
White	2.6	0.9
Black	5.4	1.2
Detroit		
White	2.5	1.0
Black	4.5	1.8

risk of developing a primary hepatocellular carcinoma. If Popper [13] contends that 75% of all cases of liver cancer occur in cirrhosis patients, this seems somewhat exaggerated. At least, this should only be true for western countries, not, however, for the African and Asian countries where the carcinoma often develops in a noncirrhotic liver [16]. From an epidemiological point of view, it should be emphasized that in numerous countries high cirrhosis rates are not associated with high rates of liver cancer and vice versa and that cohort studies with alcoholics have not shown a high risk of primary liver cancer throughout, even if the risk of cirrhosis was markedly increased (e.g., [12, 14]). Of course, one can argue that the premature death of cirrhosis patients has the effect of a competing risk factor and that these patients do not develop liver cancer simply because they die before that can occur. Falk [6] assumes that changed metabolic processes and processes of detoxication, lack of protein, and a changed immune status along with an increasing alcohol consumption will contribute to an increased risk.

Since in England in 1966 a large number of poultry died from the so-called turkey X disease, attention was drawn to the mycotoxins, especially to *aflatoxin* produced by the fungus *Aspergillus flavus*, which occurs in particular in spoiled grain and mouldy nuts. In 1971 Alpert et al. [1] were able to show that the estimated intake of aflatoxin in the countries south of the Sahara was clearly correlated with the incidence of primary liver cell carcinoma. Although it soon became apparent that aflatoxins are highly effective liver carcinogens in primates and that there are many arguments in favor of a connection between the effect of aflatoxin and liver cancer, exact proof of such a causal relationship in man is still lacking. All the same, food legislation in many countries assumed such a connection. In the German food industry, aflatoxin controls are permanent, in particular in the processing of peanuts.

The proven associations justify intervention studies with the aim of preventing aflatoxin formation as far as possible by improved methods of harvesting, drying, and storage of endangered species of grain and nuts. In 1981 Linsell [9] reported on the plans of the IARC (Lyon) to carry through such intervention studies.

The most essential risk factor for primary liver carcinoma seems to be the hepatitis B virus (which will be discussed in greater detail in the following chapters). According to Kew et al. [7], the incidence of primary liver cell carcinoma runs parallel worldwide with the infection of the population with the hepatitis B virus. Beasley et al. [3] were able to show in their prospective study in Taiwan that HBsAg-positive men are at a 200 times higher risk of developing the disease than a HBsAg-negative control group of the same age. And Linsell [9] estimated the risk of hepatitis B patients of developing liver cancer to be higher than that of heavy smokers of developing lung cancer. "If (as seems likely) vaccination reduces carriers by 90%, and if neonates in Africa, South East Asia and China could be vaccinated, then nearly 200000 cases of cancer would be avoided each year" [10]. It is to be hoped that such intervention studies can be initiated in the African and Asian populations at risk in the next few years.

Since Bernstein et al. [5] first pointed to a possible connection between the intake of androgens and the development of benign and malignant liver tumors in 1971, numerous corresponding cases have been reported on. Up to 1976 11 cases of hepatocellular carcinomas in patients on contraceptives and 14 such cases in patients undergoing therapy with anabolics were reported.

While it was also possible to generate benign and malignant liver tumors with such substances in animal experiments, even if only with certain species of animals and with excessively high doses not used in man, evidence of a causal connection between the administration of contraceptives and anabolics respectively and the development of hepatocellular carcinomas is still missing [15].

In the German Thorotrast Study [17] carried out in the German Cancer Research Center, a total of 5000 patients treated with Thorotrast in the years 1930–1951 were followed up. Up to 1981, 256 cases of malignant liver tumors were observed among 1689 deceased Thorotrast patients, while among 1280 deceased controls only 2 liver cancers were found. Eighty-five percent of these tumors were carcinomas (preponderantly of the cholangiocellular type) and 25% were hemangiosarcomas. In four cases, there were sarcomas and carcinomas at the same time.

The shortest latency period with these tumors amounted to 16 years, the longest to more than 40 years. With an increasing accumulated Thorotrast doses there was a rise in the proportion of liver tumors.

In the short space at my disposal I have been able to give you but a brief insight into the epidemiology and etiology of primary liver cancer and to broach a few problems which will be presented in greater detail and from a more detailed scientific standpoint in the following chapters.

References

1. Alpert ME, Hutt MSR, Wogan GN et al.: Association between aflatoxin content of food and hepatoma frequency in Uganda. Cancer 28 (1971) 253-260
2. Aoki K: Cancer of the liver - international mortality trends. World Health Statist 31 (1978) 28-50
3. Beasley RP, Hwang LY, Lin CC, Chien CS: Hepatocellular carcinoma and hepatitis B virus. Lancet 1981, II, 1129-1132
4. Becker N, Frentzel-Beyme R, Wagner G: Krebsatlas der Bundesrepublik Deutschland - Altas of Cancer Mortality in the Federal Republic of Germany. Berlin Heidelberg New York Tokyo: Springer 1984
5. Bernstein MS, Hunter RL, Yachnin S: Hepatoma and peliosis hepatis developing in a patient with Fanconi's anemia. New Engl J Med 284 (1971) 1135-1136
6. Falk H: Liver. In: D. Schottenfeld and J. F. Fraumeni, Jr. (eds): Cancer Epidemiology and Prevention, pp 668-682. Philadelphia London Toronto: W. B. Saunders 1982.
7. Kew MC, Gear AJ, Baumgarten J et al.: Histocompatibility antigens in patients with hepatocellular carcinoma and their relationship to chronic hepatitis B virus infection in these patients. Gastroenterology 77 (1979) 537-539
8. Krain LS: Primary liver cancer in California. Oncology 28 (1973) 117-125
9. Linsell CA Liver cell cancer - intervention studies. J Cancer Res Clin Oncol 99 (1981) 51-56
10. Muir CS, Parkin DM: The world cancer burden: prevent or perish. Brit Med J 290 (1985) 5-6
11. Parkin DM, Stjernwärd J, Muir CS: Estimates of the worldwide frequency of twelve major cancers. Bull WHO 62 (1984) 163-182
12. Pell S, D'Alonzo CA: A five-year mortality study of alcoholics. J Occup Med 15 (1973) 120-125
13. Popper H: Hepatic cancers in man: quantitative perspectives. Environm Res 19 (1979) 482-494
14. Robinette CD, Hrubec Z, Fraumeni JFJr: Chronic alcoholism and subsequent mortality in World War II veterans. Amer J Epidemiol 109 (1979) 687-700
15. Scheuer A, Lehmann F-G: Lebertumoren bei Therapie mit Kontrazeptiva und Anabolika. Internist 18 (1977) 208-214
16. Theilmann L, Gmelin K: Das primäre Leberzellkarzinom. Klinikarzt 14 (1985) 169-172
17. Van Kaick G, Muth H, Kaul A et al.: Results of the German Thorotrast Study. In J. D. Boyce, J. F. Fraumeni, Jr. (eds): Radiation Carcinogenesis: Epidemiology and Biological Significance. New York: Raven Press 1984
18. Waterhouse J, Muir C, Shanmugaratnam K et al. (eds): Cancer Incidence in Five Continents, vol. IV. Lyon: IARC 1982

Epidemiology of Primary Liver Cancer in a West German Population: The Saarland

G. Dhom and K. Rimkus

Until now no study has been performed in the Federal Republic of Germany relating primary cancer of the liver to population data. The present study is based on data from the Saarland Cancer Registry. Furthermore, cases of primary liver cancer (PLC) were obtained from two Institutes of Pathology serving the same region, which has a population of one million.

The present study is based on 321 cases from the period 1967–1981. All cases without histological examination were excluded. The annual incidence of all liver carcinomas is 1.6, of hepatocellular carcinomas (HCC) only 1.2, and of cholangiocellular carcinomas (CCC) 0.3 per 100000 population. There is a sex ratio of 3:1 in HCCs, while CCCs show an equal distribution (Table 1).

During the 15 years of the study, we have noticed an increase in incidence of HCC from 1.1 to 1.4 and of CCC from 0.2 to 0.4 per 100000 (Tables 2, 3). It is

Table 1. Incidence (per 100000) of primary liver cancer in the Saarland

	No. of inhabitants 1967–1981	All liver cancer		HCC		CCC	
		No.	*I*	*No.*	*I*	*No.*	*I*
Men	513000	167	2.2	141	1.8	25	0.3
Women	567000	92	1.1	53	0.6	25	0.3
	1080000	259	1.6	194	1.2	50	0.3

Table 2. Changing incidence (per 100000) of HCC in the Saarland

Period	Σ		Men		Women	
	No.	*I*	*No.*	*I*	*No.*	*I*
1967–1971	59	1.1	49	1.9	10	0.4
1972–1976	57	1.1	39	1.5	18	0.6
1977–1981	78	1.4	53	2.1	25	0.9

Table 3. Changing incidence (per 100000) of CCC in the Saarland

Period	Σ		Men		Women	
	No.	*I*	*No.*	*I*	*No.*	*I*
1967–1971	12	0.2	6	0.2	6	0.2
1972–1976	17	0.3	8	0.3	9	0.3
1977–1981	21	0.4	11	0.4	10	0.4

Cancer of the Liver, Esophagus, and Nasopharynx
Edited by G. Wagner and Zhang You-Hui

Table 4. Crude incidence (per 100000) and age-standardized incidence rates (ASR) in the Saarland

	Period	No. of inhabitants	Liver cancer		
			No.	*I*	ASR
Total	1967-1981	1080000	259	1.6	1.1
Urban	1967-1981	382000	130	2.3	1.6
Rural	1967-1981	698000	129	1.2	0.9
Men	1973-1977	523000	60	2.3	1.7
Women	1973-1977	577000	38	1.3	0.9

Table 5. HB-S-AG-positive cells in liver cirrhosis in primary liver cancer (orcein staining)

	N	HB-S-AG+		HB-S-AG+ with cirrhosis		HB-S-AG+ without cirrhosis	
		(n)	(%)	*(n)*	(%)	*(n)*	(%)
HCC	38	12	31.6	10/29	34.5	2/9	22.2
CCC	17	0	-	0	-	0	-

remarkable that the increase in HCC is based on a significant increase in women ($P=0.05$). The entire population of the Saarland is almost one million, and there are only 5 cities with more than 40000 inhabitants. In these urban areas, an accumulation of PLC can be seen (Table 4). Although on average only 30% of the whole population live in these 5 cities, 50% of all carcinomas were found there.

Among the autopsy patients with HCC, 88.3% had liver cirrhosis. The proportion of CCC with cirrhosis is much lower: 28.3%. Histological specimens of liver tissue from 38 HCC and 17 CCC patients were stained with orcein for the presence of hepatitis B surface antigen. In 12 cases (31.6%) of HCC, orcein-positive cells were found (Table 5), with cirrhosis in 10/29, without cirrhosis in 2/9. Chronic alcoholism was the cause of cirrhosis in 10 cases (12%) of HCC and in 2 cases of CCC.

The proportion of 31.6% HBS-AG-positive liver cirrhosis with HCC in the Saarland is a rate within the upper range in Europe. Only in one case were orcein-positive tumor cells in HB-S-AG-positive cirrhosis seen.

Risk Factors of Primary Liver Cancer in the High Prevalence Area Chongming County; Results from a 5-year Follow-up

Tu Ji-Tao, Gao Ru-Nie, Zhang Dan-Hua, Gu Bin-Chang, Xu Guan-Xiong, Fang Ru-Kang, Pan Jie-Ping, Yu He, Huang Yu-Long, and Zhou Xiao-Han

Primary liver cancer (PLC) ranks third among all cancer sites in the People's Republic of China and causes at least 100000 deaths per year. High mortality areas are concentrated in the east to south coastal region, including many coastal islands [7]. To identify the risk factor(s) responsible for the high rate is of interest.

Chongming Island is one of the high prevalence areas for PLC in China, with an age-adjusted (world standard) mortality rate of PLC for 1974–1978 of 50.8 per 100000 in males and 17.0 in females. It is a long and narrow coastal island situated at the outlet of the Yangtze river (Changjiang). The PLC mortality rate was significantly higher in the eastern than the western part of the island, and higher among commune members than among small town residents [4].

The specific aim of this prospective cohort study is to identify the risk factors responsible for the high PLC rate in Chongming Island. The possible role of hepatitis B virus (HBV) infection, exposure to aflatoxin B1, contaminated water, cigarette smoking, alcohol consumption, and the family PLC history were studied.

Preliminary results of the first 5 years (1980–1984) follow-up are presented.

Study Subject and Method

All males over 40 years of age living in 4 communes with different PLC rates were considered as potential study subjects. Two of these communes were located in the eastern part and the others in the western part of the island; 12222 men (98% of all eligible subjects) participated in the study.

Serum samples collected from each study subject were tested for HBV markers, HBsAg by reverse passive hemagglutination (RPHA), anti-HBs by passive hemagglutination (PHA), and anti-HBc by the immune adherence hemoagglutination (IAHA) method. Subjects who were positive for either HBsAg (with or without anti-HBs) and/or anti-HBc (without anti-HBs) were considered HBV carriers.

Samples of different kinds of cooked staple foods randomly collected from the families of the study subjects were tested for aflatoxin B1 contamination by the method of thin layer chromatographic assay.

Data for sources of drinking water, cigarette smoking, amount of maize consumption, alcohol habits, and family PLC history were collected by trained "barefoot doctors" using a standard questionnaire.

Primary liver cancer cases were found in the Chongming Cancer Registry. Data on all cases were reviewed by Drs. Tu and Gao at the end of each follow-up year.

Cancer of the Liver, Esophagus, and Nasopharynx
Edited by G. Wagner and Zhang You-Hui

Study subjects were stratified on the basis of their age group, HBV status (carrier or not), and exposure history of other risk factors under study. The PLC incidence rate for each group was computed by using cumulative person years as a measure. The age distribution of all study participants was used as a standard for calculating the age-adjusted rates. Differences between rates were analyzed statistically by the chi-square test [8].

Results

One hundred and six PLC cases developed within the 5-year follow-up period. The association of PLC with the different risk factors under study was as follows.

Monofactor Analysis. The results of the monofactor analysis are summarized in Table 1.

Hepatitis B Virus Infection. Of the 12222 study subjects, 1971 (16.1%) were identified as HBV carriers, and 64 of the 106 PLC cases developed among HBV carriers. The age-adjusted incidence rate of PLC in HBV carriers was 699.0 per 100000 person-years, which was 8 times higher than in noncarriers (86.9). The difference was statistically significant.

Sources of Drinking Water. Six main types of water were used as drinking water by the study participants; they are house ditch, field ditch, field well, kitchen well, river, and tap water. The water in the house ditch and the field well was rain water and permeated through the soil. It was separated from the flowing river water: thus it was stagnant water. The field ditch was temporarily connected with the river; it was semistagnant water. The river on Chongming Island is a small tributary of the Yangtze river; it flows from west to east and south to north. The source of the tap water was the flowing river. The kitchen well was a small and shallow (about 2 m deep from the surface of the earth) well dug in the kitchen room for private drinking. In order to avoid the disturbing influence of changing water types, the analysis of drinking water types was restricted to those who had drunk one type of water consistently through the previous 30 years. The PLC incidence rates of those drinking from house ditch (272.0) and field well water (254.6) were significantly higher than those drinking from river water (117.1) and tap water (103.6). No study participants entered the kitchen water group, because this type of water source began to be used only in 1974.

Maize Consumption (Aflatoxin B1 Consumption). It is difficult to examine the aflatoxin B1 consumption of each study participant directly. In 1981–1983, we collected different kinds of cooked staple food (maize, wheat, and rice) from 435 families (4% of the participating families) and examined them for aflatoxin B1 contamination. As reported from other PLC high-prevalence areas in China, maize was also more heavily contaminated in Chongming. Results showed that aflatoxin B1 contamination was three and five times higher with maize than with wheat and rice, respectively. Thus, we took the amount of maize consumed as a crude measure of aflatoxin B1 ingested. The amount of maize consumed in 4 different years (1949, 1958, 1967, and 1979) was recorded for each study subject, and an average annual amount was calculated. Study subjects were stratified into groups according to their average

Table 1. The relationship of various factors with PLC

Factor	PLC incidence		RR		HBV carrier rate (%)
	Cases	Rates			
HBV infection					
Noncarrier	42	86.9	1.0		
Carrier	64	699.0	8.0**		
Drinking water					
Tap water	2	103.6	1.0		16.20
River water	13	117.1	1.1	1.0	17.94
Field ditch water	9	184.1	1.8	1.6	19.33
Field well water	9	254.6	2.5*	2.2**	15.72
House ditch water	12	272.0	2.6*	2.3**	15.96
Maize consumption					
No	4	89.2	1.0		18.21
Yes	102	191.4	2.1*		15.85
Average amount of maize consumed					
15 kg/year	19	349.2	3.9**		16.55
45 kg/year	52	170.8	1.9		16.10
75 kg/year	29	180.5	2.0		15.11
105 kg/year	2	124.7	1.4		16.41
Cigarette smoking					
Nonsmoker	32	156.7	1.0		15.92
Smoker	74	199.1	1.3		16.31
Number of cigarettes smoked					
<300/year	8	78.0	0.5		16.93
300–599/year	23	176.7	1.1		15.19
⩾600/year	43	232.9	1.5**		16.83
Alcohol drinking					
Nondrinker	77	197.9	1.0		16.06
Drinker	29	156.4	0.8		16.24
Family PLC history					
Negative	102	173.0	1.0		15.91
Positive	4	268.2	1.6		24.91

* $P<0.05$; ** $P<0.01$

annual amount of maize consumed, and the PLC adjusted incidence rate for each stratum was calculated. Although the PLC incidence rate of the four maize-consuming groups was higher than that of those who had not eaten any maize within the previous 30 years, only those who ate 15 kg/year had a rate significantly higher not only than that of the non-maize-consumers but also than that of those who ate 45 kg, 75 kg, and 105 kg.

Cigarette Smoking. The percentage of current smokers among the 106 PLC cases was 69.8%, near that of the total study subjects (64.7%). The PLC incidence rate increased with the amount of cigarettes smoked, but only heavy smokers (exceeding 600 cigarettes/year) had a rate significantly higher than the nonsmokers.

Alcohol Consumption. Residents of Chongming Island prefer to drink a kind of locally made fermented rice wine. The PLC incidence rate of the drinkers (156.4) was 20% lower than that of the nondrinkers; the difference was not statistically significant.

Family Primary Liver Cancer History. The difference between the rates of those who had a family PLC history (268.2) and those without such a history (173.0) was not big enough to draw any conclusions.

The HBV carrier rates of each group are listed in the right column of Table 1. From the results mentioned above, the relative risk (RR) of HBV carriers to noncarriers was much higher than that of other factors. Thus, the RR of other factors might be confounded if the HBV carrier rate was much higher or lower among compared groups. A statistically significant difference of HBV carrier rates among compared groups was only found between those who had or had not a family PLC history.

Bifactor Analysis

Since the HBV carrier status was the most important risk factor for PLC, we divided all study participants into two major subgroups - HBV carriers and noncarriers - and then compared the role of other factors within the same subgroup. The results of the bifactor analysis are summarized in Table 2.

Noncarrier Subgroup. The differences of PLC incidence rates between those who drink different types of water, smokers and nonsmokers, alcohol drinkers and nondrinkers, and between those with or without a family PLC history were not statistically significant. The PLC incidence rates of those who consumed different amounts of maize showed the same pattern as seen in the monofactor analysis. The results suggested that all the factors studied, other than HBV infection, did not play an independent role in the development of primary liver cancer.

HBV Carrier Subgroup. The results from this subgroup showed a different pattern than that seen in the noncarrier subgroup. Differences in the PLC incidence rates between those who drink house ditch water and field well water and those who drink river water and tap water not only existed but were large. The RRs of those who drink field well water and house ditch water to those drinking river water was 4.0 and 3.5 and to those drinking tap water 7.8 and 6.8, respectively. Cigarette smokers had a higher rate than nonsmokers. Furthermore, as the amount of cigarettes smoked increased, so did the trend in rates. As we had found in the monofactor analysis and in the noncarrier subgroup, the PLC incidence rate of those who consumed $\geqslant$ 15 kg maize/year was significantly higher than of all other strata in this category.

Relative Risks of HBV Carriers to Noncarriers in Different Categories. Regardless of which factor we used to stratify the study participants, the PLC incidence rates of HBV carriers in different categories were all significantly higher than those of noncarriers. The relative risk of carriers to noncarriers was 2.5 in those who drunk the tap water, which increased to 13.9 and 21.4 in those who drunk house ditch water and field well water respectively.

Table 2. The relationship of various factors with PLC among HBV carriers and noncarriers

Factor	HBV carriers				Noncarriers			RR[c]
	Cases[a]	Rate[b]	RR		Cases	Rate	RR	
Drinking water								
Tap water	1	182.1	1.0		1	73.9	1.0	2.5
River water	7	355.8	2.0	1.0	6	64.5	0.9	5.5
Field ditch water	5	540.2	3.0	1.5	4	103.6	1.4	5.2
House ditch water	9	1232.2	6.8*	3.5**	3	88.5	1.2	13.9
Field well water	7	1428.4	7.8*	4.0**	2	66.7	0.9	21.4
Maize consumption								
No	3	322.1	1.0		1	31.3	1.0	10.3
Yes	61	736.9	2.3		41	91.0	2.9	8.1
Average amount of maize consumed								
15 kg/year	7	1550.8	4.8**		12	301.6	9.6**	5.1
45 kg/year	34	712.9	2.2		18	69.5	2.2	10.3
75 kg/year	18	705.8	2.2		11	81.0	2.6	8.7
105 kg/year	2	1037.7	3.2		0	0.0		
Cigarette smoking								
Nonsmoker	16	489.4	1.0		16	95.0	1.0	5.2
Smoker	48	802.4	1.6**		26	83.2	0.9	9.6
Amount of cigarettes smoked								
<300/year	8	460.4	0.9		0	0.0		
300-599/year	14	710.3	1.5		9	86.9	0.9	8.2
≥600/year	26	951.4	1.9**		17	99.1	1.0	9.6
Alcohol drinking								
Nondrinker	45	733.1	1.0		32	97.9	1.0	7.4
Drinker	19	640.2	0.9		10	63.7	0.7	10.1
Family PLC history								
Negative	60	680.8	1.0		42	88.6	1.0	7.7
Positive	4	1072.0	1.6		0	0.0		

[a] Number of PLC cases
[b] Age-adjusted incidence rate of PLC
[c] PLC incidence rate of HBV carriers to noncarriers
* $P<0.05$; ** $P<0.01$

Discussion

There are plenty of scientific reports concerning the causal factors of primary hepatocellular carcinoma. Strong evidence from many case-control and cohort studies conducted in China [1, 5, 12] suggests that HBV infection is related to PLC, but the PLC mortality rate does not always run parallel to the HBsAg carrier rate in the population studies [3]. The uneven geographical distribution of PLC in China and the inconformity of HBV carrier rates to PLC rates among populations in different parts of this country suggested that there should be other risk factors in the high prevalence areas. Research for other risk factors for PLC is of importance, since it may lead to another way of cutting down the PLC incidence rate to a certain level even before the planned HBV vaccination will become effective.

Results of our 5-year follow-up indicate that HBV infection is important for PLC. The PLC incidence rate in HBV carriers was 8.0 times higher that in noncarriers in the monofactor analysis. When the study participants were divided into different small groups according to their exposure to other factors, HBV infection consistently showed its role in the development of PLC. This means, no matter what the environment was, that the effect of HBV infection always persisted. Thus, we believe that HBV infection is the strongest risk factor for PLC in Chongming Island.

But the problem of why Chongming Island has a much higher PLC mortality rate than many other counties in China and why the PLC mortality rate of eastern Chongming Island is significantly higher than that of western Chongming Island remains unsolved. As shown in Table 3, study participants living in Kongyan, a commune situated in the eastern part of this island, had the highest PLC incidence rate but the lowest HBV carrier rate. The PLC incidence rates between subjects living in different communes showed no statistical differences among noncarriers but among HBV carriers; the PLC rate of those who lived in Kongyan commune was significantly higher than that of the other three communes. Thus, there should be other risk factors which interact with HBV infection, responsible for the high PLC incidence rate in Chongming, especially in the eastern part of Chongming Island.

Another finding from our study is that the drinking of field well water and house ditch water was another important risk factor for PLC. Study participants who drank house ditch water or field well water had a significantly higher PLC incidence rate than those who drank river water and tap water among HBV carriers. The RR of carriers to noncarriers was 2.5 among those who drank tap water and 5.5 among those who drank river water; it increased to 13.9 and 21.4 among those who drank house ditch water and field well water, respectively. These findings lead to some interesting ideas: (1) hepatocarcinogenic substance(s) should exist in these two types of stagnant water, (2) those hepatocarcinogenic substances do not act independently but interact with HBV infection, and (3) without the interactive effect of the hepatocarcinogenic substances in stagnant water the role of HBV infection in

Table 3. Hepatitis B virus carrier rate and PLC incidence rate of the study subjects living in different communes

Commune	HBV carrier rate (%)	Age-adjusted PLC incidence rate			RR[a]
		Total	Carrier	Noncarrier	
Kongyan	13.7[b]	223.0[c]	1077.4[d]	88.6	12.2
Baozhen	15.1	146.2	537.8	77.7	6.9
Sanxing	18.1	182.1	521.9	106.8	4.9
Miaozhen	18.6	158.5	618.8	60.1	10.9

[a] PLC rate of the HBV carriers to noncarriers
[b] Significantly lower than Sanxing and Miaozhen commune
[c] Significantly higher than Baozhen Commune
[d] Significantly higher than the other three communes

PLC will be limited to a lower level. The synergetic effect of HBV infection and hepatocarcinogenic substances in stagnant water might be the cause of the high incidence of PLC in Chongming Island and could be used to illustrate the geographical distribution of PLC in this island.

Professor Su suggested that hepatocarcinogenic substances existed in stagnant water - ditch water in Qidong and Haimen County - and that the PLC incidence rate dropped by changing to a relatively safe water after a 5-year period [9]. Part of our study participants had changed their drinking water 12 years (from house ditch, field ditch, and river water to field well water) or 5 years (from house ditch, field ditch, and river water to kitchen well water) before the beginning of our prospective cohort study. Examining the change in PLC incidence among these participants will be worthwhile.

Results from previous case-control studies suggested that cigarette smoking was an independent risk factor for PLC among non-HBV carriers [10, 13]. In our study, the PLC incidence rate of nonsmokers was 10% higher than that of smokers in non-HBV carriers, while among HBV carriers the PLC rate of smokers was significantly higher than that of nonsmokers. Cigarette smoking might be another, but not important, co-risk factor for PLC.

Based on the viewpoint of geographical epidemiology, Wang [11] compared the data of aflatoxin B1 contamination of maize and peanuts with the PLC mortality rates reported from different parts of China and found a positive correlation between them. Reports indicated that maize was more severely polluted by aflatoxin B1 than rice wheat in many PLC high-risk areas, and PLC mortality rates of the production brigades (communes) increased with the amount of maize produced or the average amount of maize allotted to each commune member [2]. But the result of a case-control study conducted in the same high-risk area showed that the aflatoxin B1 contamination was the same in the food samples collected from the case families and the noncase families [6]. In our study, we found many times that the exact amount of maize consumed by each study participant differed from the average amount of maize allotted to them. Many of the study participants fed their chicken and pigs with the maize or sold it on the open market. We found that part of the study subjects consumed only half or less than half of the amount of maize allotted, but they experienced the same or an even higher PLC rate than those who consumed the total amount of maize. Another fact we found is that the place where people grow maize instead of rice is usually poor in fresh water supply. The adjustment of the types of water drunk by each study subject in different maize consumption groups is necessary for the identification of the relationship of maize consumption and PLC.

In conclusion, the preliminary results of the 5-year follow-up of our prospective cohort study on the risk factors of PLC in Chongming Island indicate that a synergetic interaction of HBV infection and the hepatocarcinogenic substances existing in stagnant water (field well water and house ditch water) is responsible for the high PLC incidence in Chongming Island. The effect of cigarette smoking and maize consumption (aflatoxin B1 intake) should be further examined by multifactor analysis. Thus, vaccination with HBV vaccine and improvement of the quality of the drinking water should be adopted as the measure for primary prevention of PLC at the present time.

References

1. Beasley RP: Hepatocellular carcinoma and hepatitis B virus. Lancet 1981 II: 1129-1133
2. Cancer Research Team, Guangxi Medical College: Research on primary liver cancer incidence and risk factors. Medical Information, Guangxi Medical College, 1972. (In Chinese)
3. Cancer Research Team, Guangxi Medical College: Hepatitis B virus markers among populations in different PLC prevalence areas. Selected paper on liver cancer control and research, 1978, pp. 132-143. (In Chinese)
4. Gao RN, Tu JT, Gao YT: Preliminary report on epidemiologic research for primary liver cancer in Chongming County. Tumor 1 (1981) 148-151. (In Chinese)
5. Liu JH: Liver cancer and hepatitis B virus. Qidong Liver Cancer 1981, 17ff. (In Chinese)
6. Liu ZH: Investigation on the AFB1 contamination of the staple food collected from the case- and non-case-families in different PLC prevalence areas. Fuxui Liver Cancer Res. 1983, 42ff. (In Chinese)
7. National Cancer Control Office, Nanjing Institute of Geography: Atlas of Cancer Mortality in the People's Republic of China. Beijing: China Map Press 1979
8. Rothman KJ, Boice JD: Epidemiologic Analysis with a Programmable Calculator. NIH Publ. No. 79-1649. Washington, D.C.: U.S. Government Printing Office
9. Su DL: Drinking water and liver cell cancer. Chin. med. J. 92 (1979) 748-756
10. Trichopoulos D, MacMahon B, Sparros L et al.: Smoking and hepatitis B-negative primary hepatocellular carcinoma. J. nat. Cancer Inst. 65 (1980) 111-114
11. Wang YB: Relationship between the geographical distribution of liver cancer and the aflatoxin. Tumor 1 (1981) 193ff. (In Chinese)
12. Xu JP: Association between hepatitis B virus and primary hepatocellular carcinoma. Tumor 1 (1981) 33-37. (In Chinese)
13. Yu MC, Mack T, Hanisch R et al.: Hepatitis, alcohol consumption, cigarette smoking, and hepatocellular carcinoma in Los Angeles. Cancer Res. 43 (1983) 6077-6079

Cytopathology and Pathogenesis of Primary Liver Tumors*

P. Bannasch and Heide Zerban

Current concepts on the etiology of primary liver tumors have been discussed in other chapters of this volume [64]. It is evident from these discussions that, in addition to some chemicals, infection with hepatitis B virus (HBV) may play an important role in the development of human hepatocarcinoma. A strong statistical correlation between the incidence rate of hepatocarcinoma and HBV infection has indeed been observed in many countries [20, 30, 59]. However, this strong association has not been seen universally. Lack of correlation in geographical distribution of primary hepatocellular carcinoma and HBV infection has previously been described for a number of countries, such as Mozambique [31, 53], Egypt [25], Kenya [43], China [24], and the Asian Republics of the USSR [50]. More recently, Melbye et al. [41] reported on the basis of a long-term study in Greenland that they found a low incidence of primary hepatocarcinoma despite a high prevalence of HBsAg. Thus, our understanding of the etiology of human hepatic tumors is as yet rather incomplete. In addition, the precise pathogenetic mechanism by which HBV infection might lead to a neoplastic transformation of the hepatocytes is far from clear [61].

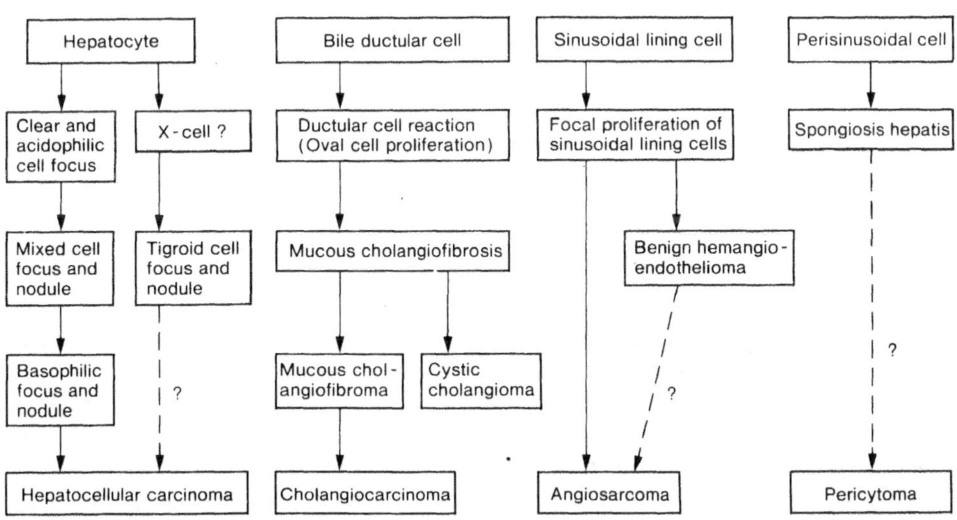

Fig. 1. Schematic presentation of sequential cellular changes in the development of epithelial and mesenchymal liver tumors

* Dedicated to Prof. Hans-Werner Altmann on the occasion of his seventieth birthday

Cancer of the Liver, Esophagus, and Nasopharynx
Edited by G. Wagner and Zhang You-Hui

Our knowledge of the pathogenesis of primary liver tumors is mainly based on investigations of experimental models, especially the rat liver treated with various chemical carcinogens. We learned from these studies that hepatocarcinogens may have at least four different types of target cells in the liver, namely the hepatocytes, the bile ductular epithelia, the sinusoidal, and the perisinusoidal cells (Fig. 1). All of these cell types may be specifically altered by the carcinogen and give rise to tumors or tumor-like lesions [7] such as hepatocellular carcinomas, cholangiocarcinomas, angiosarcomas, and pericytomas. Sequential cellular changes have been observed during the development of most of these tumor types. The detailed analysis of the different steps of tumorigenesis has considerably improved our understanding of the pathogenesis of primary liver tumors.

Hepatocellular Tumors

Hepatocellular carcinomas induced in rats by chemical carcinogens show fundamentally the same histology and cytology as the corresponding human tumors. They are usually composed of basophilic cells which are poor in glycogen. The tumors grow in trabecular, adenoid or solid formations and may be combined with liver cirrhosis.

For more than 100 years the association between liver cirrhosis and carcinoma has dominated the discussion on the pathogenesis of this tumor type [3, 32], although it had been known for a long time that human hepatic tumors may occur without any concomitant cirrhosis [33, 42, 56, 71]. A number of experiments in rats have clearly shown that the combination of cirrhosis and carcinoma as induced by chemicals depends on the dose and duration of treatment (see Bannasch [6] for literature). Fibrosis and cirrhosis develop in addition to hepatocellular carcinomas only after continuous application of high doses, which induce considerable necrotic parenchymal change, predominantly in acinuscentral parts of the liver lobule. After administration of low doses, which do not produce significant liver cell fibrosis and cirrhosis, hepatocellular tumors develop independently of liver fibrosis and cirrhosis. While there seems to be no direct causal relationship between liver cirrhosis and liver carcinoma, cirrhosis might certainly modify the action of oncogenic agents on the liver parenchyma (e.g., by eliciting DNA synthesis in hepatocytes by regenerative stimuli). Some authors have speculated that liver cirrhosis might be especially important in the frequent association of chronic liver disease due to viral hepatitis B with hepatocarcinomas in humans. However, Okuda et al. [49] concluded from a comparative study of the histopathology and frequency of hepatitis B markers that the generally held view that hepatocarcinoma in a noncirrhotic liver is caused by nonviral carcinogens and that hepatocarcinoma arising from a background of cirrhosis is due to hepatitis B virus seems untenable. Chemicals for which epidemiological studies suggested an involvement in the development of human hepatic tumors are the aflatoxins, arsenic, and combined oral contraceptives [63]. The possible interaction between chemicals and viruses in the neoplastic transformation of hepatocytes was discussed at this meeting by Tu et al. [64].

During the past 20 years, putative preneoplastic foci of altered hepatocytes have been described in different species after administration of various chemical carcinogens (for recent reviews see [11, 17, 27, 55, 68, 71]). From our own experimental experience and observations in other laboratories, we inferred that an ordered pattern of sequential metabolic cellular changes is followed during hepatocarcinogenesis [11, 17]. When we detected years ago in rat liver treated with nitrosomorpholine that the glycogen-poor hepatocellular carcinomas originated from foci storing glycogen in excess, this appeared to be a paradox [5]. In the meantime, many findings have been reported which are in favor of a sequence of cellular changes leading from the glycogenotic cells to hepatoma cells poor in glycogen, but rich in ribosomes (Fig. 1). As demonstrated only recently by microdissection and biochemical microanalysis, the early preneoplastic foci contain, on average, 100% more glycogen than the normal liver parenchyma [3]. In tissue sections stained with H & E, the glycogen storage cells appear clear or acidophilic (Tables 1, 2). The acidophilia is due to an additional proliferation of the smooth endoplasmic reticulum. The preneoplastic clear or acidophilic glycogen storage foci persist even after withdrawal of the carcinogen for weeks and months and may progress through mixed and basophilic cell foci to adenomas (neoplastic nodules) and carcinomas. This sequence has been adopted for the classification of preneoplastic liver lesions of the rat [17, 58] and appears also to be applicable to other species [7, 68]. It is important to realize, however, that under certain conditions, especially after repeated administration of high doses of one or several hepatocarcinogens, reversible foci and nodules may develop which resemble the persistent lesions in their cytology and cytochemical pattern [36, 43, 48, 60].

The biological significance of these reversible changes has not been clarified up to the present. Farber [27] emphasized that resistance to cytotoxicity of chemical carcinogens is a feature of the cell populations within reversible nodules. This type of hepatic nodule does not appear to be comparable to regenerative nodular hyperplasia as defined in human pathology. Whereas the hepatocytes in human livers usually show a phenotype which is very close to the normal state [2], the cells of the experimentally induced nodules in question are characterized by a pronounced reversion-linked phenotypic instability which is hardly compatible with the concept of a mere regenerative hyperplasia [13]. On the other hand, Thung and Gerber [62] classified human hepatic nodules as nodular "regenerative" hyperplasia which exhibited enzymatic changes similar to those observed in experimental animals.

In experimental pathology confusion with the hitherto poorly understood reversible type of lesions can be avoided by using "stop experiments" in which behavior of the preneoplastic cell populations and their progression toward neoplasms is followed after withdrawal of the carcinogen [5]. We used this experimental approach

Table 1. Morphological phenotype and classification of foci of altered hepatocytes

Type of focus	Glycogen	SER	RER/ribosomes	Mitosis
Clear cell foci	+++	+	+	+
Acidophilic cell foci	+++	++(+)	+	+
Intermediate cell foci	++	+(+)	++	++
Tigroid cell foci	(+)	+(+)	++(+)	++(+)
Basophilic cell foci	–	–	+++	+++
Mixed cell foci	Mixed	Mixed	Mixed	Mixed

SER, smooth endoplasmic reticulum; RER, rough endoplasmic reticulum

Table 2. Schematic presentation of the sequential cellular changes during hepatocarcinogenesis induced in rats by stop experiments with N-nitrosomorpholine

Stages	Cell populations		Cytology		
			Glycogen	Ribosomes	Mitoses
1	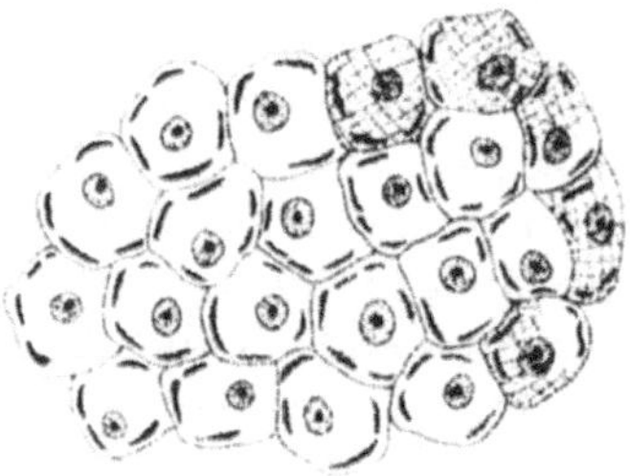	Clear and acidophilic	+ + +	+	+
2	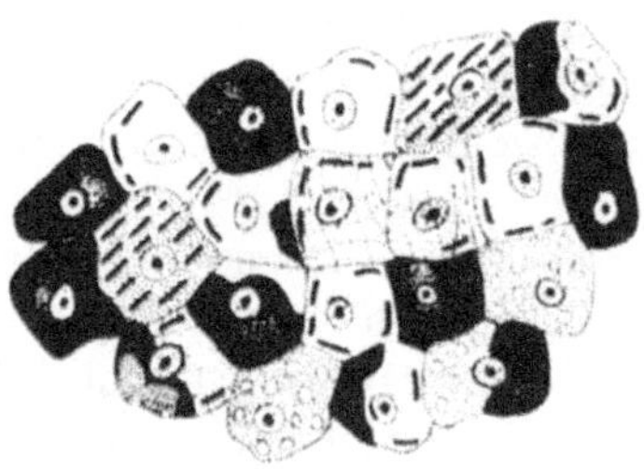	Mixed	+ +	+ +	+ +
3	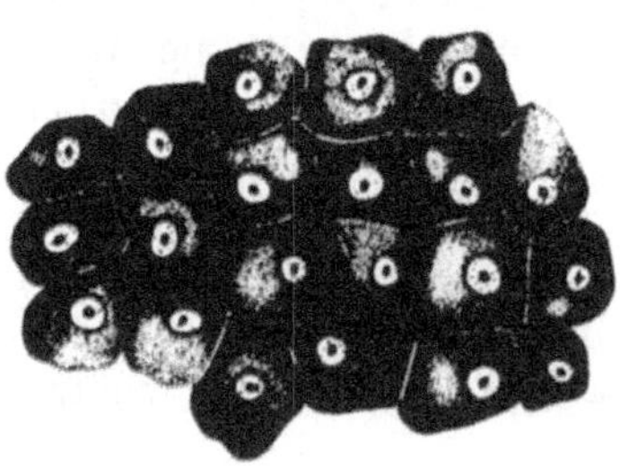	Basophilic	O	+ + +	+ + +

to study the dose dependence and sequential development of the different cell populations morphometrically in rats treated for 7 weeks with N-nitrosomorpholine (NNM) given in the drinking water in concentrations of 80, 120, 160, and 200 mg/liter [45]. The majority of the foci emerged after cessation of the carcinogenic treatment. The sequence of cellular changes outlined was confirmed at all dose levels. The first appearance and the frequency of the different lesions proved to depend on the dose of the carcinogen in a way similar to the hepatic tumors developing later on. There was no indication of any reversibility under these experimental conditions. On the contrary, the foci became larger and acquired phenotypic markers closer to neoplasia without further action of the carcinogen.

The cytomorphological and cytochemical changes described are usually closely related to a great variety of alterations in the activity of enzymes, including those of the carbohydrate metabolism [11, 17, 27, 44, 55]. Some of these enzymatic changes have also been observed in focal or nodular lesions of the human liver [28, 62, 65]. We were especially interested in the enzymes of the alternative pathways of carbohydrate metabolism and investigated by enzyme histochemistry and biochemical microanalysis some important enzymes in glycogen storage foci, neoplastic nodules, and hepatocellular carcinomas in rats treated with NNM. One of the earliest changes observed in glycogen storage foci is a reduction in the activity of the adenylate cyclase which plays an important role in the regulation of different metabolic pathways, including that of carbohydrate metabolism [26]. Some weeks after the appearance of the first glycogen storage cells, the majority of the pronounced glycogen storage foci show, in addition to this alteration, decreased activity of glycogen phosphorylase and of glucose-6-phosphatase, while the activity of glucose-6-phosphate dehydrogenase, the key enzyme of the pentose phosphate pathway, increases [29]. More detailed quantitative studies of the glucose-6-phosphate dehydrogenase revealed that there is a gradual increase in enzyme activity from the small glycogenotic foci, which show only a tendency to higher values, via the large glycogenotic to mixed cell foci [37]. The development of neoplastic nodules and hepatocellular carcinomas from the foci is associated with additional enzyme histochemical changes: the reduction of the glycogen initially stored in excess is usually correlated with an increase in the activity of the glycolytic enzyme glyceraldehyde-3-phosphate dehydrogenase, while that of the glucose-6-phosphate dehydrogenase remains high [29]. A considerable increase in the activity of glucose-6-phosphate dehydrogenase, which was combined with an enhanced cholesterol synthesis, has recently also been detected by means of biochemical methods in nodules induced with the Solt/Farber procedure [38]. These results agree with the hypothesis that the molecular changes underlying the glycogenosis might trigger an adaptation of cellular enzymes which could gradually redirect the carbohydrate metabolism toward other metabolic pathways, such as glycolysis and the pentose phosphate pathway [11]. The results of the cytochemical investigations in situ are also in line with many earlier biochemical findings in transplantable hepatomas, especially with the molecular correlation concept of Weber [70]. The tigroid cell foci (Fig. 1), which have been described as a variant of preneoplastic hepatic foci [8], and the intermediate cell foci induced in infant mice by a single dose of diethylnitrosamine [66] are not preceded by an obvious hepatocellular glycogenosis but show enzymatic changes in the alternative pathways of carbohydrate metabolism similar to the other types of preneoplastic liver lesions.

Some observations in humans suggest that the sequence of cellular changes in man and experimental animals is in principle identical [11]. Thus, foci of clear or acidophilic (ground glass) cells storing glycogen in excess have occasionally been found in the livers of patients bearing multicentric hepatocellular carcinomas [1]. The predominance of glycogen-rich cells in many adenomas and in clear cell carcinomas of the liver is well known [1, 12, 72]. According to Wu and colleagues, the clear cell variety of hepatocarcinoma may also develop in patients with persistent hepatitis B virus infection. An even more interesting aspect of human pathology pertinent to our experimental results is the appearance of hepatic tumors increasingly reported in patients suffering from inborn hepatic glycogenosis, mostly that of the von Gierke type (see [11, 34] for literature). Liver tumors could be detected by scintigrams, ultrasonograms, biopsies, or autopsies in many patients with this genetically fixed disease. Whereas the tumors were relatively rare in the 1st decade of life, they appeared in all patients who survived adolescence. Histologically, both adenomas and carcinomas were diagnosed, and in some cases the clinical course of the disease suggested transformation from adenomas into carcinomas. The observations in humans lend further support to the hypothesis that the metabolic disturbance leading to the hepatocellular glycogenosis, which is probably fixed at the genetic level in both humans and experimental animals, might also be causally related to the neoplastic transformation of the hepatocytes [5, 11].

Cholangiocellular Tumors

In addition to hepatocellular tumors, virtually all types of cholangiocellular tumors known from human pathology may be induced in rats by chemical carcinogens [9]. The tumors develop in particular after application of high doses of carcinogens such as NNM, which produce pronounced necrotic alterations of the liver parenchyma. Under these experimental conditions, a very complex sequence of cellular changes occurs in which four distinct stages can be identified (Fig. 1). The changes of the bile duct epithelia start with a ductular (oval) cell reaction which may progress to cholangiofibrotic areas, benign cystic cholangiomas, cholangiofibromas, and eventually also cholangiocarcinomas. During the second stage of tumorigenesis, the ductular cell reaction proceeds to a mucous cholangiofibrosis looking like a scar at both the macroscopic and the microscopic level. Many ductular cells are converted into goblet cells storing and secreting abundant mucus substances which contain PAS-positive neutral glycoproteins and alcianophilic acid components. The production of mucopolysaccharides in proliferated bile ducts appears to be specific for carcinogenic liver intoxications [14, 22] and might be a phenomenon analogous to hepatocellular glycogenosis. According to Chou and Gibson [21], an accumulation of mucopolysaccharides might also play an important role in the development of human cholangiocellular tumors.

In rat liver, expansively growing tumors may originate from the mucous cholangiofibrosis after long lag periods. There are two possibilities: either benign cystic cholangiomas develop which no longer synthesize mucous substances, or the cholangiofibrosis progresses to a cholangiofibroma, which is characterized by an especially pronounced production of collagenous fibers and mucopolysaccharides. The cholangiofibroma does not metastasize, but it is potentially malignant and may transform into a cholangiocarcinoma. During this process, the excessive production of mucopolysaccharides gradually disappears again. While the pathogenesis of human polycystic disease of the liver shows many similarities to that of benign cystic cholangiomas in rodents [6, 14], little is known about possible early stages of cholangiocarcinoma in man [71].

In rat liver, cholangiocarcinomas and tumors composed of both hepatocellular and cholangiocellular components may also develop without passing a cholangiofibrosis as an early stage [7]. Some observations in humans favored the concept that tumors or tumor components with a cholangiocellular phenotype may not only develop from cells of the intrahepatic biliary system but also from hepatocytes which undergo metaplasia during neoplastic transformation [2]. Recently, this concept has been supported by detailed electron microscopic and cytochemical studies of adenoid formations in epithelial tumors induced in rat liver with nitrosomorpholine in our laboratory [54]. With all the methods used, tumor cells could be demonstrated which were characterized by fine structural and cytochemical features in between hepatocellular and cholangiocellular components. Whereas transitions between preneoplastic hepatic foci and tumors of this kind were frequently observed, no sequential or topographical relationship to bile duct proliferations or cholangiofibrosis could be detected. Thus, there appears to be sufficient evidence that cholangiocellular tumors may develop from both bile ductular cells and hepatocytes [2, 54]. An origin from hepatocytes is especially likely when a mixed hepato-cholangiocellular pattern is present.

Vascular Liver Tumors

Vascular liver tumors attract considerable interest in view of their recently increased incidence in man. They arise from the sinusoidal lining cells - namely the endothelial cells - and can be induced by chemical carcinogens in various animal species (for literature see [7, 51, 57]). Maltoni [40] produced angiosarcomas in rodent liver by exposure to vinyl chloride shortly before the association of this chemical with liver angiosarcomas was recognized in man [23, 39]. Thus, vinyl chloride represents an excellent example of a chemical that not only induces malignant tumors in both animals and man but also acts at the same site and hits the same type of target cells [51].

The pathogenesis of vascular liver tumors is also linked with characteristic cellular changes. The sequential histological alterations that occur during the morphogenesis of angiosarcomas in rodents and man show many similarities [51], but the antecedent fibrosis seen in human liver does not seem to play an important role in rodents.

The sinusoidal lining cells may give rise to three types of vascular lesions occurring after treatment with chemical carcinogens, namely peliosis hepatis, benign angiomas, and angiosarcomas. Peliosis hepatis is characterized by an irregular focal dilatation of the sinuses. The classification of this lesion as a neoplastic disease or a preneoplastic condition is controversial [15]. The lining sinusoidal cells may at best show some minor alterations such as nuclear enlargement. However, in Mastomys given single or twofold intraperitoneal injections of 10 or 5 mg/kg body wt. N-nitrosodimethylamine, Wayss et al. [69] were able to observe all transitions to unequivocal angiomas. It is especially interesting that anabolic androgenic steroids, which have been related to the liver-cell adenomas frequently developing in association with peliosis hepatis in man, may induce this lesion in rats, too [46]. In the nitrosamine-treated rodents, we observed transitions from benign angiomas to angiosarcomas after very long lag periods, but this seems to be the exception rather than the rule. Angiosarcomas induced in rat liver by NNM usually develop without a preceding benign prestage. The first sign of tumorigenesis observed in this case is a proliferation of highly atypical mesenchymal cells along the liver cell plates. These cells can be nicely demonstrated by antibodies to vimentin, the intermediate filaments characteristic for normal and neoplastic mesenchymal cells. This immunocytochemical method is not only very helpful in the sometimes difficult differential diagnosis of angiosarcomas and anaplastic hepatocellular carcinomas, but it also reveals that many cells of the angiosarcomas accumulate excessive amounts of vimentin filaments [18, 19]. These vimentin storage cells most probably correspond to the polyhedral cells described in human angiosarcomas by Popper and colleagues [52] and are pathognomonic for malignant mesenchymal liver tumors, especially the angiosarcomas. The cause of the accumulation of the intermediate filaments in sarcoma cells is not known. However, it may be speculated that metabolic aberrations similar to those which lead to the storage of polysaccharides or lipids in epithelial cells hit by chemical carcinogens might be responsible [19].

Spongiosis Hepatis and Pericytoma

Finally, the perisinusoidal cells may be the target of chemical carcinogens (Fig. 1). This cell type has only been clearly identified during the past 20 years and has variously been called Ito cell, lipocyte, or fat-storing cell [67]. The perisinusoidal cells are located between the sinusoidal lining cells and the hepatocytes and have been shown to be involved in the metabolism of vitamin A and most probably also in the production of collagen. In rat liver treated with hepatocarcinogens, these cells are considered to be the site of origin of a peculiar, hitherto largely neglected cyst-like lesion for which we proposed the descriptive term "spongiosis hepatis" [10, 16]. Under the light microscope, it is evident that the holes of the sponge are not lined by epithelial or endothelial cells. In contrast to peliosis, the multilocular formations of spongiosis are not filled with blood but with a finely flocculent material rich in acid mucopolysaccharides. Electron microscopic analysis of the spongiotic areas reveals that they are composed of cells which are very similar to fibroblasts and sometimes even to typical fat-storing cells. The fibroblast-like cells show extremely elongated cytoplasmic processes which form the walls of the spongy lesions and are usually observed in close association with a thick coat resembling a basement membrane. To our knowledge, spongiosis hepatis has not been recognized as a pathomorphological entity in other species. Only in a report of human hepatic adenomas that appeared in users of oral contraceptives has a picture been published showing spongiosis-like changes within an adenoma [47]. It is still unclear whether spongiosis hepatis should be considered as a preneoplastic or as a neoplastic liver lesion. However, during the past few years we have observed a considerable cell proliferation within spongiotic areas in some rats treated with NNM after long lag periods [16]. Apparently there were also transitions into malignant mesenchymal tumors which we classified as pericytomas. In man pericytomas of the liver have only rarely been described [2, 35]. With respect to the pathogenesis of this tumor type, it is of particular interest that our experimental results suggest that the accumulation of acid mucopolysaccharides within the spongiotic formations seems to disappear during transformation of spongiosis into pericytoma. If this surmise can be confirmed, the analogy between sequential alterations of carbohydrate metabolism during neoplastic transformation of epithelial liver cells and at least one type of mesenchymal liver cell should lead to more detailed studies of these metabolic aberrations.

References

1. Altmann H-W: Pathology of human liver tumors. In H. Remmer, H. M. Bolt, P. Bannasch et al. (Eds): Primary Liver Tumors, pp. 53-71. Lancaster: MTP Press 1978
2. Altmann H-W: Neubildungen der Leber. Verh. Dtsch. Krebs-Ges. 5 (1984) 423-435
3. Anthony PP: Precursor lesions for liver cancer in human. Cancer Res. 36 (1976) 2579-2583
4. Bagshawe AF, Gagengi DM, Camerson CH et al.: Hepatitis B_S antigen and liver cancer. A population based study in Kenya. Brit. J. Cancer 31 (1975) 581-584
5. Bannasch P: The Cytoplasm of Hepatocytes during Carcinogenesis. Berlin: Springer 1968. (Recent Results in Cancer Research, Vol. 19)
6. Bannasch P: Die Cytologie der Hepatocarcinogenese. In H. W. Altmann, F. Büchner, H. Cottier et al. (Hrsg.): Handbuch der allgemeinen Pathologie, Bd. 6, Teil 7, S. 123-276. Berlin: Springer 1975
7. Bannasch P: Strain and species differences in the susceptibility to liver tumor induction. In V. Turusov, R. Montesano (Eds): Modulators of Experimental Carcinogenesis, pp. 9-38. Lyon: IARC 1983. (IARC Scientific Publications, Vol. 51)
8. Bannasch P, Benner U, Enzmann H et al.: Tigroid cell foci and neoplastic nodules in the liver of rats treated with a single dose of aflatoxin B_1. Carcinogenesis 11 (1985) 1641-1648
9. Bannasch P, Benner U, Zerban H: Cholangiofibroma and cholangiocarcinoma, liver, rat. In T. C. Jones, U. Mohr, R. D. Hunt (Eds): Monographs on Pathology of Laboratory Animals, Digestive System, pp. 52-65. Berlin: Springer 1985
10. Bannasch P, Bloch M, Zerban H: Spongiosis hepatis. Specific changes of the perisinusoidal liver cells induced in rats by N-nitrosomorpholine. Lab. Invest. 44 (1981) 252-264
11. Bannasch P, Hacker HJ, Klimek F et al.: Hepatocellular glycogenosis and related pattern of enzymatic changes during hepatocarcinogenesis. Adv. Enzyme Reg. 22 (1984) 97-121
12. Bannasch P, Klinge O: Hepatozelluläre Glykogenose und Hepatombildung beim Menschen. Virchows Arch. Abt. A 352 (1971) 157-164
13. Bannasch P, Moore MA, Hacker HJ et al.: Potential significance of phenotypic instability in focal and nodular liver lesions induced by hepatocarcinogens. In H. Brunner, H. Thaler (Eds): Hepatology: A Festschrift for Hans Popper, pp. 191-209. New York: Raven Press 1985
14. Bannasch P, Reiss W: Histogenese und Cytogenese cholangiocellulärer Tumoren bei Nitrosomorpholin-vergifteten Ratten. Zugleich ein Beitrag zur Morphogenese der Cystenleber. Z. Krebsforsch. 77 (1971) 108-133
15. Bannasch P, Wayss K, Zerban H: Peliosis hepatis, rodents. In T. C. Jones, U. Mohr, R. D. Hunt (Eds): Monographs on Pathology of Laboratory Animals, Digestive System, pp. 110-115. Berlin: Springer 1985
16. Bannasch P, Zerban H, Fuegel M: Spongiosis hepatis, rat. In T. C. Jones, U. Mohr, R. D. Hunt (Eds): Monographs on Pathology of Laboratory Animals, Digestive System, pp. 116-123. Berlin: Springer 1985
17. Bannasch P, Zerban H, Hacker HJ: Foci of altered hepatocytes, rat. In T. C. Jones, U. Mohr, R. D. Hunt (Eds): Monographs on Pathology of Laboratory Animals, Digestive System, pp. 10-30. Berlin: Springer 1985
18. Bannasch P, Zerban H, Schmid E et al.: Liver tumors distinguished by immunofluorescence microscopy with antibodies to proteins of intermediate-sized filaments. Proc. nat. Acad. Sci. USA 77 (1980) 4948-4952

19. Bannasch P, Zerban H, Schmid E et al.: Characterization of cytoskeletal components in epithelial and mesenchymal liver tumors by electron and immunofluorescence microscopy. Virchows Arch. Abt. B 36 (1981) 139-158
20. Beasley RP, Hwang LY, Lin CC et al.: Hepatocellular carcinoma and hepatitis B virus. A prospective study of 22,707 men in Taiwan. Lancet 1981, II: 1129-1133
21. Chou ST, Gibson JB: The histochemistry of biliary mucins and the changes caused by Clonorchis sinensis. J. Path. 101 (1970) 185-197
22. Chou ST, Gibson JB: A comparative histochemical study of rat livers in alphanaphthyl-iso-thiocyanate (ANIT) and DL-ethionine intoxication. J. Path. 108 (1972) 73-83
23. Creech JL, Johnson MN: Angiosarcoma of liver in the manufacture of polyvinyl chloride. J. occup. Med. 16 (1974) 150-151
24. Delong S: The relationship of hepatitis B virus infection to hepatoma: Pros and Cons. In W. Szumeness, H. J. Alter, J. E. Maynard (Eds): Viral Hepatitis, pp. 253-259. Philadelphia: The Franklin Institute Press 1981
25. Editorial: Link beween hepatoma and hepatitis B. Brit. med. J. 1978, II: 718-719
26. Ehemann V, Mayer D, Hacker HJ et al.: Loss of adenylate cyclase activity in preneoplastic and neoplastic lesions induced in rat liver by N-nitrosomorpholine. Carcinogenesis 7 (1986) 567-573
27. Farber E: Precancerous steps in carcinogenesis. Their physiological adaptive nature. Biochim. Biophys. Acta 738 (1984) 171-180
28. Gerber MA, Thung SN: Enzyme pattern in human hepatocellular carcinoma. Amer. J. Path. 98 (1980) 395-400
29. Hacker HJ, Moore MA, Mayer D et al.: Correlative histochemistry of some enzymes of carbohydrate metabolism in preneoplastic and neoplastic lesions in the rat liver. Carcinogenesis 3 (1982) 1265-1272
30. Hann HL, Kim CY, London WT et al.: Hepatitis B virus and primary hepatocellular carcinoma: Family studies in Korea. Int. J. Cancer 30 (1982) 47-51
31. Harrington JS, McGlashan ND, Bradshaw E et al.: A spatial and temporal analysis of four cancers in African gold miners from Southern Africa. Brit. J. Cancer 31 (1975) 665-678
32. Higgins GK: The pathologic anatomy of primary hepatic tumors. In G. T. Pack, A. H. Islami (Eds): Tumors of the Liver, pp. 15-37. Berlin: Springer 1970. (Recent Results in Cancer Research, Vol. 26)
33. Higginson J, Svoboda DS: Primary carcinoma of the liver as a pathologist's problem. Path. Ann. 5 (1970) 61-89
34. Howell RR, Stevenson RE, Ben-Menachem Y et al.: Hepatic adenomata with type 1 glycogen-storage disease. J. Amer. med. Ass. 236 (1976) 1481-1484
35. Keller EHJ, Roesler A, Störkel S: Therapie beim Hämangiopericytom der Leber. Tumor Diagn. Ther. 6 (1985) 244-245
36. Kitagawa T: Histochemical analysis of hyperplastic lesions and hepatomas of the liver of rats fed 2-fluorenylacetamide. Gann 62 (1971) 207-216
37. Klimek F, Mayer D, Bannasch P: Biochemical microanalysis of glycogen content and glucose-6-phosphate dehydrogenase activity in focal lesions of rat liver induced by N-nitrosomorpholine. Carcinogenesis 5 (1984) 265-268
38. Ledda-Columbano GM, Columbano A, Dessi S et al.: Enhancement of cholesterol synthesis and pentose phosphate pathway activity in proliferating hepatocyte nodules. Carcinogenesis 6 (1985) 1371-1373
39. Lloyd JW: Angiosarcoma of the liver in vinyl chloride/polyvinyl chloride workers. J. occup. Med. 17 (1975) 333-334
40. Maltoni C: Occupational carcinogenesis. In C. Maltoni (Edit.): Cancer Detection and Prevention. Proceedings of the 2nd International Symposium on Cancer Detection and Prevention, Bologna 1973, pp. 19-26. Amsterdam: Excerpta Medica 1974
41. Melbye M, Skinhøj P, Nielsen NH et al.: Virus-associated cancer in Greenland: Frequent hepatitis B virus infection but low primary hepatocellular carcinoma incidence. J. nat. Cancer Inst. 73 (1984) 1267-1272
42. Miyai K, Ruebner B: Acute yellow atrophy, cirrhosis and hepatoma. Arch. Path. 75 (1963) 609-617

43. Moore MA, Hacker HJ, Bannasch P: Phenotypic instability in focal and nodular lesions induced in a short term system in the rat liver. Carcinogenesis 4 (1983) 595-603
44. Moore MA, Kitagawa T: Hepatocarcinogenesis in the rat; the effect of the promoters and carcinogens in vivo and in vitro. Int. Rev. Cytol. 101 (1986) 125-173
45. Moore MA, Mayer D, Bannasch P: The dose-dependence and sequential appearance of putative preneoplastic populations induced in the rat liver by stop experiments with N-nitrosomorpholine. Carcinogenesis 3 (1982) 1429-1436
46. Nadell J, Kosek J: Peliosis hepatis. Arch. Path. Lab. Med. 101 (1977) 405-410
47. Nime F, Pickren JW, Vana J et al.: The histology of liver tumors in oral contraceptive users observed during a national survey by the American College of Surgeons Commission on Cancer. Cancer 44 (1979) 1481-1489
48. Ogawa K, Medline A, Farber E: Sequential analysis of hepatic carcinogenesis. A comparative study of the ultrastructure of preneoplastic, malignant, prenatal, postnatal, and regenerating liver. Lab. Invest. 41 (1979) 22-35
49. Okuda K, Nakashima T, Sakamoto K et al.: Hepatocellular carcinoma arising in noncirrhotic and highly cirrhotic livers: A comparative study of histopathology and frequency of hepatitis B markers. Cancer 49 (1982) 450-455
50. Okuda K, Peters RL (Eds): Hepatocellular Carcinoma. New York: Wiley 1976
51. Popper H, Maltoni C, Selikoff IJ et al.: Comparison of neoplastic hepatic lesions in man and experimental animals. In H.H. Hiatt, J.D. Watson, J.A. Winsten (Eds): Origin of Human Cancer, Book C, Human Risk Assessment, pp. 1359-1382. Cold Spring Harbor: Cold Spring Harbor Laboratories 1977. (Cold Spring Harbor Conferences on Cell Proliferation, Vol. 4)
52. Popper H, Thomas LB, Telles LC et al.: Development of hepatic angiosarcoma in man induced by vinyl chloride, thorotrast and arsenic. Amer. J. Path. 92 (1978) 349-370
53. Prates MD, Torres FO: A cancer survey in Lourenco Marques, Portuguese East Africa. J. nat. Cancer Inst. 35 (1965) 729-757
54. Ruan Y-B: Zytochemische und elektronenmikroskopische Charakterisierung des zellulären Phänotyps adenoider Lebertumoren. Diss. Universität Heidelberg 1985
55. Scherer E: Neoplastic progression in experimental hepatocarcinogenesis. Biochim. Biophys. Acta 738 (1984) 219-236
56. Steiner PE: Cancer of the liver and cirrhosis in Trans-Saharan Africa and the United States of America. Cancer 13 (1960) 1085-1166
57. Stewart HL: Comparative aspects of certain cancers. In F.F. Becker (Edit.): Cancer. A Comprehensive Treatise, Vol. 4, pp. 303-374. New York: Plenum Press 1975
58. Stewart HL, Williams G, Keysser CH et al.: Histologic typing of liver tumors of the rat. J. nat. Cancer Inst. 65 (1980) 179-206
59. Tabor E, Gerety RJ, Vogel CL et al.: Hepatitis B virus infection and primary hepatocellular carcinoma. J. nat. Cancer Inst. 58 (1977) 1197-1200
60. Tatematsu M, Takano T, Hasegawa R et al.: A sequential quantitative study of the reversibility or irreversibility of liver hyperplastic nodules in rats exposed to hepatocarcinogens. Gann 71 (1980) 843-855
61. Tiollais P, Pourcel C, Dejean A: The hepatitis B virus. Nature 317 (1985) 489-495
62. Thung SN, Gerber MA: Enzyme pattern and marker antigens in nodular "regenerative" hyperplasia of the liver. Cancer 47 (1981) 1796-1799
63. Tomatis L: Exposures associated with cancer in humans. J. Cancer Res. clin. Oncol. 108 (1984) 6-10
64. Tu J, Gao R, Zhang D et al.: Risk factors of primary liver cancer in the high prevalence area Chongming County - results from a five years follow-up. In G. Wagner, Zhang You-Hui (Eds): Cancer of the Liver, Esophagus, and Nasopharynx. Berlin-Heidelberg-New York-Tokyo: Springer 1987
65. Uchida T, Miyata H, Shikata T: Human hepatocellular carcinoma and putative precancerous disorders. Their enzyme histochemical study. Arch. Path. 105 (1981) 180-186
66. Vesselinovitch SD, Hacker HJ, Bannasch P: Histochemical characterization of focal hepatic lesions induced by single diethylnitrosamine treatment in infant mice. Cancer Res. 45 (1985) 2774-2780
67. Wake K: Perisinusoidal stellate cells (fat-storing cells, interstitial cells, lipocytes), their

related structure in and around the liver sinusoids, and vitamin A-storing cells in extrahepatic organs. Int. Rev. Cytol. 66 (1980) 303-353

68. Ward JM: Morphology of potential preneoplastic hepatocyte lesions and liver tumors in mice and a comparison with other species. In J. A. Popp (Edit.): Mouse Liver Neoplasia, pp. 1-26. Washington: Hemisphere Publ. Corp. 1984
69. Wayss K, Bannasch P, Mattern J et al.: Vascular liver tumors in Mastomys induced by single or twofold administration of dimethylnitrosamine. J. nat. Cancer Inst. 62 (1979) 1199-1207
70. Weber G: Differential carbohydrate metabolism in tumor and host. In M. S. Arnott, J. van Eys, Y.-M. Wang (Eds): Molecular Interrelation of Nutrition and Cancer, pp. 191-208. New York: Raven Press 1982
71. Weinbren K: Precancerous states in the liver. In R. L. Carter (Edit.): Precancerous States, pp. 254-277. London: Oxford Medical Publications 1984
72. Wu PC, Lai CL, Lam KC et al.: Clear cell carcinoma of liver. An ultrastructural study. Cancer 52 (1983) 504-507

Proliferation and Clonal Selection in Hepatocarcinogenesis*

*H. M. Rabes**

Cell proliferation, an essential prerequisite of malignant transformation, appears relevant also for liver tumor induction, at least in experimental animals, but probably also in humans. The normal adult liver is a stable organ, in animals as well as in humans. Cell proliferation runs at a low gear; less than one cell/10^3 is in DNA synthesis, less than one hepatocyte/10^4 is in mitosis. It is not surprising that in a normal adult liver the incidence of hepatomas is very low. In experimental animals this can easily be shown: A single exposure to a liver carcinogen fails in most cases to induce tumors in the intact liver. However, after continuous treatment with low dosages of a carcinogen, liver tumors develop [5]. The same effect, but with a much longer latency period, can be observed after a single dose of carcinogen if this is administered in combination with a stimulus for cell proliferation. One single exposure to various carcinogens after toxic cell loss or partial resection of the liver is sufficient to initiate the development of hepatomas [10, 35; for review see 4].

Some selected aspects of the relationship between cell proliferation and liver carcinogenesis are considered here. It is difficult to analyze the proliferation-related initiating effects of a carcinogen if there is a latency period of 1 or more years to determine the incidence of tumors under various experimental conditions. However, the liver provides an analytical advantage in this respect: It is possible to recognize and measure in this organ the development of putative preneoplastic subpopulations at a very early stage of the carcinogenic process. After carcinogen treatment, distinct and sharply demarcated subpopulations are found in enzyme-histochemical sections of the liver with an aberrant enzymatic phenotype [2, 5, 7, 15, 16, 28, 29, 36].

A positive correlation exists between the occurrence of these foci and the administered carcinogen dose, on the one hand, and the incidence of hepatocellular carcinomas on the other [11, 16]. This has led to the conclusion that these foci are involved in the carcinogenic process and represent putative, but not necessarily obligatory, preneoplastic subpopulations. Taking the frequency of ATPase-deficient foci in the liver as a marker for the initiating action of a carcinogen, it is possible to determine the initiation sensitivity of hepatocytes during specific stages of proliferation after partial hepatectomy.

Investigations in the past have shown that partial resection of the liver fails to induce a synchronous start of DNA synthesis in hepatocytes of the remaining liver. The G_1/S transit is scattered from 15 to 40 h after the operation, depending on the

* The original work reported in this paper was supported by grants from the Deutsche Forschungsgemeinschaft, Bonn, and Dr. Mildred Scheel-Stiftung für Krebsforschung, Bonn.

Cancer of the Liver, Esophagus, and Nasopharynx
Edited by G. Wagner and Zhang You-Hui

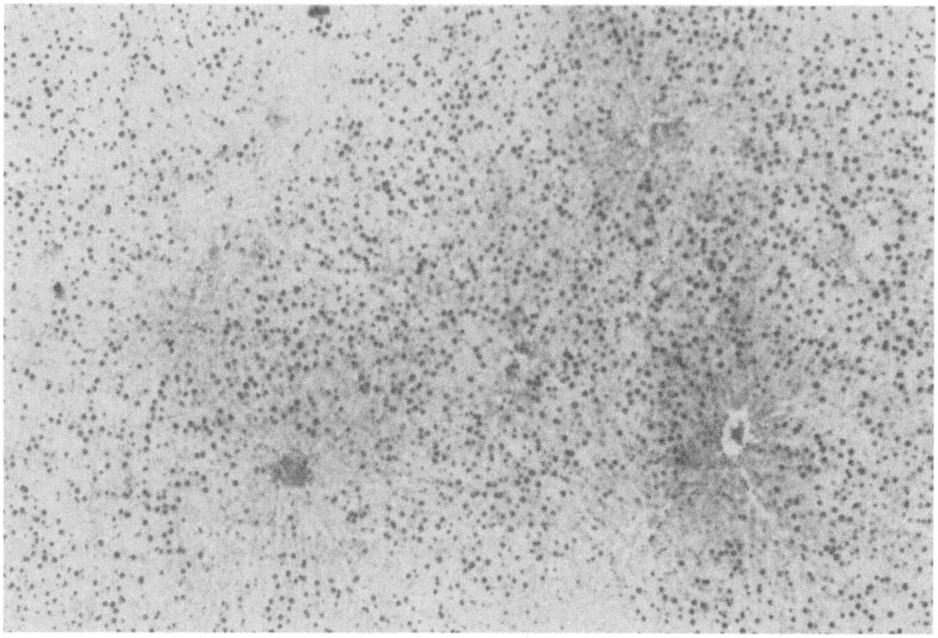

Fig. 1. Autoradiogram of regenerating rat liver 60 min after [^{3}H]-thymidine injection at 43 h after partial hepatectomy and 4 h after a continuous intravenous infusion of HU from 14 to 39 h after partial hepatectomy. About 80% of the hepatocytes are simultaneously in DNA synthesis

intralobular localization of hepatocytes [18], with periportally located liver cells being the first to enter S phase and the perivenous hepatocytes starting DNA synthesis after a delayed G_1 phase. Thus, the model of regenerating rat liver lacks a stringent prerequisite for an exact delineation of transformation-sensitive periods of the cell cycle.

In order to circumvent the heterogeneous reaction to the proliferative stimulus of partial hepatectomy, the start of DNA synthesis in regenerating rat liver was synchronized by means of a continuous infusion of hydroxyurea (HU), which reversibly inhibits the ribonucleoside diphosphate reductase and accumulates hepatocytes at the G_1/S boundary. After release from the HU block, hepatocytes proceed into DNA synthesis with a higher degree of synchrony [17]. Depending on the duration of HU infusion, up to 80% hepatocytes are found simultaneously in S phase (Fig. 1). After about 6.5 h, the cells proceed into G_2 with rapid desynchronization afterwards because of the different duration of G_2 in various parts of the liver lobule. This model provides an opportunity to determine cell cycle-related differences of transformation sensitivity more definitely than in the merely partially synchronized regenerating liver.

A single dose of the hepatocarcinogen diethylnitrosamine administered at G_0 or G_1 or during S phase reveals a striking difference in the initiating activity. In normal rats diethylnitrosamine given at a dose of 40 mg/kg results in a low incidence of ATPase-deficient preneoplastic liver foci. The same dose induces significantly more foci if injected in partially hepatectomized rats in G_1. However, a significantly fur-

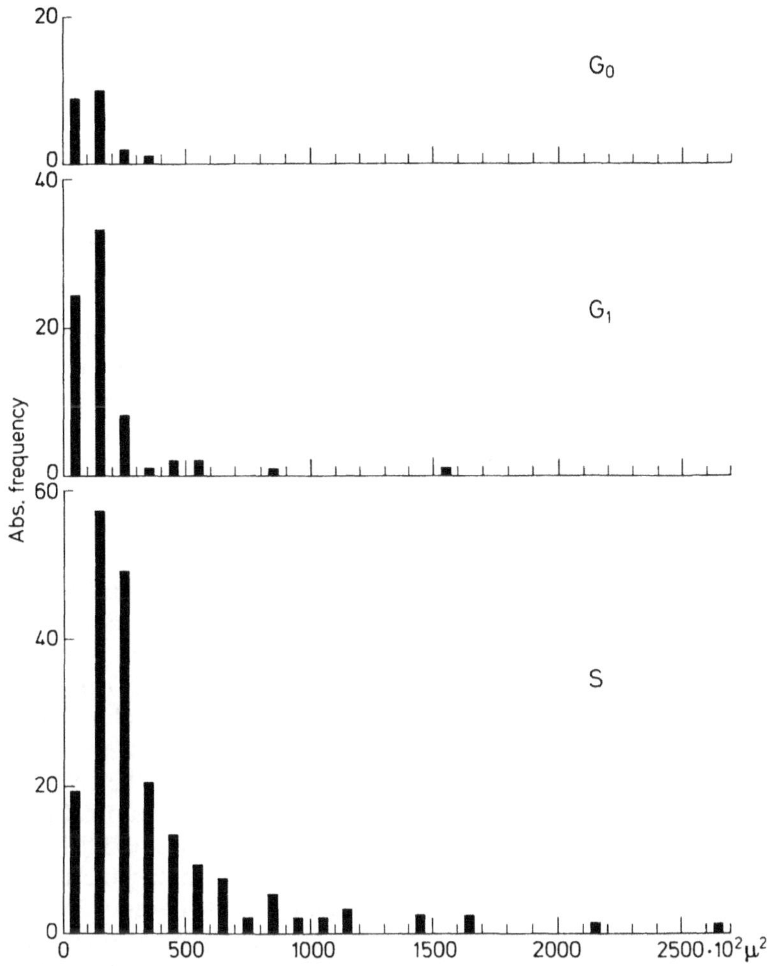

Fig. 2. Number *(ordinate)* and size ($\mu^2 \times 10^2$, *abscissa*) of ATPase-deficient preneoplastic cell populations in the liver 90 days after a single i.p. injection of 40 mg/kg diethylnitrosamine in intact rats *(G_0, top)*, 4 h after partial hepatectomy *(G_1, middle)*, or 1 h after a continuous hydroxyurea infusion from 14 to 24 h after partial hepatectomy (S phase, *bottom*). Combined results a group of five rats, with 10 cm^2 of cryostat section area evaluated in each animal

ther increased incidence of preneoplastic populations is observed after diethylnitrosamine exposure during S phase. The histograms of number and size of ATPase-deficient cell populations are shown in Fig. 2. The ratio of the frequencies is 1:3.3:8.8 for liver exposed in G_0, G_1, or S phase, respectively [9]. These results favor the hypothesis that a hepatocyte in DNA synthesis might be a preferential target cell for the initiating action of a carcinogen.

However, with the use of diethylintrosamine it was not possible to go one step further toward estimating the time of highest transformation sensitivity during the cell cycle because this carcinogen has to be metabolized to generate the actual ultimate carcinogen [13], and not much is yet known about changes of the metabolism of this carcinogen during liver regeneration. N-methyl-N-nitrosourea (MNU) is a far better suited carcinogen for an exact evaluation of cell cycle-related initiation sensitivity because this chemical is decomposed heterolytically at the physiological pH just after injection with a half life of about 7 min [34]. Electrophilic cations arise immediately which interact with nucleophilic sites of cellular constituents. If this carcinogen is given at a dose of 25 mg/kg to rats at various parts of the liver cell cycle after partial hepatectomy and HU synchronization, a preferential sensitivity of early S phase is disclosed. The number of ATPase-deficient preneoplastic foci, determined 90 days after carcinogen treatment, was low after exposure in early G_1, increased during the phase of HU-induced accumulation of hepatocytes at the G_1/S boundary, and reached a maximum after exposure in early S phase. As early as 3 h after release from the HU block, i.e., in the middle S phase, the number of ATPase-deficient foci is significantly decreased and remains low after exposure during the late part of DNA synthesis and in G_2M [25]. Determination of the size distribution of ATPase-deficient foci at various parts of the cell cycle revealed a congruent pattern. It is concluded that hepatocytes differ in their initiation sensitivity according to their peculiar position in the cell cycle during carcinogen exposure but, once initiated, the further development of foci is independent of the cell cycle position at initiation.

The question arises if cell cycle-dependent differences of initiation probability of hepatocytes are due to an increased binding of the ultimate electrophilic carcinogen to DNA, which could explain the high sensitivity of cells in early S phase. A preferential binding site for alkylating nitrosamines and nitrosamides is the N7-position of guanine, which, however, does not appear to be related to the critical initiating events of malignant transformation [34]. Besides nitrogen atoms of purines and pyrimidines in DNA, the oxygen atoms provide specific target sites for the covalent binding of electrophilic ultimate carcinogens. Among these, the 0^6-position of guanine has a significant importance as a biologically relevant alkylation site [32]. Loveless [12] argued that 0^6-alkylguanine in DNA represents a promutagenic lesion which may, because of interference with hydrogen-bonding, lead to base-mispairing during DNA replication and thus to transition mutation. In cell-free systems, the occurrence of base-mispairing has been observed with an 0^6-methylguanine-containing template in a DNA polymerase assay [1]. In consequence, the amount and the persistence of 0^6-alkylguanine in a given cellular DNA after treatment with a carcinogen has been related directly to the probability of transformation.

Biochemical analysis of DNA base alkylation in regenerating rat liver during various parts of the cell cycle disclosed no increased formation of critical DNA adducts like O^6-alkylguanine during the most transformation-sensitive parts of the cell cycle, i.e., early S phase. Treatment of rats with ^{14}C-labeled dimethylnitrosamine resulted in a peak of both N7- and O^6-methylguanine formation at 12 h after partial hepatectomy, i.e., during late G_1 phase. An unexpected pattern was seen in radiochromatographs of liver DNA hydrolysates obtained after treatment in S phase: Alkylation of the O^6-position of guanine is, 2 h after injection of [^{14}C]dimethylnitrosamine (1.43 mg/kg), smaller than after exposure in G_1. The ratio O^6-methylguanine/7- methylguanine, which corrects for the loss of alkylated bases due to DNA replication, shows the same pattern. The ratio is high during G_1 and drops considerably during the S phase [19]. This low molar fraction of O^6-methylguanine is not a result of a decreased formation of O^6-methylguanine, but is due to a

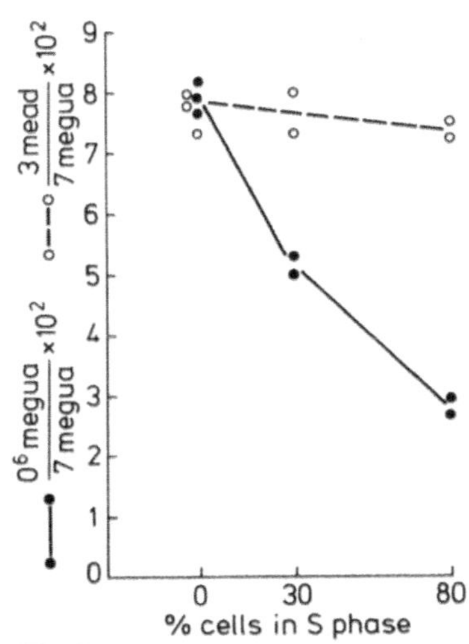

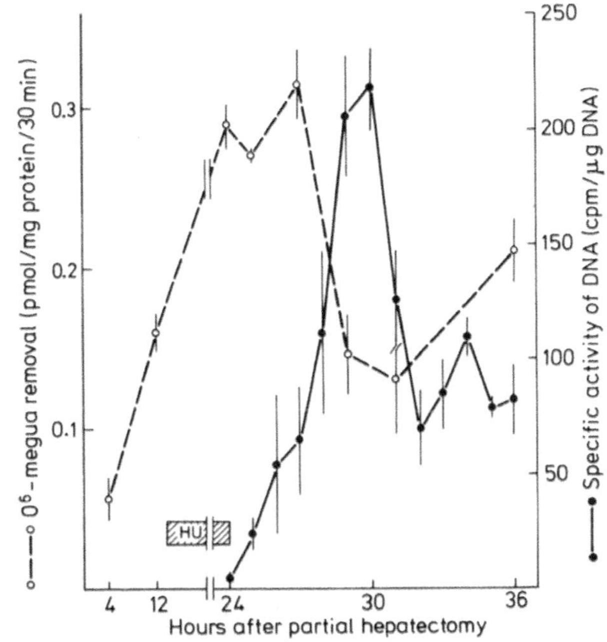

Fig. 3. Fig. 4.

Fig. 3. Correlations between the size of the S phase compartment in regenerating rat liver and the stability of O[6]-methylguanine and 3-methyladenine in relation to 7-methylguanine in liver DNA. Results from radiochromatograms of DNA hydrolysates 2 h after i.p. injection of 0.57 mg/kg [^{14}C]dimethylnitrosamine in intact rats (0% cells in S phase), 24 h after partial hepatectomy (30% cells in S phase), and 4 h after a hydroxyurea block from 14 to 39 h partial hepatectomy (80% hepatocytes in S phase).
Ordinate: O[6]-methylguanine/7-methylguanine ratio $\times 10^2$ (●); 3-methyladenine/7-methylguanine ration $\times 10^2$ (○); *abscissa:* size of the hepatocellular S phase compartment percentage hepatocytes in the S phase. *Each point* represents one experiment with the pooled liver of three rats. [24]

Fig. 4. DNA synthesis and O[6]-methylguanine repair in regenerating rat liver after partial hepatectomy and synchronization of DNA synthesis by continuous infusion of hydroxyurea. Specific activity of DNA (●—●) determined 1 h after [^{3}H]thymidine injection. Mean ±SE from four to five animals. O[6]-methylguanine repair (○—○) studied with methylated calf thymus DNA in vitro incubated in rat liver protein obtained at different time intervals after partial hepatectomy and hydroxyurea infusion form 14 to 24 h after operation. The O[6]-methylguanine elimination is given as pmol/mg liver protein/30 min. Mean ±SD from four to seven determinations at each point. [31]

rapid elimination during DNA synthesis [22, 24]. The loss of [O[6]]methylguanine increases approximately proportional to the size of the S phase compartment in the liver, whereas the removal of 3-methyladenine remains at the same level irrespective of the number of cells in S phase (Fig. 3).

A specific O[6]-methylguanine DNA transferase has been described which is capable of eliminating the methyl group from O[6]-methylguanine in double-stranded DNA by means of an acceptor protein [8, 14]. The cell cycle specificity of this important DNA repair enzyme can be demonstrated in an in vitro system. Methylated, tritium-labeled calf thymus DNA was incubated under standard conditions with protein fractions prepared from regenerating rat liver at various parts of the cell cycle. The O^6-methylguanine DNA transferase activity was measured by determining the loss of tritiated methyl groups from the O^6-position of guanine. Figure 4 shows that the O^6-methylguanine DNA transferase increases during G_1 to reach a maximum in the early S phase, but declines rapidly in the middle of the S phase before DNA synthesis reaches its peak [31].

These results suggest that the potential of hepatocytes for eliminating the promutagenic O^6-methylguanine is most intense during the period of maximum transformation sensitivity, that is during the early S phase.

Some hypothetical considerations can be summarized as follows: It has to be concluded that the relatively rare event of cellular transformation in rat liver is increased in a peculiar subpopulation located in a short part of the cell cycle, late G_1 and early S phase. It appears paradoxical that DNA repair is particularly high during this cell cycle period, but the increased capacity to eliminate the promutagenic O^6-methylguanine during early DNA synthesis might serve physiologically as a protective measure against base-mispairing during DNA replication. The action of the responsible enzyme is, however, confined to very low alkylation dosages. It is expended in the reaction and fails, after higher carcinogen dosages, to reduce effectively the amount of this promutagenic DNA lesion to prevent the initiation of preneoplastic foci. It could be argued that the persistence of O^6-methylguanine appears less important for the initiation than the peculiar cell cycle position of the target cells [23]. The increased transformation sensitivity during late G_1, early S phase might be due to the fact that the interval between alkylation at critical DNA sites and start of DNA synthesis is too short to permit effective DNA repair before base-mispairing occurs during DNA replication.

The rapid decline of transformation sensitivity during the middle and late S phase points to the importance and specificity of events during the early S phase. The preferential initiation at the early S phase might suggest a preferred replication and possible mutation in early S phase of cellular genes which are involved in malignant transformation. One tends to think about oncogenes in this connection. The identification of proliferation- and differentiation-related oncogenes proceeds rapidly, but nothing is yet known about their replication pattern during specific parts of DNA synthesis in hepatocytes. Besides mutational events, carcinogen-induced changes of the physiological methylation pattern [26] during early S phase and also gene amplification [30] or translocation processes after temporary carcinogen-induced inhibition of DNA replication could play a role in the initiation during this phase.

We have to come back to the origin and fate of those ATPase-deficient hepatocellular foci which we claimed to represent preneoplastic cell populations. There are still arguments about their preneoplastic character. The question is: Do these cell groups represent a cohort of cells simultaneously converted to this peculiar state as a result of the toxic action of the carcinogen? Then, a specific preneoplastic character would be rather unlikely. Or do these populations consist of the proliferating progeny of just one single transformed cell endowed with proliferative potential after a specific interaction with a carcinogen? The apparently hereditary phenotypic aberration combined with a stem cell potential for clonal growth would favor the assumption of a preneoplastic character.

Clonal origin has been described for a variety of human tumors [6]. However, the evaluation of preneoplastic lesions in experimental animals by a method similar to the glucose-6-phosphate dehydrogenase mosaicism in humans only became possible by a mutant mouse strain that expressed a point mutation in the phosphoglycerate kinase gene. This enzyme is encoded on the X-chromosome. By breeding males with the mutant phosphoglycerate kinase PGK-1A and normal homozygous females expressing the wild-type PGK-1B, a female offspring was produced that was heterozygous with respect to the PGK pattern. Cells of these mice contain the paternal PGK-1A-X chromosome and the maternal PGK-1B-X chromosome. In early embryogenesis, lyonization occurs, a randomized inactivation of either the paternal or maternal X-chromosome. The adult female mouse is composed of a mosaic of PGK-1A- and PGK-1B-expressing cells. By means of a recently developed microfluorimetric, electrophoretic method [3], these two allozymes can be separated and quantitatively determined in small tissue samples. These samples, which were punched from cryostat sections of the liver and other organs, always contain both allozymes, indicating that the patch size of homogeneous populations with respect to PGK expression is small (approximately eight cells in rat liver [21]. Thus, the basic substrate for an evaluation of the clonal origin of preneoplastic foci was the hepatocellular mosaic of PGK expression.

Preneoplastic foci were initiated and promoted in the liver by continuous feeding of 2-acetylaminofluorene to the mosaic mice. Small tissue samples were obtained by punching from cryostat sections of normal liver and ATPase-deficient preneoplastic foci. The microfluorimetric, electrophoretic evaluation revealed a mosaic expression of both PGK-1A and PGK-1B in normal liver tissue, but samples obtained from ATPase-deficient cell populations expressed selectively either the paternal or the maternal PGK type (Fig. 5) [21]. It is evident from these results that ATPase-deficient foci develop with high probability by clonal growth of a single initiated cell.

Such cells appear to be endowed with an increased proliferative potential as compared with the normal hepatocyte of the adult resting liver. It is completely unknown whether this potential is based on an autocrine stimulation as proposed by Sporn and others [33]. A clone is formed. This clone develops slowly at first, but with increasing speed in later stages. The cell cycle, at the beginning in the order of about 50 h, becomes short. A cell cycle time of about 20 h has been measured at an advanced stage. The population doubling time decreases and reaches values of slightly more than 2 days, with a t_S, the DNA synthesis time, of about 6 h and a labeling index of about 8% [20].

Although clonally grown from a single cell, the further development indicates a rapid loss of cellular homogeneity. Single cell cytophotometry of DNA in Feulgen-stained ATPase-deficient foci reveals three different patterns of DNA content (Fig. 6): Foci were observed with almost exclusively diploid hepatocytes, but others contained an almost pure tetraploid cell population. The presence of either 2 N or 4 N cells in several foci indicates that these clones preserved homogeneously the original cell type. However, other foci were found with a mixed ploidy pattern of 2 N, 4 N, and 8 N cells. Such a mixed pattern was also observed in advanced hepatomas. The comparison of the size of the ATPase-deficient foci with a different DNA pattern disclosed that homogeneous populations were present mainly in the small

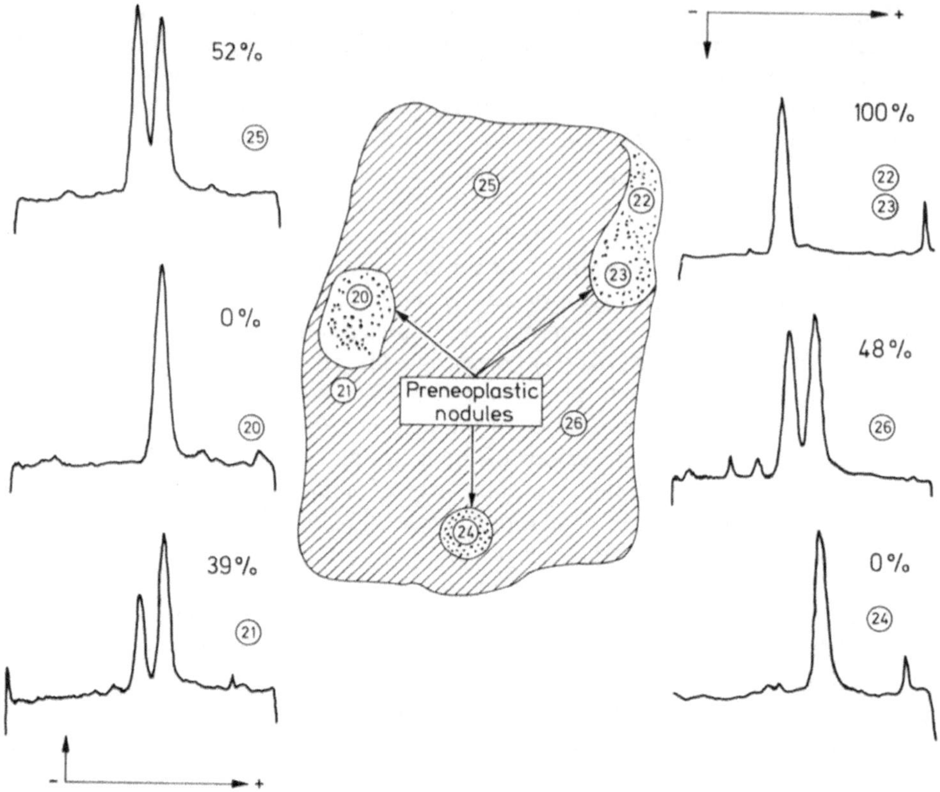

Fig. 5. Demonstration of a selective PGK-1A or PGK-1B expression in ATPase-deficient preneoplastic cell populations in contrast to the mixed PGK pattern in the adjacent liver of a female C3H mouse which was heterozygous for PGK 1A/1B. ATPase-deficient populations were induced by feeding of 2-acetylaminofluorene for 14 months. Sites of three preneoplastic populations are shown along with the position of seven samples punched out of a 40 μm frozen section. The fluorimetric records on both sides show electrophoretically fast PGK-1A (mutant enzyme) and slow PGK-1B (wild-type enzyme) in extracts of 3-nl tissue samples. *Arrows,* start of electrophoresis. *Ordinates,* PGK-1B as percentage of total PGK activity calculated from the peak areas. [21]

Fig. 6. Single cell cytophotometry of Feulgen-stained DNA in cryostat sections (20 μm) of ▶ preneoplastic liver. In early stages of development, the ATPase-deficient preneoplastic foci induced by a single exposure to 25 mg/kg *N*-methyl-*N*-nitrosourea 1 h after hydroxyurea infusion form 14 to 24 h after partial hepatectomy contain almost exclusively diploid *(bottom)* or tetraploid hepatocytes *(upper right).* Advanced, larger preneoplastic foci consist of a mixture of di-, tetra-, and octoploid hepatocytes *(upper left),* indicating an increasing heterogeneity. *Abscissa,* DNA content in arbitrary units; *ordinate,* DNA content/nuclear area ratio. (For details see [27])

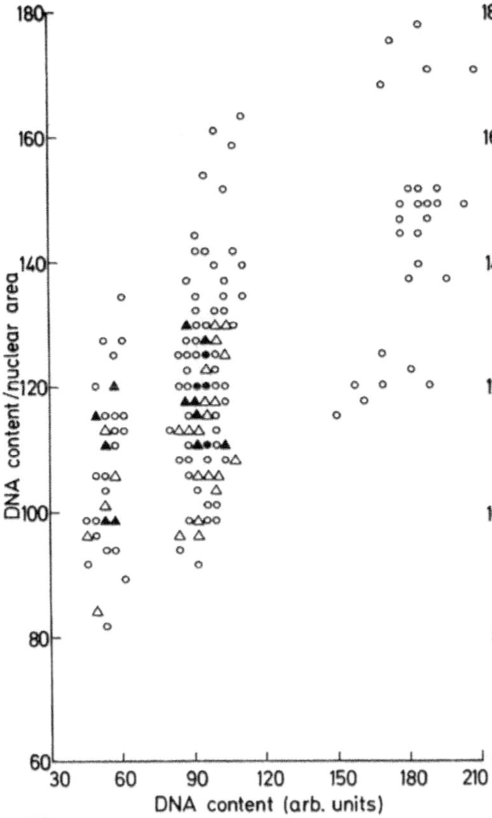
180
160
140
120
100
80
60
DNA content/nuclear area
30 60 90 120 150 180 210
DNA content (arb. units)

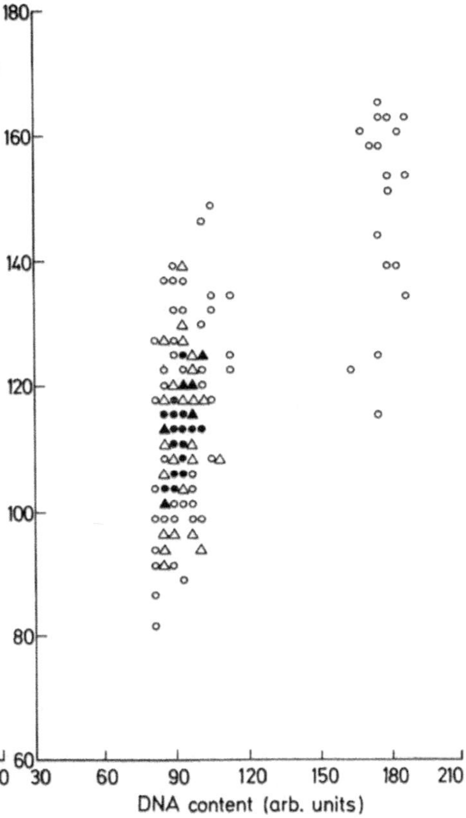
180
160
140
120
100
80
60
30 60 90 120 150 180 210
DNA content (arb. units)

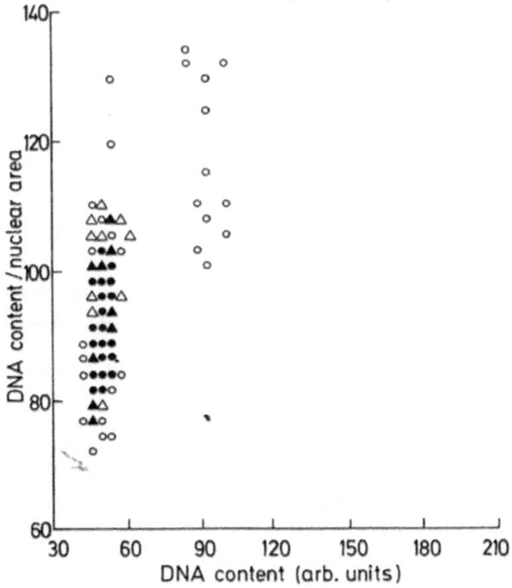
140
120
100
80
60
DNA content/nuclear area
30 60 90 120 150 180 210
DNA content (arb. units)

foci, with not much difference in the size of foci containing 2 N or 4 N cells, respectively. However, in the larger foci a heterogeneous DNA pattern prevailed which apparently ends up in the striking heterogeneity of the hepatoma [27].

These data suggest that ATPase-deficient preneoplastic foci consist of cells with an increased growth potential and might represent, though clonally derived from a single cell, a genetically unstable population prone to give rise to various subpopulations, a few of which may end up, possibly by another clonal selection, in overt malignancy.

Cell proliferation is significant at various stages of hepatocarcinogenesis. It renders a hepatocyte more susceptible to the transforming action of a chemical carcinogen, may be involved in humans with the integration of hepatitis B DNA into the genome, and could be essential for translocation and also for gene amplification. The fact that initiated cells are endowed with a proliferative advantage over normal liver cells is relevant for the development of the initial preneoplastic cell clones and, due to genetic instability, for the selection of subpopulations with an altered, possibly autonomous, malignant or even metastatic phenotype.

References

1. Abbott PJ, Saffhill R: DNA synthesis with methylated poly(dC-dG-)templates. Evidence for a competitive nature to miscoding by 0^6-methylguanine. Biochim. Biophys. Acta 562 (1979) 51-61
2. Bannasch P, Mayer D, Hacker HJ: Hepatocellular glycogenosis and hepatocarcinogenesis. Biochim. Biophys. Acta 605 (1980) 217-245
3. Bücher T, Bender W, Fundele R, Hofner H, Linke I: Quantitative evaluations of electrophoretic allo- and isozyme patterns. FEBS Lett 115 (1980) 319-324
4. Craddock VM: Cell proliferation and experimental liver cancer. In: Cameron D., Linsell A., Warwick GP (eds) Liver cell cancer, pp. 153-201. (Amsterdam: Elsevier 1976)
5. Farber E: The sequential analysis of liver cancer induction. Biochim. Biophys. Acta 605 (1980) 149-166
6. Fialkow PJ: Clonal origin of human tumours. Biochim. Biophys. Acta 458 (1976) 283-321
7. Gössner W, Friedrich-Freksa H: Histochemische Untersuchungen über die Glukose-6-Phosphatase in der Rattenleber während der Cancerisierung durch Nitrosamine. Z. Naturforsch. (B) 19 (1964) 862-863
8. Harris AL, Karran P, Lindahl T: O^6-Methylguanine-DNA methyltransferase of human lymphoid cells: Structural and kinetic properties and absence in repair-deficient cells. Cancer Res. 43 (1983) 3247-3252
9. Hartmann A, Rabes HM: Die Entstehung präneoplastischer Läsionen in der Rattenleber nach zweimaliger Karzinogenexposition in spezifischen Phasen des Zellzyklus. Verh. Dtsch. Ges. Pathol. 66 (1982) 503
10. Kaufmann WK, Kaufman DG, Rice JM, Wenk ML: Reversible inhibition of rat hepatocyte proliferation by hydrocortisone and its effect on cell cycle dependent hepatocarcinogenesis by N-methyl-N-nitrosourea. Cancer Res. 41 (1981) 4653-4660
11. Kunz W, Appel KE, Rickart R, Schwarz M, Stöckle G: Enhancement and inhibition of carcinogenic effectiveness of nitrosamines. In (H. Remmer, H. M. Bolt, P. Bannasch, H. Popper, eds), Primary Liver Tumors, p. 261-283. Lancaster: MTP Press 1978
12. Loveless A: Possible relevance of O^6-alkylation of deoxyguanosine to the mutagenicity and carcinogenicity of nitrosamines and nitrosamides. Nature 233 (1969) 206-207
13. Miller EC, Miller JA: Biochemical mechanism of chemical carcinogenesis. In (H. Busch (ed): The molecular biology of cancer, pp. 377-402. (New York: Academic Press 1974)
14. Pegg AE, Wiest L, Foote RF, Mitra S, Perry W: Purification and properties of O^6-methylguanine-DNA transmethylase from rat liver. J. Biol. Chem. 258 (1983) 2327-2333

15. Pitot HC, Sirica AE: The stages of initiation and promotion in hepatocarcinogenesis. Biochim. Biophys. Acta 605 (1980) 191-215
16. Rabes HM, Scholze P, Jantsch B: Growth kinetics of diethylnitrosamine-induced, enzyme-deficient "preneoplastic" liver cell populations in vivo and in vitro. Cancer Res. 32 (1972) 2577-2586
17. Rabes HM, Iseler G, Czichos S, Tuczek HV: Synchronization of hepatocellular DNA synthesis in regenerating rat liver by continuous infusion of hydroxyurea. Cancer Res. 37 (1977) 1105-1111
18. Rabes HM: Kinetics of hepatocellular proliferation as a function of the microvascular structure and functional state of the liver. In Porter, R., Whelan, J. (eds): Hepatotrophic factors, pp. 31-59. Elsevier-Excerpta Medica-North Holland, Amsterdam Oxford New York. Ciba Foundation Symposium 1978
19. Rabes HM, Kerler R, Wilhelm R, Rode G, Riess H: Alkylation of DNA and RNA by (^{14}C)dimethylnitrosamine in hydroxyurea-synchronized regenerating rat liver. Cancer Res. 39 (1979) 4228-4236
20. Rabes HM, Szymkowiak W: Cell kinetics of hepatocytes during the preneoplastic period of diethylnitrosamine-induced liver carcinogenesis. Cancer Res. 39 (1979) 1298-1304
21. Rabes HM, Bücher Th, Hartmann A, Linke I, Dünnwald M: Clonal growth of carcinogen-induced enzyme-deficient preneoplastic cell populations in mouse liver. Cancer Res. 42 (1982) 3220-3227
22. Rabes HM, Wilhelm R, Kerler R, Rode G: Dose- and cell cycle-dependent O^6-methylguanine elimination from DNA in regenerating rat liver after (^{14}C)dimethylnitrosamine injection. Cancer Res. 42 (1982) 3814-3821
23. Rabes HM: Development and growth of early preneoplastic lesions induced in the liver by chemical carcinogens. J. Cancer Res. Clin. Oncol. 106 (1983) 85-92
24. Rabes HM, Kerler R, Rode G, Schuster C, Wilhelm R: O^6-methylguanine repair in liver cells in vivo: Comparison between G_1- and S-Phase of the cell cycle. J. Cancer Res. Clin. Oncol. 108 (1984) 36-45
25. Rabes HM, Müller L, Hartmann A, Kerler R, Schuster Ch: Cell cycle-dependent initiation of adenosine triphosphatase-deficient populations in adult rat liver by a single dose of N-methyl-N-nitrosourea. Cancer Res. 46 (1986) 645-650
26. Riggs AD, Jones PA: 5-methylcytosine, gene regulation, and cancer. Adv. Cancer Res. 40 (1983) 1-30
27. Sarafoff M, Rabes HM, Dörmer P: Correlations between ploidy and initiation probability determined by DNA cytophotometry in individual altered hepatic foci. Carcinogenesis 7 (1986) 1191-1196
28. Schauer A, Kunze E: Enzymhistochemische und autoradiographische Untersuchungen während der Cancerisierung der Rattenleber mit Diäthylnitrosamin. Z. Krebsforsch. 70 (1968) 252-266
29. Scherer E: Neoplastic progression in experimental hepatocarcinogenesis. Biochim. Biophys. Acta 738 (1984) 219-236
30. Schimke RT: Gene amplification, drug resistance, and cancer. Cancer Res. 44 (1984) 1735-1742
31. Schuster C, Rode G, Rabes HM: O^6-methylguanine repair of methylated DNA in vitro: Cell cycle-dependence of rat liver methyltransferase activity. J. Cancer Res. Clin. Oncol. 110 (1985) 98-102
32. Singer B: Guest editorial: N-nitroso alkylating agents: formation and persistence of alkyl derivatives in mammalian nucleic acids as contributing factors in carcinogenesis. J. Natl. Cancer Inst. 62 (1979) 1329-1339
33. Sporn MB, Roberts AB: Autocrine growth factors and cancer. Nature 313 (1985) 745-747
34. Swann PF, Magee PN: Nitrosamine-induced carcinogenesis. The alkylation of nucleic acids of the rat by N-methyl-N-nitrosourea, dimethylnitrosamine, dimethyl sulphate and methyl methanesulphonate. Biochem. J. 110 (1968) 39-47
35. Warwick GP: Effect of the cell cycle on carcinogenesis. Fed. Proc. 30 (1971) 1760-1765
36. Williams GM: The pathogenesis of rat liver cancer caused by chemical carcinogens. Biochim. Biophys. Acta 605 (1980) 167-189

Oncogenes in Primary Hepatic Cancer

Gu Jian-Ren, Hu Li-Fu, Wan Da-Feng, and Hong Jing-Xing

Primary hepatic cancer (PHC) is one of the most prevalent malignancies on the east and south coasts of China. Extensive epidemiological surveys of PHC in these areas indicate that the incidence of PHC is closely correlated with HBV infection, aflatoxin contamination, and other putative carcinogenic factors in the drinking water. However, direct evidence is still lacking as to which of these factors operate in hepatocarcinogenesis and how they operate. Therefore, the identification and isolation of oncogenes in PHC will help us to elucidate the target genes which carcinogens may attack and the mechanism of carcinogenesis.

Transforming Activity of DNAs from PHC and Hepatoma 7402 Cell Line into NIH3T3 Cells

We isolated high molecular weight DNA from a specimen of hepatocellular carcinoma which was pathologically proved and contained integrated HBV DNA in genomic DNA. High molecular weight DNAs were also isolated from a human hepatoma 7402 cell line (established by Dr. Chen Rei-ming, Institute of Cell Biology, Chinese National Academy of Sciences, in 1974). The DNA transfection of NIH3T3 mouse cells was performed according to calcium phosphate precipitation methods [13, 15]. Foci of morphologically transformed cells were picked and cloned. The tumorigenicity of transformed foci was tested by subcutaneous inoculation of transformed cells ($1-2 \times 10^6$ cells/mouse) into newborn Swiss mice. The DNA from transformants was analyzed by Southern transfer and hybridization with human repetitive sequence. Only the DNAs from transformants which contained the integrated human sequence were used for the secondary and subsequent transfection.

The transformation efficiency of DNA from PHC and 7402 is illustrated in Table 1 [8]. The number of foci per microgram donor DNA was 0.016 and 0.080 respectively for primary and secondary transfection experiments of PHC DNA, and 0.016 and 0.160 for 7402 DNA. The tertiary transfection efficiency was greater than 1.0 for 7402 DNA (not listed in the table). It indicated that the putative transforming sequences were enriched after repeated cycles of transfection.

The hybridization with human repetitive sequences, when either Cot 1 [13] or total human leukocyte DNA was used as probes, showed the positive bands of human sequences in transformed NIH3T3 mouse [8].

Cancer of the Liver, Esophagus, and Nasopharynx
Edited by G. Wagner and Zhang You-Hui

Table 1. Transfection efficiency of DNA of primary hepatic cancer and hepatoma 7402 cell line

Cycle of transfection	Donor DNA	No. foci/μg^{-1} DNA/10^{-5} cells
1. Primary transfection	PHC WD-1	0.016
	NIH 3T3	0.000
Secondary transfection	T-1	0.080
	T-8	0.088
	Salmon sperm	0.001
2. Primary transfection	7402	0.016
	NIH 3T3	0.002
Secondary transfection	NIH-7402	0.160
	NIH 3T3	0.005

Transfection procedures basically corresponded to those of Shih et al. [15]. Sixteen hours before transfection 3×10^5 NIH 3T3 cells were seeded to each bottle. Seventy to seventy-five micrograms of high molecular DNA were added to 45 μg NIH 3T3 or salmon DNA and sheared by a single passage through a 20-gauge syringe needle. The DNA mixture was ethanol-precipitated and redissolved in 1.5 ml transfection buffer (0.7 mM Na_2HPO_4, 21 mM Hepes (4-(2-hydroxyethyl)-piperazine-1-ethanol-sulfonic acid) 0.145 M NaCl, pH 7.05); $CaCl_2$ was added to a final concentration at 125 mM and left at room temperature for 15–20 min. The DNA mixture was diluted ten fold with Dulbecco's modified Eagle's medium; 10% calf serum and 5 ml suspension were added to each bottle of cells. After 4–6 h, DNA medium was removed and the cells were refed. On the 3rd day after the transfection, the cells were trypsinized and seeded into two to three bottles. The cultures were fed three times per week. The foci were scored 20–21 days posttransfection. Transfection efficiency represented the number of foci per microgram donor DNA equivalent to 10^5 target cells.

The nature of the transforming foci was further confirmed by a test for tumorigenicity by subcutaneously injecting $1-2 \times 10^6$ cells into 24-h-old newborn Swiss mice. Tumor formation was observed within 2 weeks and confirmed by pathological examination. WD-1 was a specimen of a primary hepatocellular carcinoma of a 54-year-old male, with HBV integration in genomic DNA (data not shown here). T1T8 were two independent primary transformants from WD-1 DNA. 7402 was a human hepatoma cell line established by Dr. R. M. Chen. NIH-7402 was the primary transformant from 7402 DNA

Identification of Human *N-ras* in Transformants Derived from PHC and 7402 DNA

The DNAs isolated from transformants were further analyzed [7] by restriction enzyme digestion, agarose gel electrophoresis, Southern transfer, and hybridization with ^{32}P-labeled *onc* probes, which included *v-Ha-ras* (BS9), *v-Ki-ras* (Hi-Hi-3) [4], *N-ras* (R and L probes from Wigler [18], *v-myc*, and *Blym1* [3]). The results of hybridization with *N-ras* gene are shown in Fig. 1. In the untransformed NIH3T3 cell DNA, only a faint *Eco*RI 7.2-kb band was observed, whereas in human hepatocarcinoma cell DNA there were 7.2- and 9.0-kb bands after *Eco*RI restriction. In transformants following transfection with DNA from PHC and 7402, similar double bands were observed (Fig. 1: transformants 6.1, 7.8, 7.2, 7.7, 778, 782–11). From the data previously reported, the cloned human *N-ras* gene was represented by two *Eco*RI fragments, with slight variation in sizes: the left band (5') fragment was 0.2 [19], 9.0 [12], or 8.8 kb [9]; the right fragment (3') was 7.2 [12] or 7.0 kb [19]. The size of two *Eco*RI fragments in our material was 9.0 and 7.2 kb. In some of the transformed cells from 7402 DNA, the polymorphism of banding pattern was observed (Fig. 1:

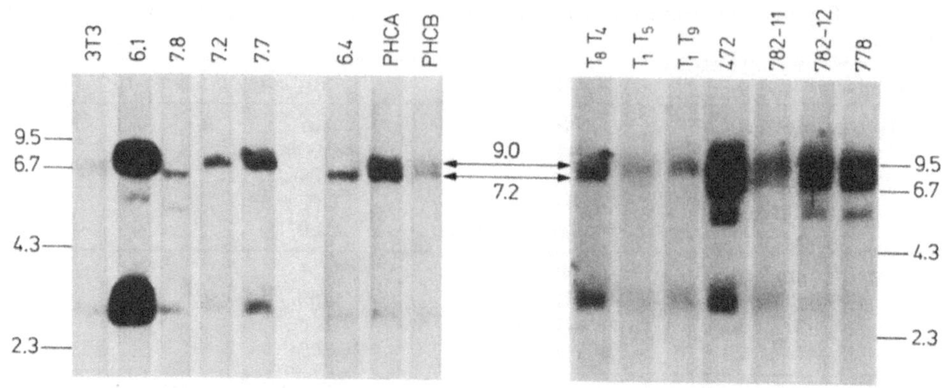

Fig. 1. Autoradiography of human *N-ras* gene in transforming cells transfected with DNAs from human primary hepatic cancer *(PHC)* and hepatoma 7402 cell line. Fifteen micrograms DNA were digested with *Eco*RI, then subjected to agarose gel electrophoresis, Southern transfer, and hybridization with human *N-ras* gene probe. 3T3 was untransformed NIH/3T3 cell; 6.1, 7.8, 7.7, and 6.4 were the secondary transformants from 7402 DNA; 778 was the tertiary transformant of 7402 DNA; 782-11 and 782-12 were the quarternary transformants from 7402 DNA; T8T4, T1T5, and T1T9 were the secondary transformants of PHC DNA; PHCA and PHAB were PHC controls. The *arrows* indicate two bands characteristic for human *N-ras* gene

lane 3, 7.8; lane 11, 472; lane 13, 782-12; lane 14, 778). In one of the transformants form 7402 DNA, 6.1 (Fig. 1: lane 2), the *N-ras* gene was amplified more than 20-fold. The polymorphism of the human *N-ras* sequence has been reported in transformants following transfection with DNAs from human neuroblastoma [18, 19] and fibrosarcoma [9]. The polymorphism and gene amplification may be the results of DNA rearrangement during the process of transfection.

Using *v-Ki-ras* and *v-Ha-ras* genes as probes, we found no human *c-Ha-ras-1* (*Bam*HI, 6.6 kb) or *c-Ki-ras-2* gene fragment (*Eco*RI 3.0-kb band) [12, 14, 17] in all the transformed cells transfected with PHC DNA. Negative results were also obtained in the hybridization with *myc* or *Blym1* probes (data not shown here).

Expression of mRNA in PHC

In order to obtain further evidence about the state of expression of oncogenes in primary liver cancer, we decided to characterize the mRNA transcripts directly from PHC. Poly$^+$(A)mRNA was isolated from 9 PHC samples, one sample of tumor-adjacent liver and one of normal liver tissue. Twenty-five micrograms of poly$^+$(A)mRNA from each sample were analyzed by formaldehyde-agarose gel electrophoresis and Northern transfer and hybridized with ^{32}P-labeled probes of different *onc,* including *v-Ha-ras, v-Ki-ras,* and *N-ras*. In six out of nine PHC mRNA samples, two bands (5.6 and 2.2 kb) were identified by hybridization with *N-ras* probe (Fig. 2). In some samples, a high molecular weight precursor band around 8.0 kb was also observed. In mRNA of three other PHCs, one normal liver, and two tumor-adjacent cirrhotic liver tissue samples, the *N-ras*-characteristic tran-

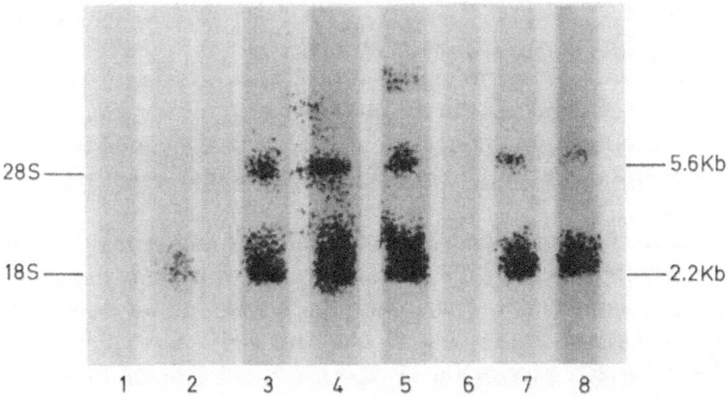

Fig. 2. Hybridization of poly(A)$^+$mRNA from PHC, tumor-adjacent normal liver and normal liver tissue with ^{32}P-labeled *N-ras* probe. *Lane* 1, normal liver; *lanes 2, 3, 4, 5, 7, 8* are from different PHC samples; *lane 6*, tumor-adjacent liver. 28s, 18s rRNA as well as denatured *Hind* III-cleaved λDNA were used as markers for calibration of the size of mRNA bands. The negative results with *v-Ha-ras, c-Ki-ras,* and others are not shown here. Only the autoradiograph of *N-ras* hybridization is presented

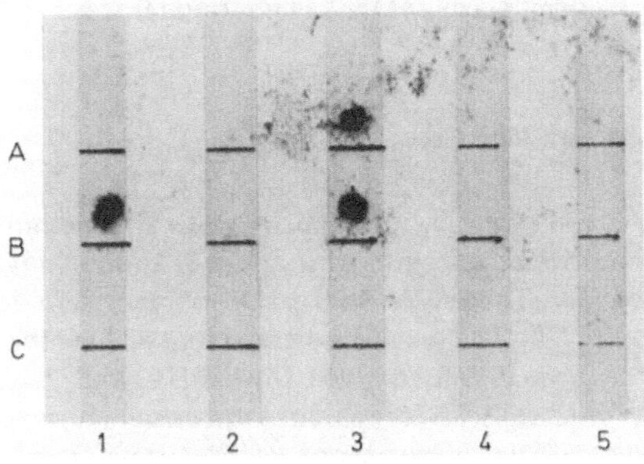

Fig. 3. Hybridization of various oncegene DNAs with ^{32}P-labeled cDNA prepared from PHC poly(A)$^+$RNA. The oncogene DNAs were spotted on the filters as follows: A_1, *v-Ki-ras(HiHi 3)*; A_2, *v-Ha-ras(BS9)*; A_3, *N-ras* (courtesy of Dr. Wigler); A_4, A_5, blank; B_1, *pAT N-ras 8.8(Hall)*; B_2, *v-abl*; B_3, *Blym 1*; B_4, *erb*; B_5, *v-fes*; C_1, *v-mos*; C_2, *v-myb*; C_3, *v-myc*; C_4, *v-sis*; C_5, *v-src*

script was too weak to be detected. No *Ki-ras-* and *Ha-ras*-characteristic transcripts were observed. One of the filters, which gave no hybridizable signals with *Ki-ras* probe, was rehybridized with *N-ras* probe. The characteristic bands appeared [11]. Therefore, in two-thirds of PHC samples the expression of *N-ras* gene was elevated compared with that of normal liver.

To further confirm the validity of the experiments, the [^{32}P]-cDNA was prepared from poly$^+$(A)mRNA of PHC samples. One to two micrograms of various *onc* DNAs, e.g., *v-Ki-ras, v-Ha-ras, N-ras* (Wigler's *R* and *L* fragment), *N-ras* (*pAT-N-ras* 8.8, A. Hall), *v-abl, Blym, erbB, v-fes, v-mos, v-myb, v-sis,* and *v-src,* were spotted on nitrocellulose filters and hybridized with [^{32}P]cDNA prepared from PHC mRNA. The results are shown in Fig. 3. We found that *N-ras* (both from Wigler and

Hall) and *Blym* were hybridized with [^{32}P]cDNA from PHC. It could further be confirmed that *N-ras* gene was remarkably expressed in PHC.

As the *ras* gene was considered a gene with constitutive expression (Shih [16], Hall et al. [9]), the expression of *N-ras* gene in the normal liver, tumor-adjacent liver, as well as one-third of PHC samples might occur, but at a low level beyond the limit of detection in our experiments. However, in 6/9 PHC samples, the *N-ras* gene was remarkably overexpressed.

Since 1983, the *N-ras* gene has been identified as the transforming gene in human neuroblastoma [18, 19], HL-60 leukemia [12], fibrosarcoma [9], rhabdomyosarcoma [9], and acute myelogenic leukemia [6]. In this report, the *N-ras* gene was identified in transformed NIH3T3 cells transfected with DNAs from PHC as well as hepatoma cell line, and the enhanced expression of *N-ras* in two-thirds of PHC was observed as compared with nontumorous liver tissue. In rat hepatic carcinogenesis, an elevated expression of *Ha-ras* was reported [5]. However, there is no evidence of the involvement of *Ha-ras* gene in our transfection experiments and no evidence of enhanced expression of *Ha-ras* gene in human PHC. Taking together the data presented strongly implies that *N-ras* is at least one of the transforming genes for PHC. This is the first report about the transforming gene and its expression in human liver cancer. The molecular cloning of *N-ras* gene and its cDNA is now under way.

Expression of p21 in Transformed Cells and 7402 Cells

Transformed cells and hepatoma 7402 cells were in vitro labeled with [^{35}S]methionine. Cell lysate was analyzed by immunoprecipitation with anti-p21 monoclonal antibodies 238, 259, and 172 (gift from Dr. Thomas Y. Shih), SDS-polyacrylamide gel electrophoresis, and autoradiography [20]. The results indicated that p21 synthesis was remarkably enhanced in transformed cells derived from PHC and 7402 DNA transfection as well as parent 7402 cells as compared with untransformed NIH3T3 cells. It provided the evidence that *N-ras* is one of the transforming sequences for hepatocarcinoma (Figs. 4–6).

Monoclonal Antibody Preparation from Transformed Cells Transfected with PHC DNA

In order to prepare antibody against p21$^{N\text{-}ras}$, Hong et al. [10] immunized Bab/c mice with transformed cells T1 derived from PHC DNA transfection. As the transformant T1 contained human *N-ras* gene and was overexpressed in p21 synthesis, it was expected that the cells should be an efficient immunogen of *N-ras* p21 for antibody preparation. The hybridoma cells were screened, and one of these clones was analyzed. Using [^{35}S]methionine-labeled 7402 cell lysate, a protein species with a molecular weight of 21000 was immunoprecipitated which comigrates at the same position as that which reacted with Anti-p21 monoclonal antibody 238 (from Dr. Thomas Y. Shih). No immunoprecipitation band was observed with normal rat and mouse sera as controls. The antibodies are reactive with various cell lines of hepato-

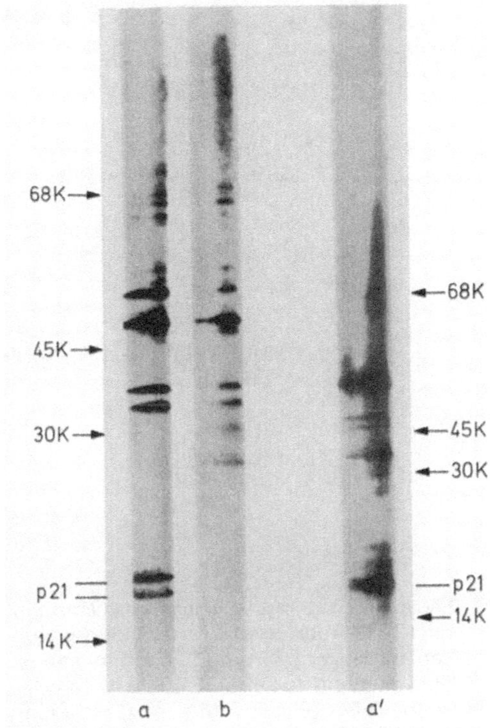

Fig. 4. p21 autoradiography of 7402 cells. *a* 7402 cells immunoprecipitated with anti-p21 259; *b* 7402 cells immunoprecipitated with normal rat serum; *a'* 7402 cells immunoprecipitated with anti-p21 238

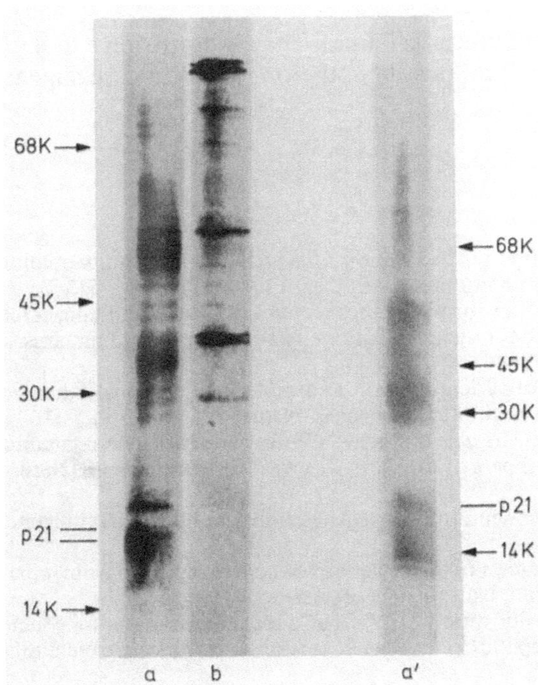

Fig. 5. p21 autoradiography of 7402 cell DNA transformed cells 782-12. *a* 782-12 cells immunoprecipitated with anti-p21 159; *b* 782-12 cells immunoprecipitated with normal rat serum; *a'* 782-12 cells immunoprecipitated with anti-p21 238

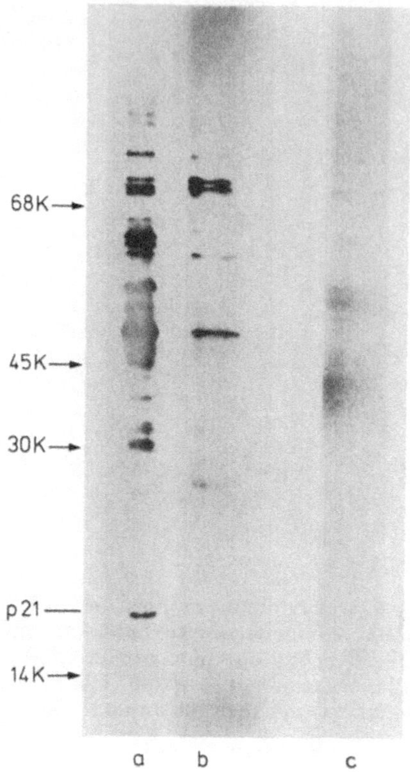

Fig. 6. p21 autoradiography of transformant cells T8T4 transfected with human primary hepatic cancer DNA. *a* T8T4 cell immunoprecipitated with anti-p21 259; *b* T8T4 cell immunoprecipitated with normal rat serum; *c* NIH/ 3T3 cell immunoprecipitated with anti-p21 259

carcinoma and also some of the lung cancer cell lines. They will provide a tool for investigating the expression of *N-ras* and possibly other *ras* genes in carcinogenesis.

References

1. Capon DJ, Seeburg PH, McGrath JP et al.: Activation of *Ki-ras 2* gene in human colon and lung carcinomas by two different point mutations. Nature 304 (1983) 507-513
2. Der CJ, Krontiris TG, Cooper GM: Transforming genes of human bladder and lung carcinoma cell lines are homologous to the *ras* genes of Harvey and Kirsten sarcoma viruses. Proc. nat. Acad. Sci. 79 (1982) 3637-3640
3. Diamond A, Cooper GM, Ritz J et al.: Identification and molecular cloning of human *Blym* transforming gene activated in Burkitt's lymphomas. Nature 305 (1983) 112-116
4. Ellis RW, DeFeo D, Shih TY et al.: The *p21 src* gene of Harvey and Kirsten sarcoma viruses originates from divergent members of a family of normal vertebrate genes. Nature 292 (1981) 506-510
5. Fausto N, Shank PR: Oncogene expression in liver regeneration and hepatocarcinogenesis. Hepatology 3 (1984) 1016-1023
6. Gamke C, Signer E, Morgni C: Activation of *N-ras* gene in bone marrow cells from a patient with acute myeloblastic leukaemia. Nature 307 (1984) 476-478
7. Gu JR, Tiang PQ, Wang X et al.: Identification of *N-ras* as a common transforming gene in human primary hepatic cancer, hepatic cell and leukemia K562 cell lines. Scientia Sinica B 5 (1985) 452-457

8. Guo G, Tiang PQ, Pan ZM et al.: Transforming activity of DNAs from human primary liver cancer and hepatoma 7402 cell lines. Chin. J. Oncol. 1 (1985) 12
9. Hall A, Marshall CJ, Spurr NK et al.: Identification of transforming gene in two human sarcoma cell lines as a new member of the *ras* gene family located on chromosome 1. Nature 303 (1983) 396-400
10. Hong J, Wei MH, Zhang X et al.: Monoclonal antibody against P21 - the product of human liver cancer oncogene *N-ras*. Tumor (Shanghai) (to be published)
11. Hu LF, Wang LP, Qui LW et al.: Expression of oncogenes in primary human hepatic cancer. Scientia Sinica B 5 (1985) 458-462
12. Murray MJ, Cunningham JM, Parada LD et al.: The HL-60 transforming sequence: A *ras* oncogene coexisting with altered *myc* genes in hematopoietic tumors. Cell 33 (1983) 749-757
13. Murray MJ, Shilo BZ, Shih C et al.: Three different human tumour cell lines contain different oncogenes. Cell 25 (1981) 335-361
14. Parada LF, Tabin CJ, Shih C et al.: Human EJ bladder carcinoma oncogene is homologue of Harvey sarcoma virus *ras* gene. Nature 297 (1982) 474-478
15. Shih C, Padhy LC, Murray MJ et al.: Transforming genes of carcinomas and neuroblastomas introduced into mouse fibroblasts. Nature 290 (1981) 261-264
16. Shih TY: Personal Communication, 1984
17. Shimizu K, Birnbaum D, Ruley MA et al.: Structure of the *Ki-ras* gene of the human lung carcinoma cell line Calu-1. Nature 304 (1982) 497-500
18. Shimizu K, Goldfarb M, Perucho M et al.: Isolation and preliminary characterization of the transforming gene of a human neuroblastoma cell line. Proc. nat. Acad. Sci. 80 (1983) 383-387
19. Taparowsky E, Shimizu K, Goldfarb M et al.: Structure and activation of the human *N-ras* gene. Cell 34 (1983) 581-586
20. Wan DF, Li HN, Gu JR: P21 overexpression in transformed NIH 3T3 cells derived from DNAs of human hepatic cancer and hepatic 7402 cell lines. Chin. J. Biochem. (to be published)

Hepatitis B Virus Sequences and Their Expression in Human Hepatoma Cells

A. Freytag von Loringhoven

We are engaged in a molecular biological analysis of the presumptive role of hepatitis B virus (HBV) in the pathogenesis of human hepatocellular carcinoma. This article is mainly about our own results obtained with the PLC/PRF/5 cell line, but I will also try to put our data in a more general context by including results from other groups, some of which were presented at a recent conference on the molecular biology by hepadnaviruses held in Cold Spring Harbor in May 1985.

First I would like to mention the architecture of the virus. It has a protein coat made up largely of the surface antigen HBsAg. The viral core contains the core antigen (HBcAg) that envelops the viral DNA, a DNA polymerase, and finally a protein that is covalently bound to the 5' end of the long strand of the viral DNA. The long DNA strand possesses a nick; the short strand has a fixed 5' end and a variable 3' end leaving a substantial gap. The small genome of 3.2 kilobases codes for 4 proteins: the surface and core antigens, the polymerase, and the HBxAg. No function has yet been assigned to this protein. It is a candidate for the protein covalently bound to the viral genome.

We have studied some 30 human hepatomas for the presence of HBV DNA by Southern blot analysis. About two-thirds of our samples contained integrated HBV sequences as evidenced by the presence of bands of higher molecular weight than the viral genome after digestion with a restriction enzyme that does not cleave HBV DNA.

To obtain a more detailed picture of the organization of integrated HBV sequences and their interaction with cellular DNA, we cloned HBV-specific sequences from the PLC/PRF/5 cell line, one of the few human hepatoma cell lines available. Out of a total of nine copies of integrated HBV sequences we obtained four [3, 4], which are shown in Fig. 1. Only one insert *(A-6.0)* contained the entire integrated copy flanked on both sides by cellular DNA. Due to an unexpected *Hind* III restriction site, the other three inserts – designated *A-10.7, A-10.5,* and *A-4.0* – were truncated by the cloning procedure yielding flanking sequences on only one side of the viral DNA. Structural analysis of our clones by restriction mapping and partial nucleotide sequencing revealed that in no case was the entire viral genome present. However, by and large the integrated sequences were colinear with the viral genome. A comparison with the HBV genome shows that *A-10.7* and *10.5* contain identical HBV sequences spanning roughly two-thirds of the genome. The S-gene is intact, whereas the polymerase and *HBx* genes are interrupted by the integration site. The same holds true for *A-6.0*. The *S*-gene is present and the polymerase and *HBx* genes are truncated. The 3' end of the *C*-gene is deleted, resulting in a fused *HBc*-polymerase reading frame. *A-4.0* is slightly

Cancer of the Liver, Esophagus, and Nasopharynx
Edited by G. Wagner and Zhang You-Hui

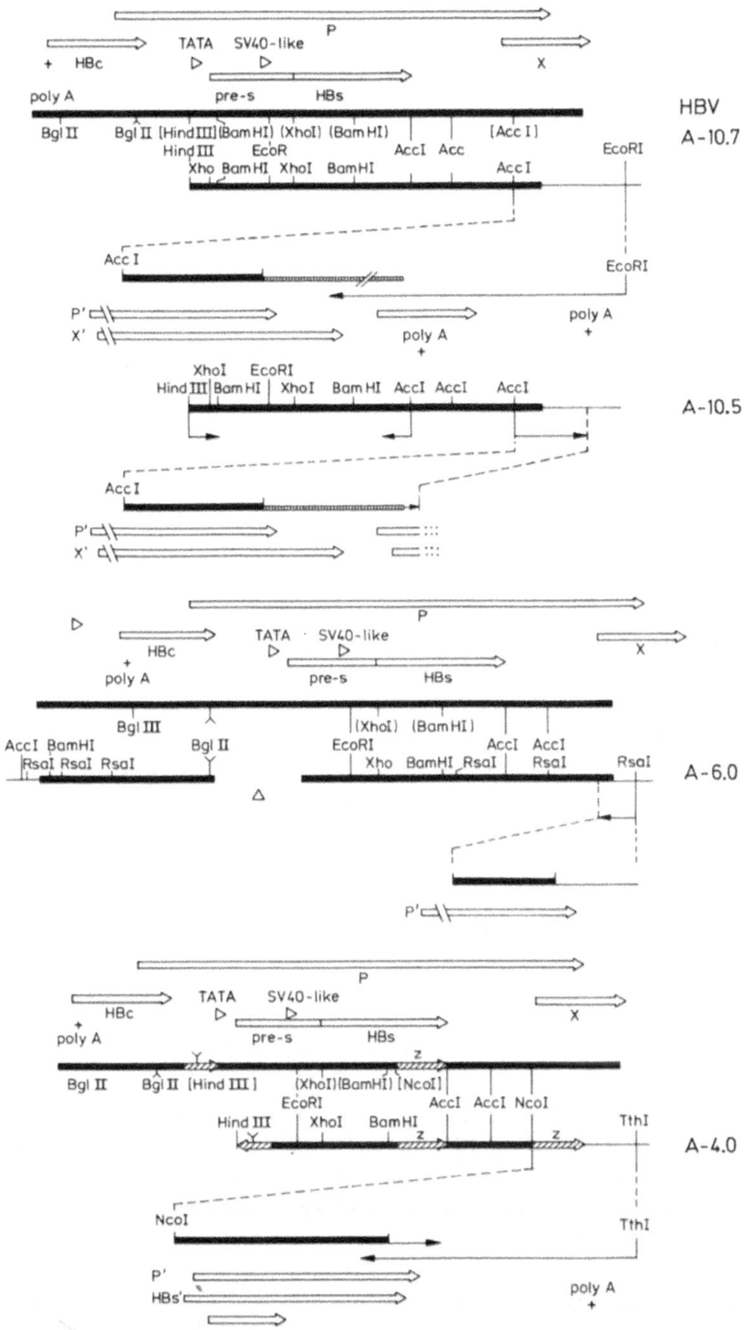

Fig. 1. Organization of HBV DNA and human flanking sequences in the HBV-specific inserts cloned from PLC/PRF/5 cells. The HBV genome (subtype adw$_2$) is aligned to HBV sequences in the cloned inserts. *Filled boxes* and *thin lines* represent HBV sequences and human DNA, respectively. Only parts of the cloned human flanking sequences are shown here (for further details see Koch et al. [3]). Duplicated *(Z)* and inverted *(Y)* HBV parts are drawn as *hatched arrows*. The hatched boxes in *A-10.7* and *A-10.5* indicate identical human flanking sequences. Reading frames are drawn as *open arrows*. Polyadenylation sites are indicated by *crosses*, promoters by *open arrowheads*

more complicated with an inversion and a duplication. Again, only the *S*-gene is intact.

From these results it emerges that only the *S*-gene is intact, whereas all other genes are truncated by viral integration. The results from Rutter's group in San Francisco, who have cloned the remaining integrated HBV copies from Alexander cells [9], confirm our conclusions. In their clones, too, the *S*-gene is preferentially included, the other genes are invariably interrupted. I should emphasize that this does not necessarily preclude expression, since fusion proteins may well be produced.

The DNA data agree with the known expression by PLC/PRF/5 cells of normal-sized HBsAg. Despite the absence of an intact *HBc* gene within the integrated viral DNA, we have demonstrated low levels of core antigen when Alexander cells are grown as nude mouse tumors, but not when cultured in vitro [5]. This shows that the expression of HBcAg is tightly regulated in PLC/PRF/5 cells. The size of this protein is not yet known. HBcAg may either be expressed as a fusion protein by integrated HBV sequences or alternatively as normal-sized protein by low levels of extrachromosomal HBV DNA present in PLC/PRF/5 cells [6]. Recently, HBxAg expression was shown in PLC/PRF/5 cells, but its size is abnormal [7]. No data are available on the expression of the polymerase. From the combined protein and DNA data of Alexander cells it appears that normal S-Ag is produced, whereas X- as well as the core antigen may be fusion proteins.

Generally, in hepatomas HBsAg is sometimes, but not always, present, whereas HBcAg has, to my knowledge, never been detected. Very little is known about HBxAg and polymerase expression. A great deal of structural information on the organization of integrated HBV sequences from hepatomas has recently become available, and what we learnt from PLC/PRF/5 cells applies by and large to other tumors, too. The S-gene is preferentially intact but not in all tumors [8]. The other genes are preferentially interrupted or deleted. No HBV gene is present intact in all tumors.

The data thus argue against a model of oncogenesis involving a transforming gene carried by HBV itself like the acutely transforming retroviruses. However, a role of fusion proteins (HBV-HBV or HBV-human) can presently not be excluded.

The very long period required (up to 10–20 years) for hepatocellular carcinomas to develop is consistent with models invoking an interaction of HBV DNA with flanking cellular sequences. It would simply take a long time for the viral DNA to integrate into the critical region of host DNA. Some of the data obtained with PLC/PRF/5 cells are consistent with models involving HBV as an insertional mutagen.

The first type of mechanism is called enhancer insertion. HBV contains an enhancer sequence, i.e. a DNA region that can stimulate the activity of a nearby promoter. This enhancer region is present near the integration site in all four inserts. One could thus envisage the stimulation of a cellular oncogene by the integrated viral enhancer.

The second mechanism is called promoter insertion. The integrated viral DNA transcribes viral as well as flanking host RNA from a viral promoter. Northern and S1 nuclease analysis of the mRNA transcribed from insert *A-10.7* has indeed shown the presence of host-virus fusion transcripts [1] (Fig. 2). These mRNAs lead to extremely high amounts of normal HBsAg. Following gene transfer into tissue-cul-

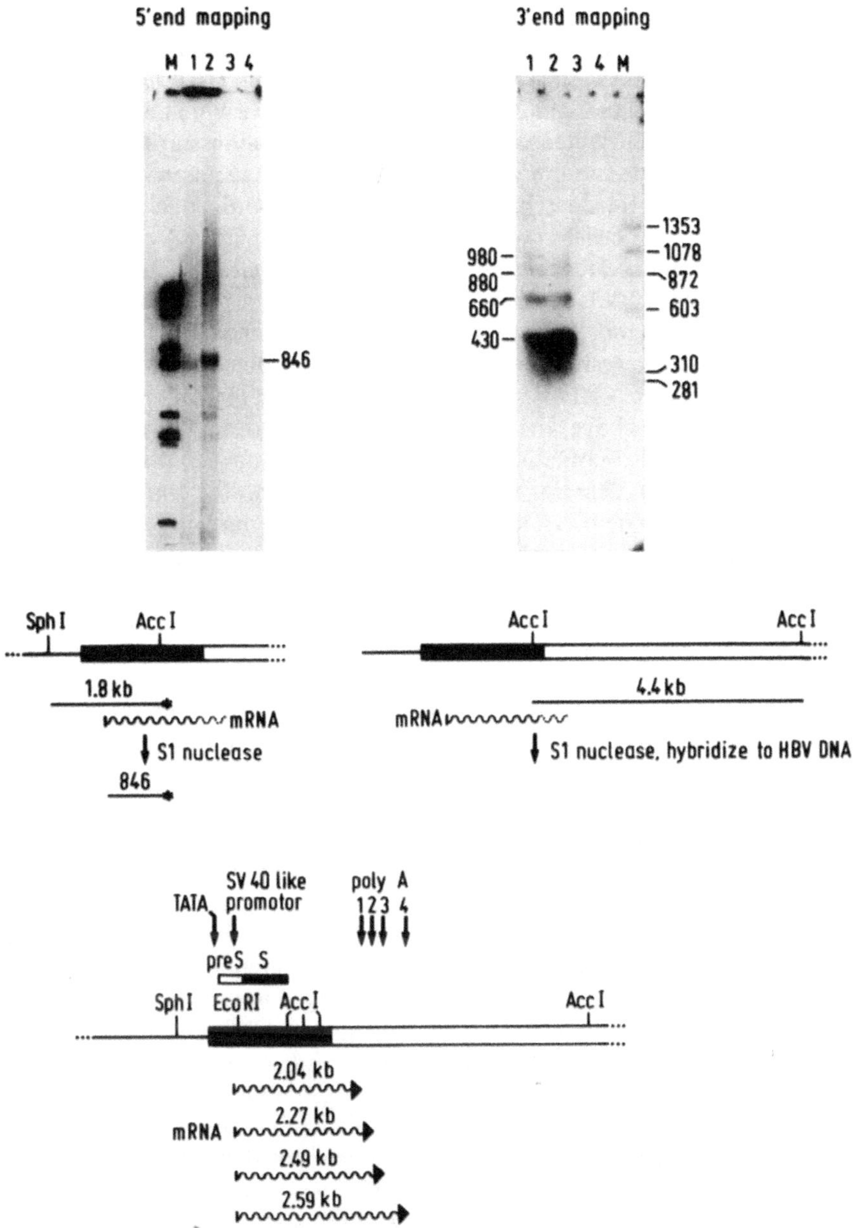

Fig. 2. HBV-specific mRNAs transcribed from insert *A-10.7.* In an excerpt of *A-10.7* the *filled box* represents HBV DNA, the *open box* human DNA, and the *thin line* plasmid DNA. *Above the locations of the preS and S gene,* the viral promoters (TATA, SV40 like) and the human polyadenylation signals are indicated. *Below* the four virus-host mRNAs are shown

tured cells, a quantitative comparison of HBsAg amounts secreted by cells transfected by *A-10.7* and genomic HBV DNA showed that the insert is nearly an order of magnitude more efficient in the production of HBsAg than HBV DNA. This may be due to a stem-loop structure at the 3' end of the messenger which may expose the poly (A) addition site. The nucleotide sequence of the region transcribed reveals fused reading frames of the viral *pol* and *X*-gene with host sequences and also one host reading frame. Unfortunately, we do not yet know if such proteins are expressed in PLC/PRF/5 cells.

The third mechanism of oncogenesis involving an interaction of integrated HBV sequences with cellular DNA consists of integration causing the inactivation of a cellular gene ("anti-oncogene") that normally suppresses the transformed phenotype. In principle, any integration event could inactivate such a gene. We also have evidence of an association of HBV integration with major rearrangements in host DNA [2]. As mentioned above, the two clones *A-10.7* and *10.5* contain identical HBV sequences. They also contain identical flanking sequences up to a position 187 bp from the junction. After this point, the host sequences are completely different. The most plausible interpretation of these data is a duplication of a region encompassing integrated viral DNA as well as flanking sequences leading to a major rearrangement of the flanking DNA.

If HBV really interacts with specific cellular sequences thus contributing to cellular transformation, one would expect a small number of cellular genes to be involved and thus to find HBV integrated in only one or at least a small number of regions in different hepatoma DNAs. By analogy, in the classic model system of promoter insertion (avian leukosis virus-induced bursal lymphomas in birds), in almost all cases the viral DNA is integrated next to the cellular *myc* gene.

Comparing different hepatomas, it turns out that HBV is not integrated into exactly the same site, as the nucleotide sequences of flanking DNA are always different. Nor is HBV integrated into the same region up to about 10 kb. This has been studied using host sequences flanking HBV integrates as probes against DNA from other tumors. Extra bands would indicate rearrangements in the same region. Thus far more than five such "flanking probes" made from different integrates have been hybridized by different labs including ours against large numbers of tumors. There is no evidence of HBV integration into the same region in different tumors.

A final possibility is preferred integration into a region larger than 10–20 kb. We, therefore, started to determine the chromosomes our cloned PLC/PRF/5 cell inserts are integrated in. This can be done by hybridizing flanking DNA probes to a panel of DNAs from mouse-human hybrid cells, each of them containing only a few human chromosomes. By correlating positive hybridization signals with the chromosomes known to be present in the hybrid cells, we assigned our insert *A-6.0* to chromosome 3. At the Cold Spring Harbor Conference, all hitherto identified chromosomal locations of HBV integrations were compiled. These results tentatively suggest a preference for chromosomes 3 and 9 (Fig. 3).

I would like to conclude by summarizing how the data on integrated HBV sequences and their expression fit different models of oncogenesis. Unfortunately, despite a lot of work the picture is still far from clear. The possibility of an HBV-transforming gene appears unlikely. A role, however, for fusion proteins cannot be excluded, since so far no extensive analysis of HBV proteins expressed in hepato-

1	2	3	4	5	6	7	8	9	10	11	12	13	14	15	16	17	18	19	20	21	22	X	Y
	+	+			+	+		+			+					+	+						
		+						+															
		+						+															
								+															

Fig. 3. Chromosomal localization of integrated HBV sequences from different hepatomas. Data were compiled at the Conference on the Molecular Biology of Hepadnaviruses held at Cold Spring Harbor in May 1985

mas exists. As a transforming mechanism transacting proteins may be considered. Some of the evidence is consistent with models of *cis* interaction with cellular sequences such as promoter or enhancer insertion or the inactivation of a cellular antoncogene, but it is intriguing to find HBV integrated in different regions in different tumors.

References

1. Freytag von Loringhoven A, Koch S, Hofschneider PH, Koshy R: Co-transcribed 3' host sequences augment expression of integrated hepatitis B virus DNA. EMBO J. 4 (1985) 249-255
2. Koch S, Freytag von Loringhoven A, Hofschneider PH, Koshy R: Amplification and rearrangement in hepatoma cell DNA associated with integrated hepatitis B virus DNA. EMBO J. 3 (1984) 2185-2189
3. Koch S, Freytag von Loringhoven A, Kahmann R, Hofschneider PH, Koshy R: The genetic organization of hepatitis B virus DNA in the human hepatoma cell line PLC/PRF/5. Nucl. Acids Res. 12 (1984) 6871-6886
4. Koshy R, Koch S, Freytag von Loringhoven A, Kahmann R, Murray K, Hofschneider PH: Integration of hepatitis B virus DNA: evidence for integration in the single-stranded gap. Cell 34 (1983) 215-223
5. Marquardt O, Freytag von Loringhoven A, Frösner G: Expression of hepatitis B virus core antigen is induced in human hepatoma cells by their growth in nude mice. J. Gen. Virol. 65 (1984) 1443-1448
6. Marquardt O, Zaslavsky V, Hofschneider PH: Evidence for non-chromosomal hepatitis B virus surface (HBsAg-) and core antigen (HBcAg-) DNA sequences in a human hepatoma cell line. J. Gen. Virol 61 (1982) 105-109
7. Moriarty A, Alexander H, Lerner R, Thornton G: Antibodies to peptides detect new hepatitis B antigen: serological correlation with hepatocellular carcinoma. Science 227 (1985) 429-432
8. Ogston C, Jonak G, Rogler C, Astrin S, Summers J: Cloning and structural analysis of integrated woodchuck hepatitis virus sequences from hepatocellular carcinomas of woodchucks. Cell 29 (1982) 385-394
9. Ziemer M, Garcia P, Shaul Y, Rutter W: Sequence of hepatitis B virus DNA incorporated into the genome of a human hepatoma cell line. J. Virol. 53 (1985) 885-892

Subclinical Hepatocellular Carcinoma

Tang Zhao-You, Yu Ye-Qin, and Yang Bing-Hui

Ten years ago, 3254 cases with primary liver cancer (PLC) in China were analyzed. The extremely high proportion of late stage patients with jaundice or ascites (52.6%), the extremely low series resection rate (5.3%), and the dismal ultimate outcome (1-year survival, 8.6%) revealed that PLC was indeed an enormous malignancy [23]. Every year, PLC causes 250000 deaths in the world [29], 100000 deaths in China [9], and 3000 deaths in Shanghai [3]. However, encouraging things have happened in China recently:

1. Hepatitis B virus (HBV), aflatoxin, contamination of drinking water, and other chemicals are considered to be etiological factors; identification of the transforming gene N-ras in PLC has been reported.
2. The concept of subclinical hepatocellular carcinoma (SCHCC) has been developed on the basis of alpha fetoprotein (AFP) serosurvey, involving a new approach to early detection, revision of the principles underlying surgical treatment, new insight into the natural history of hepatocellular carcinoma (HCC), and renewal of the prognostic concept, particularly with 5-year survival after resection of SCHCC up to 72.9% [19, 26].
3. Multimodality and aggressive approaches to the treatment of symptomatic PLC.
4. Establishment of human HCC cell lines and transplantable human HCC in immune-deficient animals.
5. More concern has been centered on the study of HCC cell membrane and its glycoprotein, glycolipid components in basic research.
6. Radioimmunodetection and radioimmunotherapy by using appropriate antibodies is also under way.

Epidemiology and Etiology of PLC in China

The standardized mortality rate of PLC in China is 14.52/100000 in males and 5.61/100000 in females. It ranks third in cancer mortality, next to gastric and esophageal cancer [9]. A trend toward increasing mortality (27.3/100000 in 1963–1965 vs. 35.8/100000 in 1976–1979) was recently observed in Shanghai [4]. The highest standardized mortality rate of up to 50.8/100000 in males and 6.0/100000 in females was recorded in Chongming County of Shanghai, an island situated on the outlet of the Yangtze River. The mortality rate in the eastern part of the county is higher than that of the west, which is correlated to the higher aflatoxin B_1 (AFB_1) concentration in cooked staple food; however, the difference in positivity of serum HBsAg

Cancer of the Liver, Esophagus, and Nasopharynx
Edited by G. Wagner and Zhang You-Hui

between these two areas is not significant [5]. Inhibition of AFB_1 on Ea rosette formation and lymphocyte mitosis [12] on T-lymphocyte proliferation [8] and natural killer activity [10] were observed, thus suggesting that it is an inhibitor of human immunity [12]. On the other hand, strong evidence of a close relation between HBV and HCC was observed in the authors' institution. In 100 cases of pathologically proven HCC, the positivities of serum HBV markers using Abbott kits were: HBsAg, 90%; antiHBs, 18%; antiHBc, 97%; HBeAg, 21%; and antiHBe, 57%. Only two cases showed negative findings in all of the HBV markers; the positivities of tissue HBV markers using Dako PAP kits were: HBsAg, 82%, and HBcAg, 25%; dysplasia was found in 73 cases. The incidence of cirrhosis was found to be 85.45% in a series comprising 220 cases with HCC [34].

A nuclear antigen (HBNA) was also reported in two human hepatoma cell lines containing integrated HBV DNA but not in three hepatoma cell lines [28]. The association of contaminated drinking water with liver cancer hyperendemicity has also been noticed in Nanhui County, a Shanghai suburb. Therefore, the common prevention catchwords that have been suggested are "control of water, control of corn, and prevention of hepatitis" [35]. Furthermore, it is postulated that increased frequency of HLA-A_3 and HLA-DRW_9, which were significantly higher than in normal controls, may have some connection with host susceptibility to HCC [11].

Definition of Subclinical HCC

A patient with SCHCC is arbitrarily defined as one without obvious HCC symptoms and signs, while clinical HCC (CHCC) exhibits both HCC symptoms and signs. SCHCC is detected principally by AFP survey or serial APF monitoring in subjects with a background of liver disease; however, CHCC is discovered in the majority of cases in patients who seek medical care because of the appearance of symptoms [19].

Materials for the Study of Subclinical HCC

A comparative study was carried out with 121 cases of SCHCC and 758 cases of CHCC in Zhong Shan Hospital during the period 1958-1984. All the patients were pathologically proven. As shown in Table 1, the mean age was around 46-48 years, the male: female ratio being 16.3:1 and 7:1 respectively. A marked liver disease background was observed in association with cirrhosis in up to 86% of the patients.

Major Features of Subclinical HCC

The special features of SCHCC as compared with CHCC could be summarized as: (1) mostly detected by AFP serosurvey (96.5% vs. 8.4%); (2) much smaller median tumor size (4 cm vs. 10 cm) and much lower median AFP level (2000 ng/ml vs. 10000 ng/ml); (3) much lower positivity of conventional diagnostic measurements, such as abnormal serum alkaline phosphatase (ALP 16.5% vs. 59.8%); (4) much

Table 1. Pathologically proven HCC ($n=879$) (Zhong Shan Hospital 1958-1984)

	SCHCC ($n=121$)	CHCC ($n=758$)
Age (range)	48 (21-67)	46 (13-82)
Male: female	16.3:1	7:1
Hepatitis history (%)	64.5	37.5
Over 5 years (%)	80.8	77.4
Cirrhosis (%)	86.3	81.3
Macronodular (%)	73.3	74.1
Cell type - HCC	98.3	93.4
Cholangio	0	2.8
Mixed	1.7	3.8

higher series resection rate (69.4% vs. 29.2%); much lower operative mortality (1.2% vs. 10.0%); and (5) much higher 5-year survival rate, particularly after resection (72.9% vs. 16.1%).

Significance in Research of Subclinical HCC

The significance of the study of SCHCC is clear. Firstly, it provides a hopeful stage for the radical cure of HCC. Curutchet [2], collecting the data of 45 authors during 1905-1970, found that only 45 five-year survivors were obtained worldwide; however, 43 cases were observed in our series, 23 of them SCHCC. Secondly, this has proved to be an important approach to improve overall HCC prognosis. As a result of an increasing proportion of SCHCC in the entire series (0% in 1958-1966, 7.2% in 1967-1975, and 21.2% in 1976-1984), a marked increase in series resection rate was observed (16.1%, 34.7%, and 39.6% respectively); this resulted in a remarkable improvement of the prognostic pattern (5-year survival rates being 1.7% and 19.5% respectively). Thirdly, this has also led to changing concepts of clinical research of HCC [26].

Problems Concerning Early Detection

In China, HCC amounts to around 90% of PLC [23]; serum AFP is detectable in the majority of HCC prior to the appearance of symptoms [7, 25]. Thus, AFP serosurveys have been employed as the principal approach for early detection of SCHCC since 1971 [16, 17, 38]. The key problem nowadays is the "cost-effectiveness." When an AFP serosurvey was performed in the total population during 1971-1980, the discovery rate was only 14.6/100000; however, it increased to 501.0/100000 in screening a high-risk population (Table 2). Subjects who had a history of hepatitis for more than 5 years or were serum HBsAg positive and aged over 40 years were considered to be in the high-risk population, the discovery rates being three to four times higher than those of their counterparts. The passive reverse hemagglutination

Table 2. Alpha fetoprotein serosurvey in a high-risk population

AFP serosurvey	Population screened	No. of HCCs detected	Discovery rate per 100000
Total population (1971-1980)	305997	45	14.6
High-risk population (1983-1984)	2997	15	501.0

Table 3. Stage patterns in survey and nonsurvey groups

Clinical stage	Survey		Nonsurvey	
	Cases	%	Cases	%
Subclinical (I)	118	64.5	3	0.5
Moderate (II)	48	26.2	493	70.8
Late (III)	17	9.3	200	28.7

assay is sensitive enough to be the initial screening test, although some false-positives will be encountered, but it is less expensive than the radioimmunoassay. Theoretically, an AFP serosurvey for a high-risk population twice a year is better; the combination with an ultrasonography survey will also increase the discovery rate; however, using a single AFP survey once a year seems to be acceptable from a "cost-effectiveness" point of view in China.

The merit of the AFP serosurvey is clear. In the survey group, SCHCC amounted to 64.5%; however, in the group not screened, moderate stage HCC amounted to 70.8% (Table 3).

Early Diagnosis

The concept of an early diagnosis of HCC has been completely changed. Instead of a combined analysis of symptoms, signs, and enzymological findings, the combined analysis of AFP and alanine aminotransferase (ALT) levels is accepted to be the principal approach to an early diagnosis of HCC [6]. Because the positive results of many conventional diagnostic measurements are too low and seem to be of no value for the early diagnosis, only ultrasonography and angiography are accepted as localization measurements (Table 4).

Alpha fetoprotein is so far the best marker for HCC; its clinical value has been thoroughly assessed [24]. However, the positivity of AFP in pathologically proven HCC was only 74.8% (558/746) in this series. Furthermore, differential diagnosis between AFP-positive HCC accompanied by abnormal ALT and chronic liver diseases in an active stage together with abnormal AFP remains a problem to be solved. Therefore, AFP variants, alpha$_1$-antitrypsin activity (A_1AT) and 5'-nucleotide phosphodiesterase isozyme V (5'-NPDase V) were also reported in China. The determination of concanavalin-A (con-A)-reactive and con-A-nonreactive AFP variants may help in the differential diagnosis of HCC [30]. A_1AT may have some

Table 4. Diagnostic value of different measurements in SCHCC and CHCC

	SCHCC (%)	CHCC (%)
Gamma-GTP over 10 units	24.8 (27/109)	74.2 (412/555)[a]
ALP over 13 units	16.5 (18/109)	59.8 (394/659)[a]
Scintigraphy (+)	42.1 (48/114)	90.5 (559/618)[a]
Ultrasonography (+)	75.4 (46/61)[a]	95.3 (202/212)[a]
Angiography (+)	82.1 (32/39)[a]	82.1 (23/28)[a]

[a] Figures were acceptable for diagnosis

diagnostic value for HCC, especially for AFP low level or negative cases; the positive results (over 157 units) were 59.8% in HCC, 5% in cirrhosis, and 3.5% in hepatitis [31]. 5'-NPDase V was claimed to be of value in the diagnosis of AFP nonproducing HCC [13]; however, it only had a limited value because of the relatively high positivity of up to 45.5% in patients with various benign hepatobiliary diseases or tumors other than hepatoma [33]. Recently, isoferritin and lipid-bound sialiac acid were shown in the authors' laboratory to be of some value for differential diagnosis of AFP-negative HCC. However, for an early detection of HCC, AFP remains the marker of choice.

For the localization of HCC, the positive results of hepatic angiography (HA), ultrasonography (US), and radionuclide imaging (RI) were 92.3%, 96.3%, and 86.5% in HCC with a diameter larger than 5 cm; 86.4%, 56.5%, and 34.8% in HCC equal to and smaller than 5 cm, 85.7%, 37.5%, and 10.0% in HCC equal to and smaller than 3 cm respectively. The lowest limit of the size of HCC for differentiation was 1 cm in HA, 2 cm in US and 3 cm in RI. US was accepted to be a noninvasive initial screening and follow-up monitoring assay for early stage HCC which seemed to be superior to computed tomography (CT) [22].

Changing Therapeutic Pattern

Resection remains the modality of choice in the treatment of both CHCC and SCHCC. Therefore, the series resection rate plays a very important role in the overall prognosis of HCC. It was encouraging that a marked increase of series resection rate was observed in comparison with the therapeutic pattern between SCHCC and CHCC (Table 5). Further analysis revealed that the type of resection was also markedly changed. Limited resection amounted to 64.3% in the resection of SCHCC;

Table 5. Therapeutic pattern of SCHCC and CHCC patients

%	SCHCC ($n=121$)	CHCC ($n=758$)
Resection	69.4	29.2
Surgery other than resection	23.2	23.4
Conservative treatment	7.4	36.3
No treatment	0	11.1

however, lobectomy amounted to 74.7% of CHCC resection. Limited resection is accepted to be the type of resection for small HCC, particularly in those right lobe cancers accompanied by cirrhosis. Limited resection has resulted in a marked increase in the resectability rate and a marked decrease in the operative mortality rate (1.2% in SCHCC resection vs. 10.0% in CHCC resection). Generally, resection with cut end 2-3 cm from the tumor is accepted to be a radical resection.

Subclinical Recurrence and Its Management

A much higher AFP normalization rate was observed after SCHCC resection as compared with CHCC resection (78.5% vs. 40.2%) and resulted in a much lower recurrence rate (39.0% vs. 83.8%). However, recurrence and metastasis remain a major problem to be solved after radical resection. Fortunately, AFP is not only of value for early diagnosis of HCC, but also of value for the diagnosis of subclinical recurrence or subclinical metastasis. We routinely performed long-term (up to 10 years) AFP follow-up monitoring in patients after radical resection of AFP-producing HCC. According to our previous experience, the reappearance of abnormal serum AFP always indicates recurrence or metastasis of HCC, provided serum ALT, bilirubin, and prothrombin time are normal. Regeneration of liver parenchyma after hepatic resection in human beings never induces abnormal serum AFP. The reappearance of abnormal serum AFP generally occurs 6-12 months prior to the establishment of a diagnosis of SCHCC and 12-18 months prior to the occurrence of HCC symptoms. In the case of clinical recurrence, further surgery is generally contraindicated; however, in subclinical recurrence, reoperation is strongly indicated, provided the liver function is in a compensated stage. In this series, 30 cases had received reoperation (14 in SCHCC group and 16 in CHCC group) for subclinical recurrence or solitary pulmonary metastasis. As has been reported, the results were most encouraging and proved to be an important approach to prolonging survival after radical resection of AFP-positive HCC [27]. According to our previous experience, the reappearance of AFP up to 200 ng/ml for 2 months is a case for thorough investigation, including ultrasonography, computed tomography, and selective angiography, if needed. Reoperation should be carried out in patients with localized findings.

Surgical Treatment of Unresectable Subclinical HCC

High-power YAG laser vaporization is an acceptable modality for the treatment of superficially located unresectable SCHCC [36]; cryosurgery using −196 °C liquid nitrogen also provides good palliation when the lesion is located near to the hepatic hilum [37]. Hepatic artery ligation or cannulation can be employed for the treatment of huge and deep-seated unresectable HCC. However, the combination of these two modalities has proved to be much better than the single procedures, and sequence second-step resection was feasible in nine cases in this series (three in SCHCC and six in the CHCC group) after a remarkable regression of the tumor [20, 21].

Table 6. Prognostic pattern of SCHCC and CHCC patients

Five-year survival (life table method)	SCHCC	CHCC
Entire series	43.9	4.2
Resected group	72.9	16.1
Unresected group	0	0

Changing Prognostic Pattern of Subclinical HCC

The prognosis of HCC has rarely changed in the past decades, with an overall 5-year survival not exceeding 3% [1, 14, 32]. However, as mentioned above, the series 5-year survival has increased from 1.7% in 1958–1966 to 19.5% in 1976–1984. This has principally been a result of an increasing proportion of SCHCC in the entire series, of increasing series resection rate, and particularly of the dramatic increase of 5-year survival after resection of SCHCC. As shown in Table 6, 5-year survivors were observed neither in the unresected group of SCHCC nor in CHCC; however, a much higher 5-year survival rate was obtained after SCHCC resection as compared with CHCC resection (72.9% vs. 16.1%) and resulted in a tenfold higher 5-year survival rate in the entire series of SCHCC than in the CHCC group [19]. In this series, 79 cases have survived more than 3 years, 38 of them being SCHCC. Of the 79 cases, 43 cases have survived more than 5 years, and SCHCC amounted to 23 cases. The majority of long-term survivors have returned to their original work, some young patients have got married after removal of small HCC 10 years ago, and some can even play football again.

Therefore, HCC is no longer an incurable disease if the patient is discovered in the subclinical stage with a relatively small tumor and early radical resection can be carried out.

The Changing Concept of the Natural History of HCC

The study of SCHCC has provided clues for the understanding of the natural history of AFP-producing HCC. Contrary to the previous opinion of a relatively short average survival time of HCC (around 2–5 months) [4, 6, 15, 23], a relatively long natural history of around 2 years does exist [18]. Generally, at the very beginning of the onset of HCC, when no changes can be found except a slight elevation of AFP, diagnosis is difficult. In the subclinical stage, the mean size of HCC is around 4 cm; early diagnosis is feasible based on an analysis of AFP and localization findings; symptoms and signs will appear 8–9 months later. There is no difficulty in diagnosing moderate stage HCC with obvious symptoms and signs; the mean period is around 4 months. The late stage characterized by ascites, jaundice, or distant metastases, particularly with emboli in the main trunk of the portal vein, seems to be irreversible and lasts 2 months until death [19]. From a clinical viewpoint, a radical cure of HCC by resection is possible before marked spreading occurs when the tumor grows to around 5 cm; effective prolongation of survival is feasible by other combination treatment before tumor emboli occur in the portal trunk.

Conclusion

The study of SCHCC has opened a new era of HCC surgery [21]. The role of surgery in the treatment of HCC has become more important. In SCHCC, surgery may provide a radical cure for the disease; in moderate stage CHCC, surgery may merely prolong survival. Therefore, endeavors should be made for an earlier diagnosis and earlier resection. More specific nonsurgical treatment is also needed for SCHCC with uncompensated liver function. The problem of multicentric origin in some HCC patients remains a challenge for future investigation.

References

1. Axtell IM, Cutler SJ, Myers MH: End results in Cancer. Report No. 4, pp. 72-76, US Department of Health, Education and Welfare, Public Health Service, NIH, NCI, Bethesda, MD 1972
2. Curutchet HP, Terz JJ, Kay S et al.: Primary liver cancer. Surgery 70 (1971) 467-479
3. Dept. Epidemiology of Shanghai Cancer Institute, Shanghai Sanitary-antiepidemic Center: Analysis of cancer incidence, mortality and survival rates in Shanghai urban area during the period 1972-79. Tumor 2 (1982) 385. (In Chinese)
4. Ervasti J: Primary carcinoma of the liver - a pathologic and clinical study of 100 cases. Acta chir. scand. 334 (1964) 1s-65s.
5. Gao RN, Tu JT, Gao YT: A preliminary report of etiological and epidemiological studies on primary liver cancer in Chongming County of Shanghai. Tumor 1 (1981) 148-151. (In Chinese)
6. Gustafson EG: An analysis of 62 cases of primary carcinoma of the liver based on 24,000 necropsies at Bellevue Hospital. Ann. intern. Med. 11 (1937) 889-900
7. Heyward WL, Lanier AP, Bender TR et al.: Early detection of primary hepatocellular carcinoma by screening for alpha-fetoprotein in high-risk families - a case report. Lancet 1983, II: 1161-1162
8. Hong JX, Zhang QJ, Liu LW et al.: Study on the function of normal human B lymphocytes in the culture with aflatoxin B_1. In 1984 Tumor Scientific Reports Abstract, p. 21. Shanghai Cancer Institute, WHO Collaborating Centre for Research on Cancer, 1985
9. Li B, Li JY: National survey of cancer mortality in China. Chin. J. Oncol. 2 (1980) 1-10. (in Chinese)
10. Lin TZ, Zhang QJ, Len YW et al.: Study on immunological mechanism of carcinogenesis of primary liver cancer. In 1984 Tumor Scientific Reports Abstract, p. 33. Shanghai Cancer Institute, WHO Collaborating Centre for Research on Cancer, 1985
11. Liu YX, Yu XS, Gao RN et al.: Association of HLA antigen and HCC. Cancer Res. Prev. Treatm. 11 (1984) 65-67. (in Chinese)
12. Liu YX, Yu XS, Yang YQ et al.: In vitro effect of aflatoxin B_1 on human peripheral blood lymphocytes. Tumor 1 (1981) 249-250. (In Chinese)
13. Lu HM, Chen J, Jiang KL et al.: The value of serum 5'-nucleotide phosphodiesterase isozyme in the diagnosis of primary liver cancer. Nat. med. J. China 61 (1981) 219-221. (In Chinese)
14. Okuda K, The Liver Cancer Study Group of Japan: Primary liver cancers in Japan. Cancer 45 (1980) 2663-2669
15. Rosenberg DML, Oshsner A: Primary carcinoma of the liver - an analysis of fifty five autopsied cases, the record of a case with resection, and a review of the recent literature. Surgery 24 (1948) 1036-1068
16. Shanghai Coordinating Group for Research on Liver Cancer: AFP sero-survey in diagnosis and screening of hepatocellular carcinoma. Nat. med. J. China 53 (1973) 455-457. (In Chinese)
17. Shanghai Coordinating Group for Research on Liver Cancer: Diagnosis and treatment of

primary hepatocellular carcinoma in early stage - report of 134 cases. Chin. med. J. 92 (1979) 801-806
18. Tang ZY: A new concept on the natural course of hepatocellular carcinoma. Chin. med. J. 94 (1981) 585-588
19. Tang ZY (Edit.): Subclinical Hepatocellular Carcinoma. Beijing: China Academic Publ.; Berlin: Springer 1985
20. Tang ZY: Current status of treatment of hepatocellular carcinoma. Chin. med. J. 98 (1985) 257-264
21. Tang ZY: Hepatocellular carcinoma - When should we stop surgery? (Guest editorial). J. exp. clin. Cancer Res. 4 (1985) 5-9
22. Tang ZY, Lu JZ, Zhou NQ et al.: Small hepatocellular carcinoma (HCC). VI. Value of hepatoarteriography, B-scan ultrasonography and liver scintiscan in the localization of small HCC - a comparative study based on operative findings. Acta acad. med. primae Shanghai 9 (1982) 101-105. (In Chinese)
23. Tang ZY, Yang BH: Primary liver cancer - clinical analysis of 3254 cases (from 11 provinces, 21 hospitals, in China). Cancer Res. Prev. Treatm. 2 (1974) 207-215. (In Chinese)
24. Tang ZY, Yang BH: Clinical evaluation of alpha-fetoprotein as tumor marker for hepatocellular carcinoma. Chin. J. Oncol. 3 (1981) 205-209. (In Chinese)
25. Tang ZY, Yang BH, Tang CL et al.: Evaluation of population screening for hepatocellular carcinoma. Chin. med. J. 93 (1980) 795-799
26. Tang ZY, Ying YY, Gu TJ: Hepatocellular carcinoma - changing concepts in recent years. In H. Popper, F. Schaffner (eds): Progress in Liver Diseases, Vol. 7, pp. 637-647. New York: Grune & Stratton 1982
27. Tang ZY, Yu YQ, Zhou XD: An important approach to prolonging survival further after radical resection of AFP positive hepatocellular carcinoma. J. exp. clin. Cancer Res. 3 (1984) 359-368
28. Wen YM, Mitamura K, Merchant B et al.: Nuclear antigen detected in hepatoma cell lines containing integrated hepatitis B virus DNA. Infect. Immun. 39 (1983) 1361-1367
29. World Health Organization: Prevention of Liver Cancer. WHO Techn. Rep. Ser. No. 691. Geneva 1983
30. Xu KL, Yu EX, Lu LN et al.: Alpha-fetoprotein variants and their clinical significance. Chin. med. J. 97 (1984) 538-542
31. Xu SK, Guan SF, Wang GL et al.: Assay of alpha$_1$-antitrypsin activity in the diagnosis of hepatocellular carcinoma - determination of serum trypsin inhibitor capacity. Tumor 1 (1981) 245-248. (In Chinese)
32. Yang BH, Tang ZY: Primary liver cancer - a clinical analysis of 1045 cases. In Z. Y. Tang (Edit.): Primary Liver Cancer, pp. 366-374. Shanghai: Shanghai Sci. Techn. Publ. 1981. (In Chinese)
33. Yang BH, Tang ZY: Evaluation of 5'-nucleotide phosphodiesterase isozyme V for the diagnosis of primary liver cancer. Acta acad. med. primae Shanghai 9 (1982) 275-278. (In Chinese)
34. Ying YY, Zhou WR, Sung QL et al.: The relationship between hepatitis B virus, liver cirrhosis and primary hepatocellular carcinoma. Tumor 1 (1981) 49-53. (In Chinese)
35. Yu SZ: Epidemiology of primary liver cancer. In Z. Y. Tang (Edit.): Subclinical Hepatocellular Carcinoma, pp. 188-211. Beijing: China Academic Publ.; Berlin: Springer 1985
36. Yu YQ, Tang ZY, Zhou XD et al.: Treatment of primary hepatic cancer by YAG laser, a preliminary report. Acta acad. med. primae Shanghai 8 (1981) 29-31. (In Chinese)
37. Zhou XD, Tang ZY, Yu YQ et al.: Cryosurgery for liver cancer - experimental and clinical study. Chin. J. Surg. 17 (1979) 480-483. (In Chinese)
38. Zhu YR, Lu BX: Clinical implication of AFP sero-survey. Chin. J. Oncol. 5 (1983) 38-40. (In Chinese)

Effects of 13 Mutagens on Rat Hepatic Microsomal Enzymes

Liu Yu-Gu

Hepatic microsomal enzymes are the important enzymes involved in the biotransformation of carcinogens. It is known that many drugs, insecticides, and toxic metals are inhibitors of microsomal enzymes and that they can influence the microsomal metabolism of various drugs, mutagens, carcinogens, and other toxic compounds in the body. The purpose of the present study was to examine the effect of cadmium, mercury, lead, arsenic, chromium, DDT, chlordimeform, trichlorfon, benzo(a)pyrene, aflatoxin B_1, dimethylnitrosamine, cyclophosphamide, and mitomycin C on the activities of hepatic microsomal enzymes in rats.

Male Wistar rats weighing about 200 g were used in the present study. Each compound was administered once daily. Dose and treatment duration for each compound are shown in Table 1. The control animals received an equivalent volume of corn oil i. p. or per os.

Rats were killed by decapitation 24 h after the last dosage. The liver was quickly removed and homogenized in 150 mM sucrose, 10 mM Tris-HCl buffer, pH 7.4. Microsomes were prepared by Schenkman's method [4]. The concentrations of cytochrome P-450 and b_5 were determined by the method of Estabrook [1]. Aniline hydroxylase activity was measured by a method established by O'Brien [3]. Aminopyrine and ethylmorphine N-dimethylase activities were assayed by Yang's method [5], and the concentration of microsomal protein was determined by Lowry's method [2].

Table 1. Dose, treatment duration, and route of administration in rats treated with 13 mutagens

Treatment	Dose (mg/kg)	Duration of treatment (days)	Route of administration
Cadmium	2.4	1	i.p.
Mercury	4.0	1	i.p.
Lead	100.0	1	i.p.
Chromium	17.0	1	i.p.
Arsenic	4.0	1	i.p.
Benzo(a)pyrene	10.0	7	i.p.
Aflatoxin B_1	7.2	7	i.p.
Dimethylnitrosamine	5.0	7	i.p.
Cyclophosphamide	40.0	5	i.p.
Mitomycin C	0.29	5	i.p.
DDT	2.0	7	p.o.
Chlordimeform	50.0	7	p.o.
Trichlorfon	62.5	7	p.o.

Cancer of the Liver, Esophagus, and Nasopharynx
Edited by G. Wagner and Zhang You-Hui

Table 2. Effects of 13 mutagens on rat hepatic microsomal enzymes

Treatment	Microsomal protein	Cytochrome		Aniline hydroxylase	Amino-pyrine *N*-demethy-lase	Ethyl-morphine *N*-demethy-lase
		P-450	b_5			
Control	100 (10)	100 (10)	100 (10)	100 (10)	100 (10)	100 (10)
Cadmium	92 (7)	56 (7**	81 (7)*	54 (7)**	43 (7)**	34 (7)**
Mercury	92 (7)	79 (7)**	96 (6)*	85 (6)*	73 (6)**	73 (6)*
Lead	99 (8)	76 (8)*	88 (8)	74 (8)**	60 (8)**	70 (8)*
Chromium	96 (7)	101 (7)	91 (7)	101 (7)	94 (7)	111 (7)
Arsenic	95 (7)	95 (7)	97 (7)	96 (7)	78 (7)	101 (7)
Benzo(a)pyrene	103 (8)	142 (8)*	-	136 (8)	-	-
Aflatoxin B1	102 (8)	86 (8)	-	90 (7)	-	-
Dimethylnitrosamine	92 (8)*	62 (8)***	-	66 (8)***	-	-
Cyclophosphamide	117 (9)**	109 (9)	-	103 (8)	-	-
Mitomycin C	112 (6)**	83 (6)	-	72 (6)	-	-
DDT	107 (11)	224 (11)***	132 (11)***	279 (11)***	191 (11)***	163 (11)***
Chlordimeform	99 (11)	84 (11)**	100 (11)	88 (11)*	84 (11)	66 (11)**
Trichlorfon	113 (6)**	70 (6)	-	67 (6)*	-	-

Figures are expressed as percentages of control values, and figures in parentheses represent the sample number; significant differences from control: * $P<0.05$; ** $P<0.01$; *** $P<0.001$

The results of the present study are shown in Table 2. Cadmium, lead, mercury, and chlordimeform significantly decreased the concentration of cytochrome P-450 and b_5 and inhibited the activities of aniline hydroxylase, aminopyrine, and ethylmorphine N-dimethylase; dimethylnitrosamine, trichlorfon, and mitomycin C decreased the concentration of cytochrome P-450 and inhibited the aniline hydroxylase activity by varying degrees. These results indicate that cadmium, mercury, lead, chlordimeform, dimethylnitrosamine, trichlorfon, and mitomycin C are inhibitors of the hepatic microsomal enzymes in rats. DDT and benzo(a)pyrene increased the cytochrome content and the activities of the microsomal enzymes assayed, showing that they are inducers of the hepatic microsomal enzymes. No effect whatever on microsomal enzymes was observed of chromium, arsenic, aflatoxin B_1, and cyclophosphamide.

References

1. Estabrook RW, Werringloer J: The Measurement of Difference Spectra: Application to the Cytochromes of Microsomes. In S. Fleischer, L. Packer (Eds): Biomembranes, Part C, pp. 212-220. New York: Academic Press 1978. (Methods in Enzymology, Vol. 52)
2. Lowry OH, Rosebrough NJ, Farr AL, Randall RJ: Protein Measurement with the Folin Phenol Reagent. J. biol. Chem. 193 (1951) 265-275
3. O'Brien PJ, Rahimtula AD: A Peroxidase Assay for Cytochrome P-450. In S. Fleischer, L. Packer (Eds): Biomembranes, Part C, pp. 407-412. New York: Academic Press 1978. (Methods in Enzymology, Vol. 52)
4. Schenkman JB, Cinti DL: Preparation of Microsomes with Calcium. In S. Fleischer, L. Packer (Eds): Biomembranes, Part C, pp. 83-89. New York: Academic Press 1978. (Methods in Enzymology, Vol. 52)
5. Yang CS, Strickhart FS: Inhibition of Hepatic Mixed Function Oxidase Activity by Propyl Gallate. Biochem. Pharmacol. 23 (1978) 3129-3138

Four Hundred Cases of Hepatic Resection for Primary Liver Cancer

Wu Men-Chao, Zhang Xia-Chua, Chen Han, Yao Xiao-Ping, Xu Guan-Nan, Wu Bo-Wen, and Yang Jia-Mei

Clinical research in primary liver cancer has made rapid progress in the past 2 decades. Especially in the past decade operative results have been greatly improved along with the development of current diagnostic technique, the innovation of surgical operation, and the extensive application of therapy combining Chinese traditional and Western medicine. Operative mortality has been reduced from 25% in the 1960s to less than 10% now. Operative results in small cancer are even more encouraging not only with low operative mortalities but also with a 5-year survival rate as high as 55%–60% [1]. In our hospital, 1745 patients with primary liver cancer were admitted from January 1960 to April 1984; 937 patients (53.7%) were explored operatively. Of these patients, 400 were given resections, a resection rate of 42.7%. In the following we report on our experience in the hepatectomies of these 400 patients.

Methods and Materials

Sex and Age. Of the 400 patients who underwent liver resection, 361 were males and 39 females, a sex ratio of 9.3:1. The age of the patients ranged from 6 months to 71 years, with 84.5% between 30 and 59 years old, 6.5% under 30 years old, and 9% over 60 years old.

Pathological Examination. Microscopy revealed liver cell carcinoma in 378 cases (94.5%), bile duct cell carcinoma in 14 cases (3.5%), and mixed type tumors in 8 cases (2%). Three hundred and eleven cases (77.8%) were combined with cirrhosis, among them 11 being associated with schistosomiasis. Tumors larger than 5 cm in diameter were found in 330 cases, those equal to or less than 5 cm in 70 cases.

Type of Operation. Of the 400 patients, right extended hemihepatectomy was performed in 11, right hemihepatectomy in 106, left hemihepatectomy in 64, middle lobectomy in 12, left lateral lobectomy in 112, and partial resection in 95.

Control of Bleeding During Surgery. In this series, six different methods were adopted: (1) The extrahepatic vessel ligation was used for left and right hemihepatectomy in 18 cases. (2) Contraction of the tumor-bearing lobe with rubber tube was adopted in ten cases. (3) A liver clamp was used in seven cases, this method being particularly suitable for partial liver resection. (4) Digital compression of the liver was mainly used for left lateral lobectomy or extirpation of small or marginal

Cancer of the Liver, Esophagus, and Nasopharynx
Edited by G. Wagner and Zhang You-Hui

Table 1. Correlation of operative mortality, cirrhosis and type of operation

Operation	Cirrhotic cases			Noncirrhotic cases			Total		
	No.	Deaths	%	No.	Deaths	%	No.	Deaths	%
Extended right lobectomy	5	1	20.0	6	0	–	11	1	9.0
Right hemi-hepatectomy	77	10	12.9	29	0	–	106	10	9.4
Left hemi-hepatectomy	46	3	6.5	18	0	–	64	3	4.6
Middle lobectomy	8	0	–	4	0	–	12	0	–
Left lateral lobectomy	86	2[a]	2.3	26	1[b]	3.8	112	3	2.6
Partial resection	89	0	–	6	0	–	95	0	–
Total	311	16	5.1	89	1	1.1	400	17	4.2

[a] One case died of massive bleeding from injury of the left vein. Another case died of septicemia from subphrenic infection

[b] Died of massive bleeding from injury of the left hepatic vein

tumors in 82 cases, and for some of the patients the technique of interruption of the porta hepatis was supplemented. (5) Normothermic total hepatic vascular exclusion was employed in three cases, and it was only applicable to massive size tumors close to large vessels. Its advantages were that no loss of blood occurred during liver resection. (6) Intermittent interruption of the porta hepatis was performed in 280 cases, ranging from 1 to 6 times for different cases, twice on average; each interruption usually lasted 10–20 min. In cases of severe cirrhosis, each interruption should not exceed 15 min.

Operative Mortality. In this series, 17 patients died within 1 month after operation, amounting to 4.2% of the total mortality rate. Judging from the type of operation, the mortality for 193 patients with a resection of over half of the liver was 7.2% (14 cases), while for 207 patients who underwent left lateral lobectomies or partial resection the mortality was 1.4% (3 cases). There was a significant difference in mortality between cirrhotic and noncirrhotic cases, the former being 5.1% (16/311) and the latter being 1.1% (1/89). Comparing the group with lobectomy with the group with partial resection, the mortality of the former was 5.6% (17/305) and that of the latter (95 cases) was zero. Judging from the date of operation, operative death in the 1960s occurred in 13 out of 88 cases (14.8%) and in the 1970s in 4 out of 164 cases (2.4%); since 1980 no operative death has occurred in 148 cases (Table 1). Of the 17 operative deaths, 14 died of hepatic failure accompanied by obvious cirrhosis with a resection of over half of the liver; two patients died of massive bleeding from an injury to the left hepatic vein during the operation, and one died of septicemia due to subphrenic infection.

Results. Of the 400 resectable cases, 348 were followed up, not counting 17 deaths within 1 month after operation; 25 were followed for less than 1 year, and 10 were noncommunicable cases. The 5-year survival rate was 25.8%; in these survivors a

Table 2. Postoperative results

Tumor size	No. of cases	Survival rate (%)				
		1 year	2 years	3 years	4 years	5 years
⩾5 cm	283	55.1	41.0	33.5	25.1	21.0
<5 cm	65	83.1	81.5	73.9	70.3	64.0
Total	348	60.3	48.1	40.4	31.9	25.8

tumor size of more than 5 cm was found in 21%, while a tumor size equal to or less than 5 cm was found in 64% (Table 2). One patient has survived for 19 years and is still enjoying good health. In view of the relationship between the type of operation and the survival rate, the 1- to 5-year survival rate in 253 patients undergoing entire lobectomies was 50.6%, 36.5%, 28%, 22.2%, and 18% respectively, while that in 95 patients undergoing partial resection was 86.3%, 81.3%, 77.1%, 70,9%, and 66.6% respectively. The latter survival rates had a close relation to the tumor being small, early in stage, localized, and encircled by a complete capsule.

Discussion

Surgical Indication. All the patients diagnosed as having primary liver carcinoma should not miss the opportunity to undergo operative exploration as long as their general condition permits, i.e., the liver function should be well compensated (no jaundice, no ascites, and the ratio of albumin to globulin should be unreversed), there should be no trace of extrahepatic metastasis, and the tumor lesion should be confined to one lobe or only half of the liver. Of the 973 patients explored, 400 (42.7%) were resected. Tumor size is not the only parameter for determining whether or not to explore; sometimes tumor location, pathological type, and porta hepatis are the decisive factors [2]. If the tumor is situated in the left lateral lobe or in the inferior portion of the right lobe protruding toward the abdominal cavity with a distinctive margin and an encircling capsule, it is still resectable in spite of its large size. Pathologically, in cases of well-differentiated tumors with poor blood supply and no cancer cell embolism in the main trunk of the portal vein, resection should be attempted. In one case of this series the tumor mass extended 7 cm below the right costal margin without cirrhosis; this case underwent extensive right hepatic lobectomy successfully. The resected specimen was 21 × 18 × 10 cm, weighing 1750 g. It was encircled by a capsule 0.15 cm thick. Followed up for 19 years, the patient remained alive and kicking.

For cirrhotic cases, only in those with compensated liver function is exploration indicated. If local excision is performed care should be taken to avoid resection of more than half of the liver. In our series, all of the 14 cirrhotic cases with moderate damage to liver function preoperatively died of hepatic failure after right hemihepatectomy or extended right hepatic lobectomy. There were another 65 small liver cancers associated with cirrhosis. All of them underwent local excision and had an uneventful course postoperatively. Thus, it became quite obvious that, in cases of association with cirrhosis, liver resection is not a contraindication. However, the type of operation to be performed should depend upon the capacity of the patient's liver function preoperatively. We recommend curative limited resection. Otherwise, the limited amount of remaining cirrhotic tissue would hardly be sufficient for the necessary physiological function of the body and would certainly lead to poor results.

In treating massive malignant liver tumors with multiple blood supply located near the porta hepatis, the tumor should generally be resected, if possible. But in the case of technical difficulty, the best way is to perform hepatic artery ligation or intraoperative embolization as a pretreatment, and the tumor resection should be completed by a secondary laparotomy when the tumor has been reduced in size [3]. We had five such cases with a pretreatment of hepatic artery ligation or intraoperative embolization. The tumors were reduced and thus easy to resect when reoperations were performed between 4 and 11 months after the first operation and AFP was negative postoperatively.

In recent years, more attention has been concentrated on the subject of reoperation for liver cancer recurrence. Our clinical practice had proved that further prolongation of survival time could be obtained in patients after curative resection and that liver cancer recurrence and solitary metastases can be detected at an early stage by serial AFP and B ultrasonogram [3, 4]. Twenty-one cases were explored due to reappearance of AFP in the serum, and 14 were resected, a secondary resection rate of 66.6%. For the 14 resectable cases, the survival rate of more than 1 year was 71.4% (10/14). In one of our cases reappearance of AFP was detected in the 32nd month after right hemihepatectomy. Since the first operation this patient has survived for 5 years and 9 months, enjoying good health without tumor recurrence. If the time of survival is counted from the secondary resection, it is 36 months so far.

For early asymptomatic cases with single AFP positive prior to exploration, it is necessary to rule out active hepatitis, liver cirrhosis, or other factors which could induce the elevation of AFP and then to determine the tumor site by means of a B ultrasonogram, CT, or hepatic arteriography. Sixty-one cases in our series underwent exploration and 51 were resectable with a resection rate of 83.6%. If the tumor site was difficult to confirm preoperatively, we considered the intraoperative use of real-time scanning, which had proved suitable for accurately detecting the tumor position and, consequently, a great improvement in the resection rate was ensured [5].

Improvement in Operative Technique. In the past we used to adopt extrahepatic vessel ligation for anatomical hepatectomies, but this technique is time-consuming and causes enormous blood loss; thus, we seldom use it. As to the technique of bloodless hepatic resection, though it has the advantage of less blood loss, it is contraindicated in patients with serious cirrhosis, cardiovascular diseases, and renal insufficiency [6]. In order to simplify the operative technique and improve the operative results, we have improved the operative technique through the clinical practice of the past 20 years:

1. An abdominal, curved ipsilateral subcostal incision should be used if possible. In performing a right lobectomy, the curved incision is made from the xiphoid process to the costal margin into the thorax with a division of the diaphragm; this approach can reduce postoperative complications.

2. We prefer the technique of an intermittent interruption of the porta hepatis during liver resection. First, the lobe to be resected is mobilized by dividing the peritoneal attachments and adhesions, and then the liver is rendered ischemic by a complete interruption of the gastroduodenal ligament with a rubber tube. The tumor-bearing lobe is resected along a preplanned incisional line. All the vessels and ducts encountered are clamped, severed, and ligated individually. The porta hepatis is intermittently interrupted, each interruption lasting 10–20 min. As mentioned above, the interruption time should be as short as possible. In cirrhotic cases, the time of interruption should not exceed 15 min. With this technique we performed hepatic lobectomy of various types in 280 cases. No complication resulted from the interruption of the porta hepatis. The advantages of the technique proposed here are simplicity, less blood loss, and short operative time. Thus, this technique is applicable to all types of lobectomy.
3. Any bleeding from a biliary leakage at the raw surface should be treated with silk suture and irrigated with a mixture solution of 500 mg 5-FU plus 100 ml normal saline. Routinely, we take a piece of free omentum to cover the raw surface with silk sutures at the peripheral and central area.
4. Adequate and free drainage of the abdomen with continuous or intermittent sump suction should be secured.
5. We apply an infusion of 250–500 mg 5-FU via the peripheral and portal vein as soon as the tumor has been resected.

Management of Cirrhotic Patients. In our series of 400 cases, 311 (71.8%) were accompanied by cirrhosis. Among them, 16 died within 1 month after operation, the operative mortality amounting to 5.1%, while only one patient (1.1%) died out of 89 noncirrhotic cases. In cirrhotic cases, the operative mortality was 20% of extended right hemihepatectomies, 12.9% of right hemihepatectomies, and 6.5% of left hemihepatectomies. No death occurred in ipsilateral resections in noncirrhotic cases. There were no deaths in 95 local excisions, whether with or without cirrhosis. Of the 17 deaths in our series, 14 (82.3%) died of hepatic coma; 2 died of massive bleeding, and only 1 died of septicemia from subphrenic infection. Thus, it is clear that operative mortality in cases with cirrhosis is higher than in noncirrhotic cases. The more liver tissue is resected, the higher the mortality [7]. Probably it is interrelated with the serious degree of preexisting cirrhosis and the large amount of liver tissue resected. Therefore, strict observance of surgical indication and proper control of the amount of liver resection in cirrhotic cases play an important role in reducing operative mortality.

Based on the fact that most of the patients in China with cirrhosis are detected in the stage of subclinical hepatocellular carcinoma, which means a higher proportion of single nodules with integrated capsules, a lower incidence of tumor embolism, well-differentiated cancer cells, more lymphocyte infiltration around the tumor, and the patient in a better immune status [1, 4], we have planned a policy for treating cirrhotic cases in recent years. It is local resection or left lateral lobectomy for left side tumors and curative limited resection for right side tumors and solitary recurrence of tumor. In treating massive size tumors seated in the right lobe, which are technically difficult to resect, we advocate hepatic artery ligation or intraoperative embolization as the first choice of surgery; the tumor is resected in the secondary laparotomy by the time it has been reduced in size. The above-mentioned operative measures could preserve as much liver tissue as possible and ensure that the patients have an uneventful postoperative course.

Case Detection. Early discovery, early diagnosis, and early resection are the key points for improving the operative results. Recently, the diagnostic value of AFP for primary liver cancer has been universally accepted. It has proved to be positive in more than 80% of cases and it is used to detect early small liver cancers which cannot be diagnosed by other tests. In China, a great many early cases have been discovered by active survey in the high-risk Qidong district. During 1974–1977 1 223 012 of the population were screened. Of 475 liver cancers detected, 167 were in a subclinical stage (accounting for 35.2%), of whom the 2-year survival rate after tumor resection was 69% [8]. Moreover, in the clinical study of liver cancer it was observed that incidence of primary liver cancer was higher in people with a history of liver diseases than in those without, the former amounting to 80% [9]. In our series, patients with cirrhosis were more numerous than those without (77.8% vs. 22.2%). The sex ratio of males to females was 9.3:1, and the age of incidence between 30 and 59 years was 84.5%. So it can be seen that more early cases may be discovered by screening a multitude of male and middle-aged persons having a history of chronic liver diseases, using the AFP test at regular intervals. However, 20–30% of patients suffering from primary liver cancer were still AFP-negative or low-level positive; their diagnosis is still very difficult. Recently, we have used enzymological tests of A_1AT(a_1-antitrypsin test) for this category of patients, the diagnostic positivity of A_1AT being 80%. If A_1AT plus AFP is used, the positivity may reach 96% [10]. Moreover, hepatic angiography, B ultrasonography, and CT have contributed a lot to the investigation of the tumor localization in early cases. Of these techniques, especially the B ultrasonogram has the advantages of being painless, safe, and convenient for repeated examinations. Consequently, AFP combined with B ultrasonogram, angiogram, or CT, if necessary complemented by an A_1AT test, has become more important for early diagnosis.

All the patients should be explored as soon as their liver cancers are discovered and a diagnosis made as long as their general condition permits. Because small cancers were commonly found in a single nodule, with complete capsule, good differentiation of cancer cell, more lymphocyte infiltration around the tumor, better immune status of the patient, and no tumor embolism, early curative resection is favored, especially local resection if the tumor is combined with cirrhosis and situated in the right lobe. It seems that a local excision of primary liver cancer with 1–2 cm surrounding liver tissue can lead to curative resection. In our series, 85 early patients were explored, of whom 70 were resectable, with a resection rate of 64%. In China, a 5-year survival rate of 49.3% in 42 early cases was reported by Huang [11] and of 64.4% in 48 patients by Tang [4]. These facts amply indicate that early discovery, early diagnosis, and early resection have an important bearing on the improvement of operative results.

References

1. Chen H et al.: Experiences in Re-operation of Liver Resection of Primary Liver Cancer. Acad. J. second milit. med. Coll. 5 (1984) 9
2. Huang XY et al.: Results of Surgical Treatment of Carcinoma of Liver: Report of 181 Cases. Chin. J. Surg. 20 (1982) 68
3. Iwatsuki S, Shaw BW, Starzl TE: Experience with 150 Liver Resections. Ann. Surg. 197 (1983) 247-253
4. Karematsu: Early Diagnosis and Treatment of the Minute Liver Cancer. Jap. J. Surg. 13 (1983) 32
5. National Coordination Group of Pathology of Liver Cancer: Relationship between Hepatocellular Carcinoma, Liver Cirrhosis and Hepatitis B: A Pathological Study. Nat. med. J. China 62 (1982) 257-261
6. Tang ZY et al.: Surgical Treatment of Subclinical Hepatocellular Carcinoma (HCC) and its Ultimate Outcome. J. exp. Clin. Cancer Res. 3 (1983) 261
7. Wu MC: Present Status of the Liver Cancer Research. Acad. J. second milit. med. Coll. 5 (1984) 73
8. Wu MC, Chen H, Zhang XH et al.: Primary Hepatic Carcinoma Resection over 18 Years. Chin. med. J. 93 (1980) 723-728
9. Wu MC et al.: Hepatic Resection: A 24 Year Experience. Acta Acad. Med. Wuhan 13 (1984) 379
10. Xu SK, Guan SF, Wang PL et al.: Assay of Serum a_1-Antitrypsin Activity for the Diagnosis of Primary Hepatocellular Carcinoma. Chin. Med. J. 96 (1983) 607-610
11. Zhu YR: AFP Sero-survey and Early Diagnosis of Liver Cell Cancer in the Quidong Field. Chin. J. Oncol. 3 (1981) 35-38

III Cancer of the Esophagus

Epidemiology of Esophageal Cancer in China

Li Jun-Yao

Introduction

Ancient Chinese records from about 2000 years ago noted several unique epidemiological features and possible risk factors for esophageal cancer in China. Recent epidemiological studies on this form of cancer have indicated that there are a few striking features of the distribution of esophageal cancer within China, and several risk factors have also been identified. A detailed analysis of this could open up approaches to the prevention and control of this malignancy.

This paper reviews some recent epidemiological findings on esophageal cancer in China, paying special attention to recent advances from descriptive, analytical, and operational studies.

Descriptive Epidemiology

Incidence Rates

The annual age-adjusted rates, truncated rates, and cumulative rates of esophageal cancer incidence in different areas of the world are given in Table 1, which is abstracted from the fourth volume of *Cancer Incidence in Five Continents* [7] and the Shanghai and Linxian cancer registration [2]. High rates among Chinese, particularly in Linxian and Shanghai, are noteworthy.

Mortality Rates

According to the death statistics, China has the highest death rates from esophageal cancer. In China, 18 of the 29 provinces, municipalities, and autonomous regions have a higher esophageal cancer mortality rate than all other countries, including Singapore, whose elevated risk for this disease is known to be the world's second highest (Fig. 1). Esophageal cancer accounts for 26.5% in males and 19.7% in females of all cancer deaths in China, respectively [4].

Detected Rates

The detected rates of esophageal cancer in different areas of China have been identified by mass screening, using balloon cytological methods (Table 2) [5]. A large number of cases of epithelial dysplasia and early carcinoma of the esophagus have

Cancer of the Liver, Esophagus, and Nasopharynx
Edited by G. Wagner and Zhang You-Hui

Table 1. Age-standardized and cumulative (0-74) incidence rates of esophageal cancer in selected areas

Area	World		Truncated		Cumulative	
	Male	Female	Male	Female	Male	Female
Senegal, Dakar	0.2	0.2	0.5	0.7	0.0	0.0
Brazil, Sao Paulo	14.1	2.8	25.7	4.5	1,7	0.3
Canada, Alberta	2.6	0.9	4.2	1.6	0.3	0.1
Canada, British Columbia	3.5	1.8	4.3	2.5	0.4	0.2
Colombia, Cali	3.1	1.7	3.5	2.8	0.3	0.2
Cuba	5.3	2.2	6.7	2.2	0.7	0.3
Jamaica, Kingston	7.1	3.0	5.9	3.6	0.9	0.4
Netherlands Antilles	16.7	8.7	14.5	6.3	1.8	1.1
Alameda						
White	3.6	1.6	5.2	3.0	0.5	0.2
Black	9.8	3.2	20.1	6.7	1.1	0.4
Bay Area						
White	4.0	1.9	5.4	3.4	0.5	0.3
Black	11.7	3.6	19.9	8.5	1.5	0.4
Chinese	6.9	2.1	10.9	5.2	0.8	0.2
Japanese	8.4	0.7	4.8	0.0	1.1	0.2
Los Angeles						
White	2.9	1.4	4.4	2.5	0.4	0.2
Spanish	3.1	1.1	2.9	1.8	0.4	0.1
Black	11.8	3.9	19.1	8.5	1.6	0.5
Japanese	3.9	0.8	4.9	0.0	0.4	0.1
Chinese	5.4	0.0	4.2	0.0	0.9	0.0
Connecticut	5.3	1.7	8.4	3.3	0.7	0.2
Atlanta						
White	3.2	1.2	4.7	1.7	0.4	0.2
Black	19.3	2.7	45.8	7.7	2.3	0.3
Iowa	3.1	0.8	5.4	1.4	0.4	0.1
New Orleans						
White	3.6	0.6	6.5	1.2	0.4	0.1
Black	13.8	3.0	31.2	7.3	1.5	0.3
Detroit						
White	4.8	1.4	6.6	2.4	0.6	0.2
Black	13.9	4.3	29.3	10.8	1.8	0.5
New Mexico						
Spanish	1.7	1.4	2.7	1.2	0.2	0.2
Other White	2.5	1.2	3.6	2.1	0.3	0.2
Amerindians	1.2	0.0	2.5	0.0	0.1	0.0
New York State	4.8	1.4	7.1	2.3	0.6	0.2
Puerto Rico	13.1	5.2	18.2	6.7	1.6	0.6
Utah	2.4	0.4	3.8	0.8	0.3	0.0
Seattle	3.3	1.3	5.2	2.4	0.4	0.2
Shanghai	24.7	8.0	37.8	10.9	3.0	1.0
Linxian	212.7	137.2	420.4	276.5	32.5	20.4
Hongkong	18.6	5.5	33.8	9.0	2.3	0.7
India, Bombay	15.7	10.7	21.6	19.8	1.6	1.3
India, Poona	13.1	10.4	19.4	20.2	1.6	1.2
Israel, All Jews	2.2	1.5	2.1	1.5	0.2	0.2
Japan, Fukuoka	8.4	2.0	12.2	2.1	1.1	0.3
Japan, Miyagi	13.8	3.2	16.1	2.8	1.7	0.3

Table 1. (continued)

Area	World		Truncated		Cumulative	
	Male	Female	Male	Female	Male	Female
Japan, Nagasaki	8.4	1.9	11.7	3.1	0.8	0.2
Japan, Osaka	8.6	2.1	11.2	2.5	1.1	0.2
Singapore						
Chinese	18.9	4.1	22.4	4.5	2.2	0.5
Malay	1.2	3.0	2.2	3.5	0.1	0.3
Indian	6.1	7.7	10.6	16.9	0.9	1.0
Czechoslovakia	2.5	0.4	4.3	0.6	0.3	0.0
Denmark	3.0	1.2	3.9	1.4	0.3	0.1
FRG, Hamburg	3.7	0.8	5.4	0.8	0.4	0.1
Finland	4.0	3.1	4.4	3.0	0.4	0.3
France, Bas-Rhin	17.0	0.8	38.6	1.4	2.0	0.1
GDR	2.8	0.6	4.1	0.6	0.3	0.1
Hungary, Szabolcs	1.2	0.2	2.6	0.4	0.2	0.0
Italy, Varese	7.8	1.4	11.2	1.0	0.9	0.1
Norway	2.7	0.7	3.7	0.8	0.3	0.1
Poland, Cieszyn	4.3	0.0	4.3	0.0	0.7	0.0
Romania, County Cluj	1.4	1.0	1.8	1.2	0.2	0.1
Spain, Navarra	6.3	1.2	8.7	1.5	0.8	0.1
Sweden	2.9	1.1	3.5	0.9	0.4	0.1
Switzerland, Geneva	7.2	0.9	10.1	1.5	1.0	0.1
UK, Birmingham	5.5	2.9	7.6	4.0	0.6	0.3
Yugoslavia, Slovenia	5.9	0.9	10.2	1.2	0.7	0.1
Australia, South	5.1	1.2	6.4	1.4	0.6	0.1
New Zealand						
Maori	6.4	1.2	12.1	2.0	0.7	0.2
Non-Maori	5.3	2.3	7.3	2.7	0.7	0.2
Hawaii						
Hawaiian	18.3	2.6	22.7	4.9	2.4	0.4
White	2.4	1.9	4.4	3.6	0.3	0.2
Chinese	6.3	0.6	11.0	2.1	0.7	0.1
Filipino	6.7	1.0	6.4	1.4	0.8	0.0
Japanese	4.5	0.6	4.7	0.3	0.5	0.0

been discovered, which is advantageous in terms of treatment and prevention. Areas with a high esophageal cancer risk also have concomitant high rates of dysplasia of epithelial cells of the esophagus. Over time, a progression from mild to severe dysplasia and, hence, to cancer has been observed, and the changes caused by hyperplasia can also revert to normal.

Secular Trends

The age-adjusted death rates of esophageal cancer in Shanghai have gradually been declining since 1963 (Fig. 2), but the trends of esophageal cancer mortality and incidence in Linxian showed little fluctuation from 1958 to 1982 (Fig. 3).

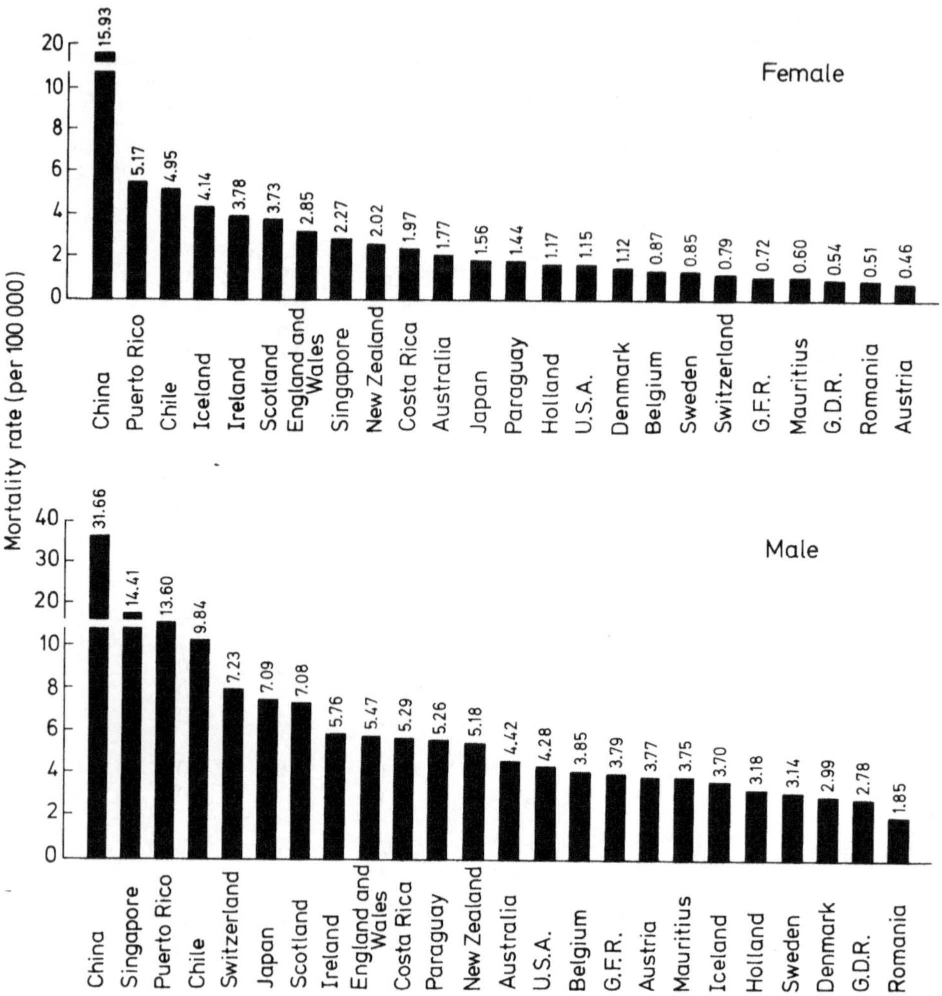

Fig. 1. Age-adjusted rates for esophageal cancer in selected countries [age-adjusted to world population (UICC 1970)]

Geographical Differences

There is a 35-fold difference in the mortality rates of esophageal cancer in both sexes between countries with the highest and lowest rates; the highest rates are 254.8/100000 for male and 161.1/100000 for females. Also, esophageal cancer shows a marked geographical gradient in mortality between areas in fairly close proximity. The areas in China with a high risk for esophageal cancer give an impression of irregular concentric belt distribution.

Table 2. Results of cytological sreening of esophagenal cancer in selected areas in China, 1971–1983[a]

Area	Province	Year of screening	No. of persons screened	Examination results					
				Carcinoma		Severe dysplasia		Mild hyperplasia	
				No.	%	No.	%	No.	%
Rencun,	Henan	1983	4297	95	2.21	278	6.47	1689	39.31[b]
Linxian								950	22.11[c]
Yaocun,	Henan	1983	3527	66	1.87	183	5.19	1295	36.72
Linxian								676	19.17[c]
Donggang,	Henan	1983	4879	89	1.82	284	5.82	1777	36.42
Linxian								937	19.20[c]
Heshun,	Henan	1983	4677	79	1.69	295	6.31	1726	36.90
Linxian								969	20.72[c]
Manasxian	Xinjiang	1974	579	11	1.90	33	5.70	160	27.63
Yaocun, Linxian	Henan	1974	14002	221	1.58	460	3.29	5750	41.06
Yangchengxian	Shanxi	1974	3316	48	1.45	39	1.18	413	12.45
Linxian	Henan	1971	7212	78	1.08	135	1.87	1626	22.54
Yentingxian	Sichuan	1972	5697	52	0.91	78	1.36	1420	24.93
Zhongxian	Hubei	1974	13613	60	0.44	136	1.00	1151	8.46
Anyang prefecture	Henan	1973	17471	88	0.50	48	0.27	1372	7.85
Longzhong xian	Sichuan	1975	5169	27	0.52	16	0.31	642	12.42
Shanghai city	Shanghai	1971	878	0	0	3	0.34	114	12.98
Zhongxiang (natives)	Hubei	1974	6909	3	0.04	16	0.23	611	8.84

[a] Source: Data are from reports of the results of cancer screening in various provinces
[b] Mild hyperplasia data
[c] Severe dysplasia, grade I

Experiences among Migrants

The results from a recent Chinese migrant study suggest that risk levels of esophageal cancer are successively lower from Guangdong to Hongkong, and from idai to erdai in American Chinese (Fig. 4), a phenomenon not to be found for any other cancer site [3]. Further studies would be the next step required for the elucidation of the displacing reasons, with emphasis on the birthplace of migrants and environmental changes in host countries.

Gullet Cancer in Chicken

Several studies in China revealed that areas of elevated risk for human esophageal cancer also have a high incidence of gullet cancer in chicken. This animal tumor shows clinical and pathological features comparable to those of human neoplasms. Also, the gullet cancer rates in chickens raised by migrants are often higher than those in chickens raised by the native host population.

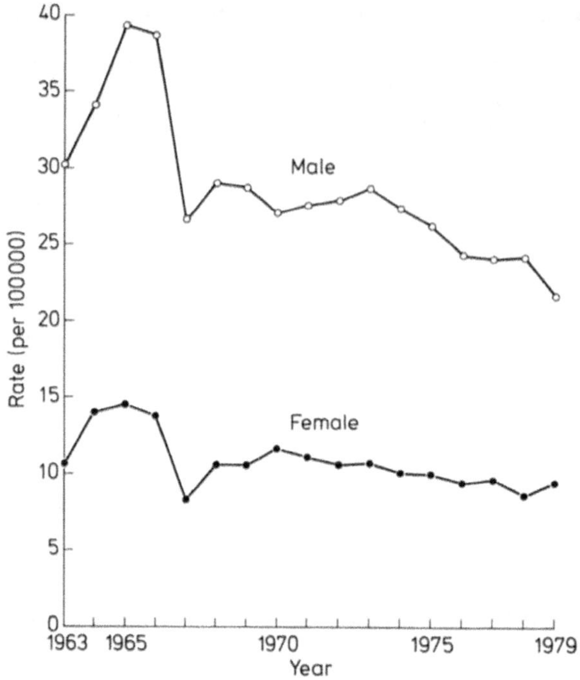

Fig. 2. Secular trends of the age-adjusted death rates of esophageal cancer in Shanghai (1963–1979)

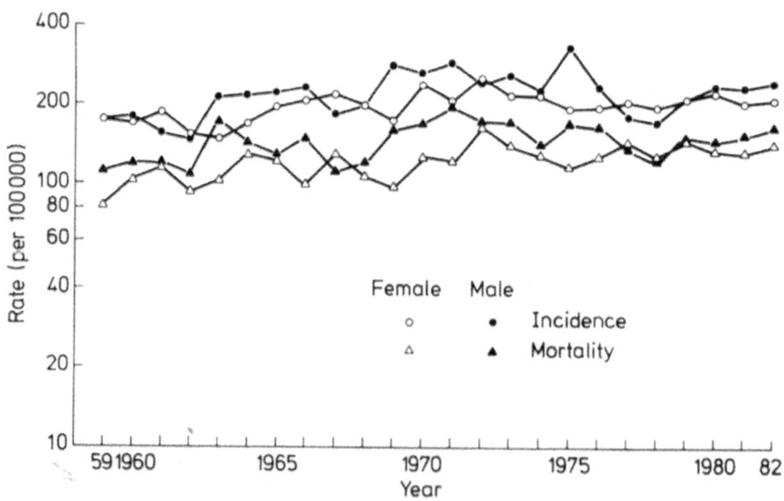

Fig. 3. Age-adjusted incidence and mortality rates of esophageal cancer in Linxian, China, 1959–1982

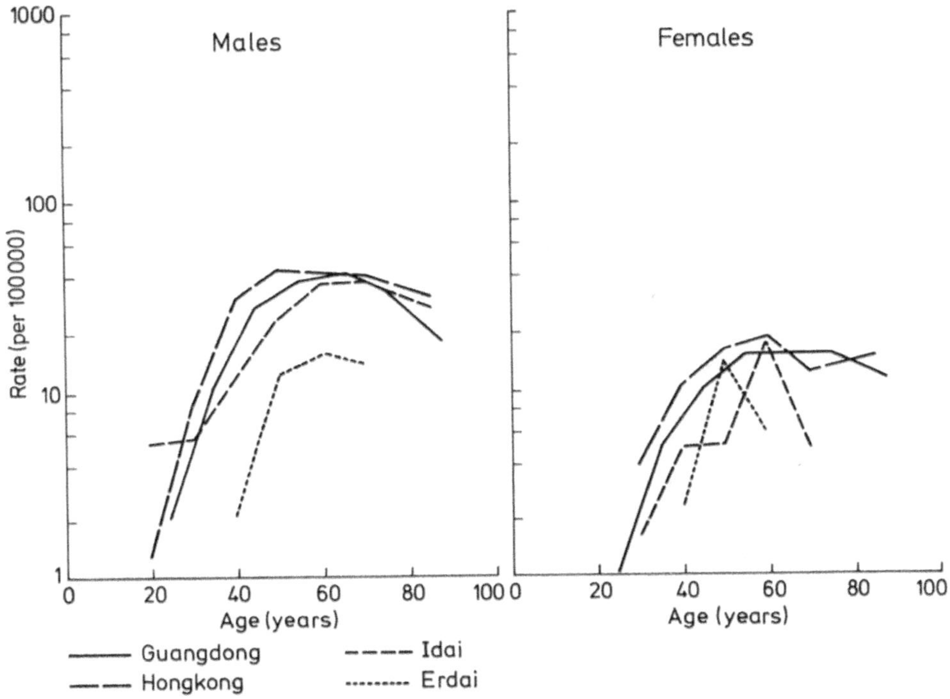

Fig. 4. Age-specific death rates of nasopharyngeal cancer among Chinese, by sex and area: Guangdong 1973-1975; Hongkong 1968-1973; United States 1969-1972

Variation in Rates by Sex

Esophageal cancer in China is more common among males than among females. In high-risk areas, the sex ratio is often low and vice versa for low-risk areas, with the exception of some counties in Guangdong province.

Ethnic Differences in Mortality

Among the minority nationalities (ethnic groups) in China, mortality from esophageal cancer is highest among the Kazaks in Xinjiang Autonomous Region, i.e., it is 2-43 times higher than among other ethnic populations, including the neighboring Uygur and Mongol groups in the same region.

Analytical Epidemiology

Correlation Studies

The data collected from the nationwide cancer survey were used to carry out correlation studies to reveal the relationship between esophageal cancer mortality and environmental factors, and demographic variables, especially diet and nutritional status in different areas. According to several studies the consumption of pickled vegetables was positively associated with an elevated mortality rate for esophageal cancer. Mortality rates were higher among communes in which a large proportion of members consume pickled vegetables or ingest such foods for a great part of the year ($r = 0.7172$ and 0.6962; $P < 0.001$) [1].

Recently, a collaborative research project by American scientists from Cornell University and Chinese scientists from China has been organized to evaluate a large number of dietary and nutritional factors thought to be related to cancer risk. So far, the preliminary results from this correlation study, showing nitrate, nitrosoproline, total nitroso compound level in urine, copper level in plasm, salt consumption, and calcium and iron intake from foods, were positively associated with an elevated mortality for esophageal cancer; and selenium, glutathione peroxidase, retinol, ascorbic acid level in plasma, vitamin A intake from foods, and legume consumption were negatively associated with the mortality rates of esophageal cancer in 65 counties of China.

Studies in Sichuan Province also showed that the amount of fresh vegetables in the diet was inversely correlated with esophageal cancer rates ($r = 0.78$, $P < 0.001$). Comparative studies conducted among the Kazak, Uygur, and Mongol groups, all residents of the same area, showed similar clear-cut results: the greater the amount of sour milk, moldy bread, smoked meat, moldy smoked meat, and moldy cheese consumed, and the larger the number of individuals having a family history of esophageal cancer, the greater the risk of cancer of the esophagus. However, this risk is lower for individuals who consume more fruit and vegetables [6].

Therefore, the close relationship between geographical variation of diet and nutritional intake and esophageal cancer has been demonstrated by correlation studies by comparing counties, communities, and groups with regard to these variables. These correlates or inverse correlates of esophageal cancer risk justify reasonable hope that further investigation of them will lead to the identification of a few truly causative or truly protective factors which can be used in the prevention and control of this disease.

Case-Control Studies

The case-control study is the most commonly used method in cancer epidemiology to develop etiological hypotheses and to put them to test. The associations of consuming fermented and moldy foods, cigarette smoking, alcohol drinking, and low socio-economic level with esophageal cancer were identified by the findings of several case-control studies in Xinjiang and Jiangsu. The influence of diet and nutrition on esophageal cancer in China was also studied in detail by a series of case-control studies.

Esophageal cancer is a disease of the poor in most areas of the world. Not all impoverished populations have a high rate of the disease, but where the disease is common, the economic level of the population is frequently lower (educational level, annual income, occupation, and housing conditions). The case-control studies conducted in Jiangsu province have shown that a lower socio-economic level is associated with this type of tumor (relative risk = 1.9–2.5).

Evidence suggests that genetic factors may play a role in the causation of esophageal cancer in Linxian, a high-risk area for this disease. Family studies suggest that genetic susceptibility does exist, and the relative risks increase manyfold among blood relatives as compared with nonblood relatives of esophageal cancer patients. The case-control studies in Jiangsu province have also indicated an increased risk for esophageal cancer among people with a family history of this disease.

Cohort Studies

In analytical epidemiology the cohort study is a powerful tool for identifying risk factors of cancer. A retrospective cohort study was designed to delineate the natural history of esophageal cancer in the population. In 1974, a cohort of about 14000 residents aged 30 years and over in Yaocun Commune of Linxian was examined by balloon cytology. The progression from mild to severe dysplasia could also revert from mild hyperplasia to normal epithelium. The follow-up study conducted in Linxian confirmed that there were different risks of esophageal cancer in cohorts with various degrees of esophageal cytological morphology (Fig. 5).

Dr. Wang Long-De analyzed the dietary status from one million American cohort study data and clearly revealed the importance of diet and nutrition in changing the risk of esophageal cancer. For example, the daily intake of green-yellow vegetables and fruit could reduce the risk of cancer of the esophagus.

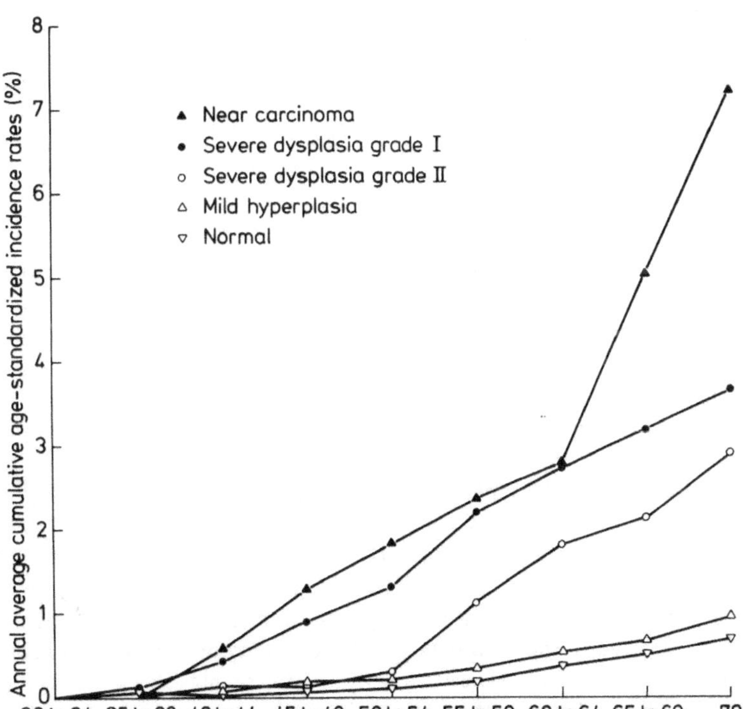

Fig. 5. Annual average cumulative age-standardized incidence rates of the cohorts with different cytologic categories

Operational Epidemiology

The intervention trial is the principal method used to study the effectiveness of preventive measures proposed. It is also an important way to evaluate the real significance of any risk factors in human carcinogenesis. According to the health policy of the Chinese Government – putting prevention first –, prophylactic measures directed against cancer risk factors have been taken in a number of high incidence areas.

In an intervention trial of severe dysplasia (precancerous lesion) of the esophagus, using cases with severe dysplasia of the esophagus detected by cytological examination in 1974, a total of 753 subjects were divided into two groups; one group were given chemopreventive drugs (vitamin C, B_2, anticancer B_3 – a traditional Chinese herb – and tilorone); another acted as a control. In 1982, preliminary results were obtained. In Table 3 the age-specific incidence rates of esophageal cancer of the general population and the treated and untreated groups of severe dysplasia in Yaocun Commune during 1974–1981 are shown. In almost all age groups the incidence rates of esophageal cancer in the treated group were lower than those in the untreated controls, except in the age group of 30 years and less, in which only one case of esophageal cancer was diagnosed. The cumulative incidence rates of esophageal cancer in the treated and untreated groups in Yaocun Commune in the same period were also different. To further confirm the effectiveness of the intervention, corresponding controls were randomly selected from the general population, matched by age and sex with the treated and untreated groups, and compared with their rates of esophageal cancer (Table 4).The results showed no difference between the treated group and the control group, but the difference between the untreated group and the control group was significant ($P < 0.001$). Unfortunately, because it was not a randomly allocated controlled trial and there was a big difference as to the rates of esophageal cancer in both groups before intervention, it would be difficult to evaluate these results (Fig. 6).

To repeat this trial and to test the hypothesis that esophageal cancer is related to nutrient intake and that supplementation by multi-vitamin-mineral pills could decrease the incidence of this disease, two intervention trials are being conducted in collaboration with the NCI in the United States to examine the effects of daily vitamin-mineral supplements on the age-specific incidence and death rates of esophageal cancer among patients with esophageal dysplasia and the general population who have not previously had cancer. In addition, these two studies will also evaluate the effects of those supplements on the regression/progression of dysplasia, age-specific incidence, and death rates of all cancers and all causes of death. Intervention trials will be two 5-year randomized, double-blind, placebo-controlled trials among about 3400 participants with esophageal dysplasia and about 30000 adults (aged 40–69 years) from the general population. The dysplasia trial is a simple two-group design with the subjects randomly assigned to intervention (vitamin-mineral pills in doses two to three times the RDA) or placebo groups. For the general population trial, a fractional factorial design is used with the four factors in doses one to two times the RDA. Over the 5-year study period, there will be a power of more than 90% to detect a 40% reduction in the cancer rate among treated dysplasia subjects and similar power to detect a 20% reduction in the treated group

Table 3. Age-specific incidence rates (‰) of esophageal cancer of the general population, the treated and untreated groups of severe dysplasia cases of esophageal mucosa in Yaocun during 1974–1982

Age group	General population			Severe dysplasia group					
				Treated			Untreated		
	Person -years	No.	‰	Person -years	No.	‰	Person -years	No.	‰
30–	16192	7	0.43	224	1	4.46	224	–	–
35–	16808	12	0.71	288	3	10.42	292	6	15.31
40–	16808	41	2.44	392	1	2.55	424	4	9.43
45–	15056	58	3.85	448	2	4.46	384	9	23.44
50–	14488	85	5.87	568	1	1.76	480	12	24.59
55–	11848	86	7.26	456	5	10.96	584	25	42.81
60–	8336	84	10.08	288	3	10.42	320	9	28.13
65–	4760	57	11.97	112	2	17.86	312	16	51.28
70–	1472	16	10.87	16	1	62.50	96	6	62.50
75–	256	1	3.91	–	–	–	8	1	125.00
80–	40	0	0	0	0	0	0	0	0
Total	106064	447	4.21	2792	19	6.81	3232	88	27.23
Cumulative rates		3.37%			5.45%			21.78%	

Table 4. Cumulative rates of esophageal cancer in the treated and untreated groups compared with matched controls

Group	No. of persons	No. of esophageal cancers	rate (%)
Treated	349	19	5.44
group	698	27	3.87
	$\chi^2 = 1.38$	$P > 0.05$	
Untreated	404	88	21.78
control	808	39	4.83
	$\chi^2 = 82.55$	$P < 0.001$	

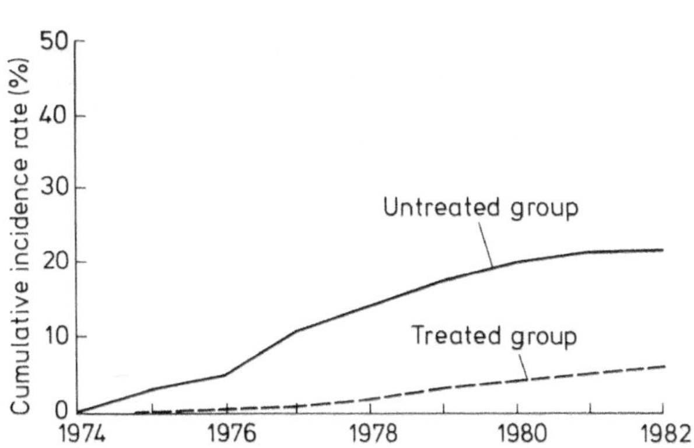

Fig. 6. Cumulative incidence rates of esophageal cancer in treated and untreated groups in Yaocun commune

of the population. To increase the effectivity of the trials, sera from every subject of both trials have been taken and stored in a freezer (−80 °C) for future analyses. The primary end points to be measured include not only the final incidence and death rates, but also several intermediate tests, i.e., the ability of the tritiated thymidine incorporation, the micronucleus test of exfoliated cells, and perhaps quantitative fluorescence image analysis. Compliance will be assessed by pill counts for all participants and biochemical tests for a sample of them. A pilot study was undertaken to assess the feasibility of a large-scale intervention in 1983. The results indicated that participants can be identified and recruited, compliance is excellent, nutritional deficiencies are common, and low-dose vitamin-mineral supplementations improve the nutritional status of the participants.

Conclusions

Several epidemological features of esophageal cancer have been identified in China. There is now a mass of evidence that exogenous factors and poor nutrition are involved and that control of theses factors would lead to a great reduction of the disease. A particularly promising area for future research is the organization of intervention studies to test etiological hypotheses and effective prevention strategies.

References

1. Department of Cancer Epidemiology of Cancer Institute of Chinese Academy of Medical Sciences (CICAMS):
   Preliminary Investigation of the Epidemiological Factors of Esophageal Cancer in China. Res. Cancer Prev. Treatm. 2 (1977) 1-8
2. Esophageal Cancer Institute of Linxian:
   Linxian Cancer Registration. 1983. (Unpublished Results)
3. King H, Li JY, Locke FB, Pollack ES, Tu JT: Patterns of Site-Specific Displacement in Cancer Mortality among Migrants: The Chinese in the United States. Amer. J. Publ. Hlth 75 (1985) 237-242
4. Li JY: Epidemiology of Esophageal Cancer in China. In Third Symposium on Epidemiology and Cancer Regstries in the Pacific Basin, Maui, Hawaii, 1981, pp. 113-120. Bethesda, MD: Nat. Cancer Inst. 1982. (Nat. Cancer Inst. Monogr., Vol. 62)
5. Li JY: New Advances on the Epidemiologic Studies of Esophageal Cancer. 1985. (In press)
6. Liu B: Investigation of the Risk Factors of Esophageal Cancer. Chin. J. Oncol. 6 (1984) 295
7. Waterhouse J, Muir C, Shanmugaratnam K, Powell J (Eds): Cancer Incidence in Five Continents, Vol. IV. Lyon: IARC 1982. (IARC Sci. Publ., No. 42)

Cancer of the Esophagus in Migrants from Different Areas in China

Liang Hao-Cai and Yu Song-Ling

Migrant studies in different regions of the world have supplied important information to research on the causes of cancer with regard to the impact of the environment on carcinogenesis (e.g., [2-4]). We had a chance to submit some groups of migrants within China to closer investigation with respect to the frequency of occurrence of esophageal carcinomas.

Material and Methods

The investigations took place in three settlement areas of Hubei Province, i.e., in the community of Dachaihu in the county of Zhongxiang, in the county of Jinmen, and on Tonghsihu farm. In all three regions, they included migrants from Henan Province as well as native inhabitants.

From the end of 1966 to the beginning of 1969, the Government settled numerous inhabitants from Xichuan county in Henan Province, where esophageal carcinoma is very frequent, in Dachaihu, and in Jinmen County - regions with a low incidence of esophageal carcinoma. At the end of 1957, workers from other regions (most of them from Shangchew county in Henan Province where esophageal carcinoma is not as frequent as in Xichuan) came to Tonghsihu, a very large farm near Wuhan. These migrant populations as well as corresponding controls in the native population were examined by a team of qualified physicians and medical students and data on births, deaths, causes of death, etc. were collected in personal interviews or with relatives of deceased persons. The data thus acquired were checked with the aid of excerpts from registries of the local hospitals. Official demographic data of the year 1964 were used as reference standards.

Results

Dachaihu. The area of this community remained uncultivated for years following a flood. It is divided into six regions, four of which are inhabited by migrants and two by natives. At the end of 1973, the number of immigrants was 50600, the number of natives 25900. From 1969 to 1983 the mean age-adjusted mortality rate from esophageal carcinoma was 15.4/100000 in the native population, but 75.8/100000 in the immigrants, which means that the rate was five times as high with the immigrants (Table 1). Since then every case of esophageal carcinoma has been recorded in a special registry.

Cancer of the Liver, Esophagus, and Nasopharynx
Edited by G. Wagner and Zhang You-Hui

Table 1. Mortality rates of esophageal cancer per 100000 population among native inhabitants and immigrants in Dachaihu (1969–1983)

Year	Native population			Immigrants		
	No. of deaths	Mortality rates		No. of deaths	Mortality rates	
		Crude	Age-adjusted		Crude	Age-adjusted
1969	5	21.72	21.80	20	43.95	45.31
1970	2	8.45	7.74	31	66.13	90.58
1971	5	20.50	18.10	43	89.25	89.31
1972	4	15.64	12.00	40	81.18	76.93
1973	7	29.78	22.00	45	97.88	92.52
1974	2	7.68	7.12	38	74.02	68.89
1975	1	3.83	3.10	37	69.79	66.64
1976	5	18.81	14.67	37	68.68	58.71
1977	4	17.21	15.42	38	67.85	57.64
1978	2	6.85	4.89	37	67.08	57.42
1979	4	14.30	13.32	44	74.67	68.37
1980	1	3.49	2.81	40	66.59	58.93
1981	4	13.75	12.17	40	58.00	58.00
1982	2	6.85	4.03	38	42.01	52.46
1983	2	6.61	4.00	36	38.05	50.07

Table 2. Mortality rates of esophageal cancer among native inhabitants and immigrants in Jinmen County (1968–1977)

Year	Native population Mortality rates		Immigrants Mortality rates	
	Crude	Age-adjusted	Crude	Age-adjusted
1968	4.95	5.32	91.06	82.96
1969	7.24	7.69	92.45	90.42
1970	0	0	65.19	61.07
1971	0	0	103.39	95.83
1972	4.39	3.90	95.53	90.41
1973	4.29	5.15	82.67	78.69
1974	8.42	7.00	71.52	70.96
1975	8.30	5.46	131.10	126.26
1976	12.27	10.53	97.89	93.87
1977	22.16	19.54	104.62	100.95
Average	7.40	7.13	94.03	98.30

Jinmen County. The migrants to Jinmen County arrived at the same time and from the same area as those in Dachaihu; unlike these, however, the families are spread over the whole area. Here data collection took place by means of the matched pair method, i.e., for every migrant family investigated two neighboring native families were examined and interviewed as controls. The number of natives in this county was 49600 at the end of 1977, the number of immigrants 23900. For the years 1968–1977, the mean age-adjusted death rate from esophageal carcinoma was 7.1 in

Table 3. Esophageal cancer among Henan and Non-Henan immigrants in Tonghsihu farm (1959-1978)

Age group (years)	Henan immigrants			Non-Henan immigrants		
	Persons	No. of deaths	Annual rate per 100000	Persons	No. of deaths	Annual rate per 100000
<40	220144	0	0	197573	0	0
40-49	23367	5	21.4	17834	7	39.3
50-59	13193	7	53.1	11740	10	85.2
60-69	7719	17	220.2	7064	15	212.3
70-79	2523	4	158.5	2267	8	252.9
80+	357	3	840.3	420	3	714.3
Total	267303	36	13.5	236898	43	18.2
Age-adjusted rate			20.0			24.8

the native population, but 98.3 in the immigrants, corresponding to a 1:13 ratio (Table 2).

Tonghsihu. Up to the end of 1978, 25114 migrants from Henan Province and 55579 farm workers, who had come from other regions, were examined on Tonghsihu farm. The annual age-adjusted mortality rates from esophageal carcinoma were 20.0 in the former and 24.8 in the latter (Table 3). This difference is not statistically significant.

Discussion

Our epidemiological studies yielded the following results:

1. In Dachaihu and in Jinmen County, the incidence and mortality from esophageal carcinoma are considerably higher with the immigrants than with the native population. In both regions the migrants come from Xichuan county, where there is evidence of a particularly high risk for this form of cancer [1]. In Tonghsihu, on the other hand, death rates were considerably lower; there was no appreciable difference between the two population groups. All migrant groups originated from regions with a low risk of esophagus cancer.
2. The mean age-adjusted mortality rate from esophageal cancer in Xichuan Province, the home of the migrants to Dachaihu and Jinmen, was 55.4/100000 prior to 1975. Even after eliminating sex and age differences, the mortality rate in Dachaihu as well as in Jinmen is still higher than in the home province. It must be taken into consideration that the life style of the immigrants to Dachaihu did not change greatly, while those settled in Jinmen were spread among the native population and thus largely adapted to the local life style.
3. There is a steep rise in death figures from esophageal cancer in migrants in Dachaihu and Jinmen with increasing age; with immigrants in Tonghsihu this trend is considerably less marked (Fig. 1).

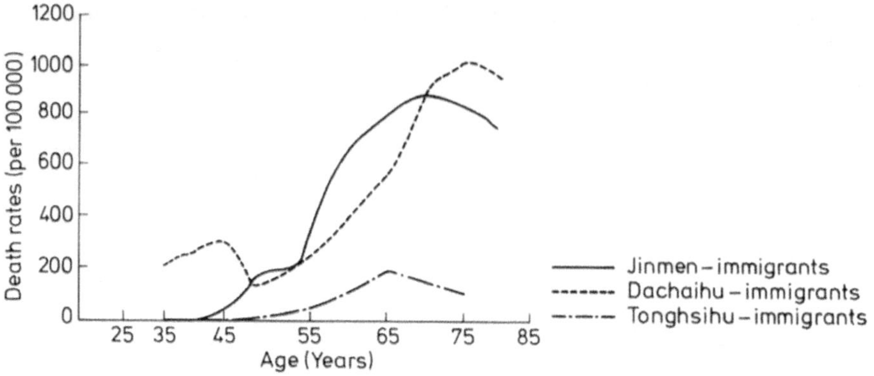

Fig. 1. Age-specific mortality rates in the different groups of immigrants

4. It is worth mentioning that in Dachaihu among 5484 chickens kept by immigrants 12 cases of esophageal carcinomas were found; however, there was not a single case among 2371 chickens kept by native inhabitants. This would indicate that the carcinogenic factor seems to have been imported by the migrants. One is tempted to think of the garbage fed to the chickens.

References

1. Department of Public Health, Xichuan County: Survey of Cancer Mortality during 1974-1976 in Xichuan County. (Unpublished communication)
2. Haenszel W: Cancer mortality among the foreign-born in the United States. J. nat. Cancer Inst. 26 (1961) 37-132
3. Haenszel W, Kurihara M: Studies of Japanese migrants. I. Mortality from cancer and other diseases among Japanese in the United States. J. nat. Cancer Inst. 40 (1968) 43-68
4. Staszewski J: Cancer of the upper alimentary tract and larynx in Poland and in Polish-born Americans. Brit. J. Cancer 29 (1974) 389-399

Cocarcinogens of the Diterpene Ester Type as Principal Risk Factors of Cancer in Curaçao and Possibly in South China:

Identification of Second Order Risk Factors of Cancer in Multifactorial Carcinogenesis

E. Hecker

Introduction

Besides curing diseases of all kinds, traditionally the old culture of China has also been committed to the idea of prevention of diseases, as reflected in the Chinese saying: „Treat a person before he has fallen ill and not only when he is already sick" [50]. Indeed, major aspects of research pursued in my laboratory group at the German Cancer Research Center are guided by the idea of contributing to the prevention of cancer by the identification of the risk factors involved, especially of cocarcinogens of the promotor type. Another important aspect is the investigation of the biochemical mechanism of action of such risk factors to provide clues for their chemical redesign to medicinally useful anticancer drugs.

Concerning the etiology of environmental cancer in experimental and epidemiological oncology, the concept of multifactorial carcinogenesis has become widely accepted. It visualizes exposure of the host to a multitude of environmental risk factors of cancer (e.g., [26]) and integrates classical and unifactorial carcinogenesis (e.g., [17, 20]). As regards the risk of cancer, such a concept comes closer to the realities of everyday human life than the classical, exclusively unifactorial concept. From the point of view of cancer research and cancer prevention including corresponding legislative action, the „multifactorial" concept of environmental cancer (tumor) etiology adds considerably to the scientific and practical complexity of cancer risk assessment and management. To retain an overview in this situation and as a heuristic means, a comprehensive but simple basic concept of carcinogenesis may be useful (e.g., [14, 21, 22]).

Prototype Processes of Carcinogenesis: Experimental and Etiological Models

As in the case of classical unifactorial carcinogenesis, it appears appropriate also in multifactorial carcinogenesis to consider certain risk factors involved and certain specific protocols of combined exposure as prototype processes of carcinogenesis. Thus, the environmental risk factors and certain specific dose/time pattern on the one hand and the host (with his possible hereditary or acquired predisposition for cancer) on the other hand are considered independent variables [17, 18]. In this way, a current and comprehensive etiological concept of environmental cancer(tumor) etiology may be developed including well-defined prototypes of risk factors, i.e., solitary and cocarcinogens defining prototype processes of carcinogenesis such as unifactorial *solitary carcinogenesis* and multifactorial *pluricarcinogenesis* and *cocar-*

Cancer of the Liver, Esophagus, and Nasopharynx
Edited by G. Wagner and Zhang You-Hui

Table 1. Uni- and multifactorial prototype processes of carcinogenesis. For cocarcinogenesis the protocol of initiation/promotion is described

Specific protocol (dose/time)	Effects (tumors)	Prototype processes, stages
■	0	Stage: initiation
■ ■ ■ ■ ■	+	*Solitary carcinogenesis*
□ □ □ □	0	Stage: promotion
■ □ □ □ □	+	*Cocarcinogenesis* as initiation/promotion

■, solitary carcinogen (initiator); □, cocarcinogen (promoter)

Table 2. Examples of uni- and multifactorial life style cancer

Life style	Cancer	Carcinogenic process involved or suspected	Distribution
Excessive sunbathing	Melanoma, skin	Solitary carcinogenesis	Worldwide
Petrol-contaminated water combined with Welensali tea	Esophagus	Cocarcinogenesis	Local (Curaçao)
Smoking cigarette	Lung	Multifactorial	Worldwide
pipe	Lips	Multifactorial	Worldwide
bhidi	Oral cavity	Multifactorial	Regional (India)
Chewing betel nut	Oral cavity	Multifactorial	Regional (India)
Warming by kangri	Skin	Multifactorial	Regional (Himalaya)

cinogenesis. Any one of these prototype processes of carcinogenesis, be it in experimental animals or in human beings, is started by "initiation," which is considered the key event of carcinogenesis also at the cell and molecular levels (see Table 1, line 1). Typically, it is elicited by subcarcinogenic dose(s) of a solitary carcinogen but not by a cocarcinogen, e.g., by a promotor of initiation [21, 22].

Prototype processes of carcinogenesis are best made clear by typical experimental models employing (a) physiochemically well defined risk factors for cancer, (b) specific but simple dose/time protocols operating in defined stages, and (c) experimental animals with (preferably) nonpredisposed target tissue(s) as visualized, for example, in Table 1. The stage of „initiation“ and the corresponding prototype process of solitary carcinogenesis (Table 1, line 2) require no further explanation. The prototype process of cocarcinogenesis in its special version of initiation/promotion is represented by combined exposure of the host to a solitary carcinogen followed by a cocarcinogen, i.e., a "per se essentially noncarcinogenic amplifier" of carcinogenesis such as an initiation (or tumor) promoter [21, 22]. Since in cocarcinogenesis of such a general understanding amplification of initiation involves noncarcinogens, the etiological and mechanistic problems encountered differ in principle from those in solitary (or pluri-) carcinogenesis [21, 22].

In human cancer, certain occupational, iatrogenic, or life style cancers (Table 2)

Table 3. Age-standardized annual incidence rates of esophageal carcinoma in Curaçao and in some regions of Central America related to 100000 of the European and world population

Region	European standard		World population		References
	Male	Female	Male	Female	
Curaçao[a,b]	32.3	19.4	21.2	12.9	[7]
Venezuela					
Caracas	–	–	–	–	[10]
Falcon, Coro	c	c	c	c	[38]
Puerto Rico	21.5	8.1	14.8	5.4	[43]
Cuba	8.7	3.7	5.7	2.4	[43]
Jamaica					
Kingston	13.4	6.6	9.1	4.7	[43]

[a] Data refer to the Netherland Antilles (islands of Aruba, Curaçao, Bonaire, St. Maarten, Saba, St. Eustatius) *without* Aruba and cover the period 1962–1973. Ninety percent of the population of the Netherland Antilles live in Curaçao
[b] Limited data for Aruba: in the period 1963–1966, 5 male and 2 female patients out of a population of about 60000 suffered from esophageal carcinoma [36]
[c] Approximately 15 esophageal carcinomas in 28 months out of a population of about 45000

may be considered to be etiological (epidemiological) models [e.g., 27] reflecting more or less precisely the prototype processes postulated and defined experimentally.[1]

Experimental analyses of such model situations may employ the experimental prototypes and are indispensible for providing the scientific background of assessment of the risk of cancer, aiming at appropriate measures of primary prevention. So far, complete experimental analyses of etiological models of multifactorial life style cancers are lacking. Recently, an etiological model situation of cocarcinogenesis was analyzed completely for the first time. It established as principal sources of the cancer risk involved a combination of pollution of drinking water by petrol for a limited period and exposure to promoters by certain local habits in everyday life [19–21, 24].

Cancer of the Esophagus in Curaçao: The First Etiological Model of Local Life Style Cocarcinogenesis by Diterpene Ester Promoters

The black and creole population of the Caribbean island of Curaçao (Netherlands Antilles) is burdened by an exceedingly high incidence rate of esophageal cancer (Table 3). Epidemiological investigations of the population at risk provided evidence of exposure to drinking water contaminated with petrol in the period 1940–1965, suggesting limited exposure of the esophagus to solitary carcinogens of the polycyclic aromatic hydrocarbon (PAH) type. Furthermore, it was established

[1] In this context, it may be pointed out, for example, that terms such as "promoter" are meaningful only under well-defined dose/time-effect pattern as verified in experimental models. In the case of etiological (epidemiological) models with their poorly defined dose/time-effect pattern, less-specific descriptive terms such as cocarcinogen (in the broad sense) are considered more adequate [20, 22].

by similar investigations that, as part of local life style on Curaçao, plant-derived preparations from about 100 different species, including two species of spurge (Euphorbiaceae), are utilized preferably for food, beverages, and folk medicine. This habit is not common on the neighboring islands (Bonaire, Aruba) or in other parts of the region where the incidence rate of esophageal cancer is average. Extracts of the 23 most frequently used plant species were assayed by the National Cancer Institute (NCI), United States, for solitary carcinogenetic activity. Five species out of the 23 were found active but not the two Euphorbiaceae species. These findings may be interpreted by an etiological hypothesis of "solitary carcinogenesis" or, if the combination with the exposure to PHA in petrol-contaminated drinking water is accounted for, of "pluricarcinogenesis." So far, however, hypotheses of this kind have not been substantiated, e.g., by rigorous chemical identification of the solitary carcinogen(s) possibly involved and by verification of the carcinogenic processes postulated in corresponding typical experimental models (see [24]).

According to the inquiries mentioned above, the Euphobiaceae species utilized in Curaçao are the bushes *Croton flavens* L. (tribus *Crotoneae*), locally known as "Welensali," and *Jatropha gossipyfolia* L. (tribus *Cluytieae*), locally called "bellyache bush." The fresh aromatic leaves of "Welensali" are used to prepare a "bush tea" as an everyday beverage ("Welensali tea"). Also other habitual utilizations of the leaves and of other parts of the bush, especially of the roots (for chewing), are widespread. Parts of the "bellyache bush" are used for a great variety of indications as folk medicinal drugs [2, 36, 37]. On the other hand, Euphorbiaceae species are generally suspected (e.g., [13, 15, 17]) of containing irritants, many of which are potent promoters in the experimental protocol of initiation/promotion, e.g., of mouse skin but also of other organs and in other experimental animals [17]. Therefore, it was considered most likely that, in the "Curaçao case", there was a situation of environmental cocarcinogenesis (etiological "cocarcinogen hypothesis" [24]). Experimental assessment of such a hypothesis became the program of a corresponding research project [25, 34].

Investigations of roots and fresh green leaves of the Welensali bush revealed that their extracts are moderately irritant on the mouse ear and that they contain 17 and 28 irritant "Welensali factors," respectively (Table 4). Their number may be subdivided essentially into two activity types, F and F'. Together, F- and F'-types represent an estimated minimal content of 1.4% and 0.06% by weight of the extracts, respectively. Individually, the Welensali factors were identified as diterpene-12,13-di-(F-types) and -12,13,20-triesters (F'-types), respectively. The polyfunctional diterpene parent alcohols involved were shown to be the tetracyclic tigliane structures 16-hydroxy- and 4-deoxy-16-hydroxyphorbol (see [24]). As a typical example, in Table 5, Welensali factor F_1, most abundant in roots and leaves, and one of its corresponding 20-esters, F_1-20-decanoate, are specified together with other Welensali factors.

As promoters of initiation in our highly standardized model on the back skin of NMRI mice, F-types exhibit in small doses a strong cocarcinogenic activity [with 7,12-dimethylbenz[a]anthracene (DMBA)] as initiator and, for example, $p = 10$ nmol Welensali factor F_1 as promoter (Fig. 1; [24]). Qualitatively and quantitatively the cocarcinogenic activity of Welensali factors of the F-type is comparable to that of the chemically related, well-established diterpene ester 12-*O*-tetradeca-

Table 4. Extracts from roots and leaves of Welensali with irritant activity, total number of Welensali factors, minimum content determined, and typical Welensali Factor F_1 together with corresponding cryptic form F_1-20-decanoate [24]. Irritant activity on the mouse ear expressed as irritant dose 50 (ID_{50}^{24}) in μg/ear

Typical extracts or factors	ID_{50}^{24} (μg/ear)[a]	Welensali factors		
		Type of activity	Identified factors (total number)	Minimal content of factors (%)[b]
Roots, methanol extract (223 g)	6.4	F, F'	17	1.4
Leaves, ethylacetate fraction (1265 g)	90	F, F' (F'')	28	0.06
Welensali factor F_1	0.022	F	–	–
F_1-20-decanoate (F'_1)	0.09	F'	–	–

[a] Standard deviation, 1.3; $P=0.05$; TPA: ID_{50}^{24}, 0.01 μg (0.016 nmol)/ear
[b] By weight of extract

Table 5. The two mixtures of Welensali factors activity type F and F' contained in Welensali tea and minimal contents as determined and estimated in one cup of tea. [24]

Welensali factors F
$R^2=OH$; $R^3=H$
$R^1=CO(CH_2)_{14}CH_3$:F_1
$R^1=CO(CH_2)_{12}CH_3$:F_3
$R^1=CO(CH_2)_{16}CH_3$:F_5

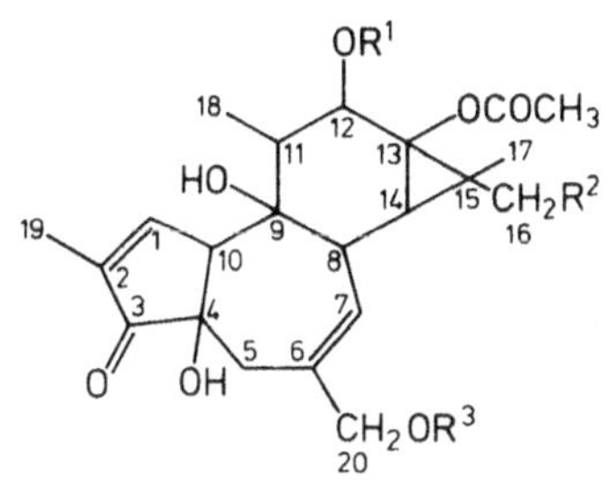

Welensali factors F'
$R^2=OH$; $R^3=Ac$
R^1 for F'-types see F_1, F_3

parent alcohol: 16-hydroxyphorbol

Activity type	Mixture composition (Welensali factors)	Minimal content in one cup of Welensali tea					
		Determined[a]			Estimated[b]		
		Absolute (μg)	Ratio (F/F')	Rel. total (ppb)	Absolute (μg)	Ratio (F/F')	Rel. total (ppb)
F	F_1 F_3 F_5	0.06			0.27		
			0.5/1	0.75		2.2/1	1.6
F'	F_1-20-octanoate F_1-20-decanoate F_3-20-cecanoate	0.12			0.12		

[a] As compared with methanolic extracts of Welensali leaves in aqueous extracts, i.e., in Welensali tea, hydrophilic contaminations carried in the latter complicate the quantitative determination of the F-types but not of F'-types
[b] For a realistic estimation of the true minimal content of the F-types in the tea, the amount of the F'-types was used as an internal standard

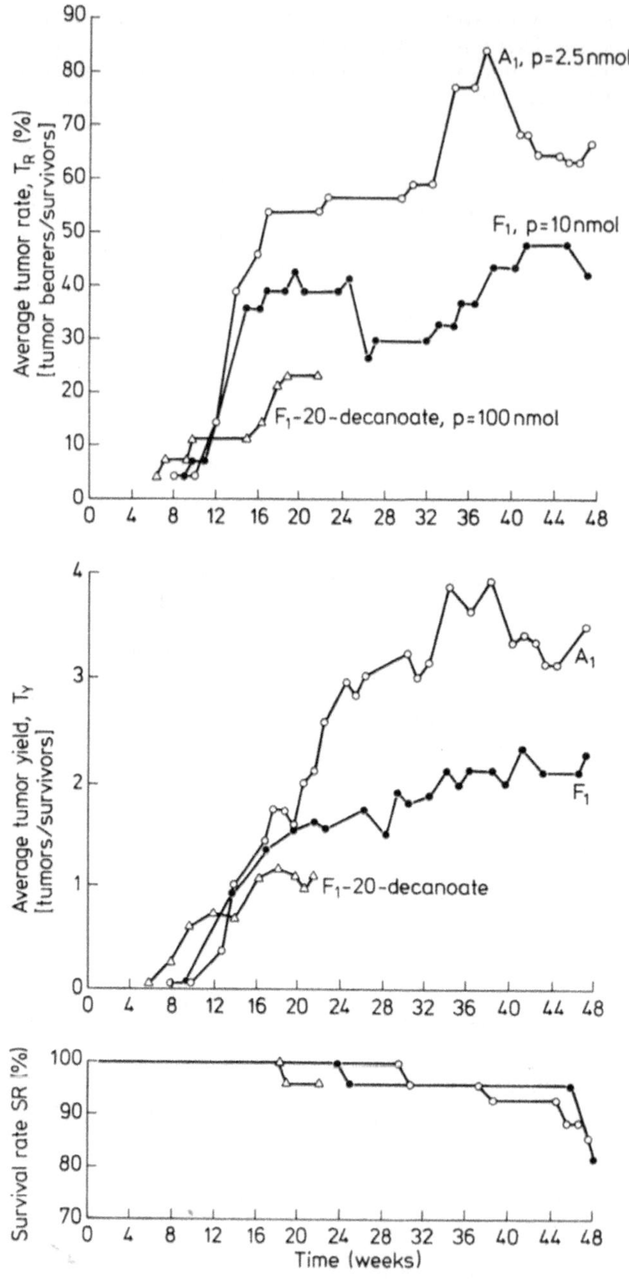

Fig. 1. Cocarcinogenic initiation- (or tumor-) promoting activity of typical Welensali factors F_1 and its 20-decanoate in the standardized assay on the back skin of NMRI mice in comparison with croton oil factor A_1 (TPA). *Initiator:* DMBA, $i = 100$ nmol; 28 females/group. *Promoter:* A_1, F_1, and F_1-20-decanoate, solvent; doses p as indicated

noylphorbol-13-acetate (TPA, see Tables 4,7). F'-types are less active as irritants (and as promoters) than corresponding F-types. Yet, due to the specific chemical substructure of F'-types regarding their 20-ester group, they may be specifically activated chemically or metabolically, e.g., by lipases or esterases, to yield corresponding highly active Welensali factors F. Therefore, F'-types are considered "cryptic irritants and promoters." In chronic exposures of mouse skin solely to a promotional protocol of F- and F'-types (see Table 1, line 3), the Welensali factors F and F' proved not to exhibit any solitary carcinogenic activity [24].

Welensali tea – the plant preparation of *Croton flavens* most frequently consumed on Curaçao – contains a mixture of activity type F and F' factors amounting to an estimated relative total (minimal) content in one cup of the tea of 1.6 ppm (Table 5, last column). It comprises two mixtures of Welensali factors F and F', each represented by three of the individual factors (Table 5, first double column). Of the three Welensali factors type F, the estimated (absolute) minimal content in one cup is 0.27 µg (Tables 5, 6). This amount (expressed in nmol F_1) exceeds more than ten times the irritant dose 50 on the mouse ear, for example, of the typical promoter Welensali factor F_1 (Table 6). The corresponding estimated (absolute) minimal content of Welensali factors type F' in one cup is 0.12 µg (Tables 5, 6). In nmoles, this amount is practically identical with the irritant dose 50 of the typical "cryptic" promoter F_1-20-decanoate (Table 6). Thus, regarding irritants and cocarcinogens in the tea the estimated (absolute) total of active principles F and F', i.e., a minimal content of 0.39 µg/cup of tea, may be considered a "basal dose". The comparison with the irritant doses 50 on the mouse ear of Welensali factors F_1 and F_1-20-decanoate (Table 6) would then suggest as an extrapolation to the human situation: with only one cup of the tea per day the dose required to maintain chronic irritation in the human esophagus may be exceeded considerably. As a rule, in fact, people on Curaçao consume more than one cup daily [37], quite apart from many other utilizations of the plant parts of Welensali (and of "bellyache bush").

The conclusions drawn from the extrapolation of the experimental data received by the etiological model are confirmed by the findings in biopsies obtained and registered in the only hospital on Curaçao, dealing with about 90% of all clinical cases on the island: in patients over 50 years of age without manifest cancer, a severe chronic inflammation of the esophagus is frequently observed [24]. Therefore, for the population at risk, chronic inflammation caused by Welensali factors – an

Table 6. Comparison of the estimated minimal content of Welensali factors activity types F and F' *in one cup of Welensali tea* and irritant dose 50 of the prototype Welensali factors F_1 and F_1-20-decanoate. [24]

Mixture of activity types	Estimated minimal content per cup		Prototype Welensali factors	ID_{50}^{24a} (nmol)	Ratio[b]
	(µg)	(nmol)			
F	0.27	0.41	F_1	0.033	~12/1
F'	0.12	0.15	F_1-20-decanoate	0.11	~1.4/1

[a] On the mouse ear
[b] For example, estimated minimal content of mixture of factors type F over irritant dose 50 of F_1 in nmoles

important element also of mouse skin promotion by diterpene esters – may be considered a principal local risk factor for cancer of the esophagus [24]. Corresponding investigations of plant parts of the "bellyache bush" *(Jatropha gossipyfolia)* are under way in our laboratory; they have already shown that this plant contains irritants of the tigliane type ("*Jatropha* factors" [2]).

The experimental analysis of the "Curaçao case" would not have been complete without testing the solitary carcinogens and cocarcinogens postulated to be involved in corresponding experimental models. Therefore – according to the specific initiation/promotion protocol (see Table 1) – a single, subcarcinogenic dose of the PAH-type solitary carcinogen DMBA was administered as initiator to NMRI mice by stomach tube, followed by repeated intubations of the cocarcinogenic diterpenester type promoter TPA. In this way, tumors of the forestomach were generated (see [17, 24]). Independently and in quite a different context, similar results were obtained in mice (and also in rats) by other scientists using analogous protocols, yet different initiators and promotors. Taking all the experimental data together, it appears most likely that in the "Curaçao case" previous limited exposure to initiators of the solitary carcinogenic PAH-type by petrol-contaminated drinking water and simultaneous or especially subsequent chronic exposure to promoters of the cocarcinogenic diterpene ester type by Welensali tea represent the principal risk factors in this life style cancer.

Experimental prototype models mimicking etiologies of human cancer are indispensable for assessing the principal risk factors of cancer as well as the specific (combination) pattern of exposure involved. No doubt, however, and for good reasons, in experimental models the complex reality of everyday human life is intentionally oversimplified. Due to the diversity of individuals and their personal habits, it is highly unlikely that in real life, for example, a "pure and simple" pattern of combined exposure, e.g., to just one initiator and one promotor (see Table 1) would prevail. It may be emphasized, therefore, that the experimental analysis presented above for the "Curaçao case" does not exclude the possibility that, under the specific conditions on the island, besides the principal local solitary and cocarcinogens as suggested here, other local risk factors may also contribute to the excessive risk of esophageal cancer such as, for example, condensed tannins (see [39]) or preparations of those five plants which exhibited solitary carcinogenic activity (see above). Also, contributions by those risk factors usually suspected to be involved in esophageal cancer, i.e., consumption of food which is too hot (see [11]), excessive consumption of alcohol (see [41]) and/or cigarettes (see [45]), nutritional deficiencies (see [46]) cannot be excluded. Furthermore, in other high-risk areas of esophageal cancer in the world, e.g., in China, "local" risk factors and/or combination patterns of exposure quite different from those postulated to be typical for the "Curaçao case" may be operative [9].

As a final step in the scientific evaluation of the "Curaçao case," it appears desirable to investigate the etiological cocarcinogen hypothesis by prospective epidemiological research [19, 24]. However, independently, the results of the experimental analysis presented here may already now provide the scientific basis for risk assessment by local health authorities in an effort to defray adequate measures of primary prevention.

Cancer of the Nasopharynx in South China: Another Etiological Model of Cocarcinogenesis by Diterpene Ester Promoters?

It is of particular interest to note that Welensali factor F_1, identified as a local risk factor for esophageal cancer in Curaçao, is chemically identical with the diterpene ester called HHPA obtained from another Euphorbiaceae species *(Aleurites fordii).* In a manner similar to TPA and many other promoting diterpene esters of the tigliane-, ingenane-, and daphnane-type [16, 51, 52], Welensali factor F_1 (or HHPA) was shown to activate Epstein-Barr virus in immortal lymphoblastoid cells [31, 32]. Moreover, in the rodent *Mastomys natalensis* a synergism for the generation of skin papilloma was shown to exist involving endogenous papilloma virus (HPV) and TPA [5].

Induction of Epstein-Barr virus (EBV) synthesis in certain human lymphoblastoid cell lines by the initiation-promotor TPA (Fig. 1) originally was detected [16, 40, 52] and measured by the number of cells carrying virus capsid (VCA) or early antigen (EA): apart from "producer" cell lines (which produce the virus spontaneously at a low rate such as, e.g., P3HR-1 and B 95-8 (Fig. 2), the synthesis of virus-related proteins is stimulated by TPA and congeners also in "nonproducer" cell lines such as NC 37 and Raji. The number of cells carrying the antigen reaches a maximum about 5 days after exposure to TPA (Fig. 2). The irritant and promoting activities in mouse skin of selected diterpene esters covering the three principal structural types correlate well with their capabilities to induce EA of EBV in NC37 and Raji cells (Table 7). Recently, it was shown that the new indole alkaloid type promoters also induce EBV synthesis in much the same way as TPA [47, 48].

The tumor viruses activated by diterpene ester promoters are related to human cancers, such as EBV to Burkitt's lymphoma and anaplastic nasopharyngeal carcinoma (NPC) [28, 31, 32, 49, 53], or HPV to genital cancers [12]. Thus, it may be sus-

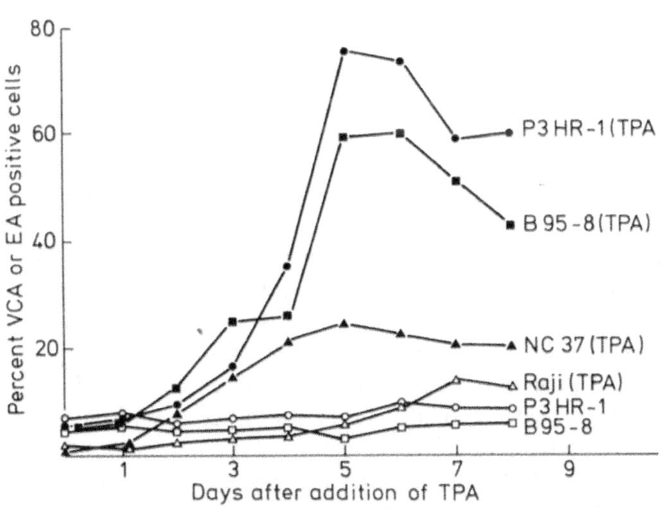

Fig. 2. Induction of synthesis of virus capsid antigen *(VCA)* in P3HR-1, B-95-8 and/or early antigen *(EA)* in NC37 and Raji in cell lines with latent genome of Epstein-Barr virus, with and without $3 \times 10^{-8} M$ TPA

Table 7. Skin irritant and promoting activities of tigliane, ingenane, and daphnane type diterpene esters in vivo and their ability to induce synthesis of EB-viral early antigen (EA) in the human lymphoblastoid NC 37 and RAJI cell< [16]

Compound	Irritation ID_{50}^{24} (nmol)[a]	Promoting activity (rel. potency)[b]	EA induction at 3×10^{-8} M NC 37[c] (% of cells)	Raji[d]
		Tigliane types		
TPA	0.016	+ + + +	13.2	5.2
4-O-MeTPA	2.3	(+)	14.1	10.2
PDD	0.01	+ + +	10.0	4.9
4α-PDD	> 150	0	0.2	< 0.01
12-Deoxyphorbol-13-decanoate	0.017	+ + +	13.4	5.8
Phorbol	> 270	0	0.3	< 0.01
		Daphnane types		
Hippomane factors $M_1 + M_2$	0.02	+ + +	14.9	8.3
Pimelea factor P_2	0.003	+ + +	11.0	7.8
		Ingenane types		
Ingenol-3-hexadecanoate	0.086	+ + +	12.8	6.5
Ingenol	> 287	0	0.1	< 0.01

[a] Irritant dose 50 (ID_{50}^{24}) on the mouse ear after 24 h
[b] Initiation/promotion standard assay on the back skin of female NMRI mice with DMBA as initiator
[c] Spontaneous EA induction 0.1%
[d] Spontaneous EA induction 0.01%

pected that geographcal regions of frequent utilization of Euphorbiaceae-derived materials, e.g., as ethnomedicinal therapeutics [1, 16, 17, 28, 49] or tung oil [31, 32], may be identical with regions of high incidence of NPC. Indeed, in recent investigations by Zeng et al. [49, see also this volume pp. 162–167], an extended program of prospective investigations of environmental materials for the activation of EBV was covered.

Key Problems in the Assessment of Cancer Risk in Multifactorial Carcinogenesis

However complex the multifactorial etiology of cancer (tumors) may be, one of the most important tasks of basic cancer research has been and still is to develop generally valid criteria for the classification of environmental carcinogens – and possibly for grading the risk imposed on humans, especially by mechanistic investigations. With the background of the progress made during the past years, there might already be a general consensus that classical solitary carcinogens will have to be considered as first order carcinogenic risk factors of cancer.

In contrast, cocarcinogens – collectively considered "per se essentially noncarcinogenic amplifiers" of carcinogenesis – which produce cancer essentially only in an appropriate combination with either initiators or predisposed tissues, may be classified as second order carcinogenic risk factors (e.g., [17, 21, 22] and previous publications). By classifying physicochemically well defined environmental risk factors in solitary carcinogens and in cocarcinogens, an acceptable grading of the risk of cancer may be achieved, allowing in the future for a more refined assessment of cancer risk [17, 35]. For health authorities this may be helpful in finding in practice (remember, for example, the saccharin case) a scientifically more appropriate balance between an overprotective legislation aiming at absolute safety and an all-permissive absence of restriction, both of which are disadvantageous to the human individual.

No doubt, established mechanisms of action of solitary carcinogens and cocarcinogens at the cell and/or the molecular level will provide the ultimate criteria for the assessment of risk imposed on the human environment [20, 29]. However, in practice, risk assessment can hardly wait until the final mechanisms of carcinogenesis have been explored. Therefore, at the present stage and from the scientific point of view, it appears appropriate to use for an assessment of environmental risk factors of cancer certain descriptive (empirical) criteria seemingly available from dose/time-effect relationships such as "irreversibility" of a process, e.g., of solitary carcinogenesis, and "reversibility" of a process, e.g., of cocarcinogenesis, especially initiation/promotion, see, for example, [17, 23, 33]. Furthermore, such criteria may suggest generally valid but specific biochemical criteria of processes of carcinogenesis to be established for a quick and inexpensive assessment of risk in appropriate short-term assays (for recent reviews on solitary carcinogens see [4], on cocarcinogens see [8, 22]). However, at the present stage of research, it would seem premature of materialize the grading of cancer risk intended based solely upon criteria such as, e.g., genotoxic (solitary carcinogen-related) versus nongenotoxic activity (cocarcinogen, specifically promoter-related) [35], and to build guidelines for legislatory action on such grounds, simply because for solitary carcinogens short-term mutagenicity assays are available [e.g., 3, 6, 20, 29, 30, 42, 44].

References

1. Adolf W, Chanai S, Hecker E: 3-*O*-Angeloylingenol, the toxic and skin irritant factor from latex of *Euphorbia antiquorum* L. (Euphorbiaceae) and from a derived Thai purgative and anthelmintic (vermifuge) drug. J. Sci. Soc. Thailand 9 (1983) 81-88
2. Adolf W, Opferkuch HJ, Hecker E: Irritant phorbol derivatives from four *Jatropha* species (Euphorbiaceae). Phytochemistry 23 (1984) 129-132
3. Albert RE: Carcinogen policy at EPA. Science 219 (1983) 796-798
4. Ames BN: Dietary carcinogens and anticarcinogens - oxygen radicals and degenerative diseases. Science 221 (1983) 1256-1264
5. Amtmann E, Sauer G, Volm M et al: Synergism between latent papillomavirus genomes and a tumor promoter in the rodent *Mastomys natalensis*. In Abstracts of the International Symposium of the Role of Co-carcinogens and Promoters in Human and Experimental Carcinogenesis, Budapest, May 16-8, 1983, p. 1.
6. Benbrook CM: Carcinogen policy at EPA. (Letter). Science 219 (1983) 798
7. de Boer SY: Frequentia van Kanker van Mond-Tong-Pharynx-Slokdarm en de Nederlandse Antillen. Diss. Landslaboratorium voor de Volkszondheit, Afdeling Pathologisch Anatomisches Laboratorium Curaçao, Niederländische Antillen, 1979
8. Bohrmann JS: Identification and assessment of tumor-promoting and cocarcinogenic agents: state-of-art in vitro methods. Critic. Rev. Toxicol. 11 (1983) 131-167
9. Cheng JS, Sala M, Li MH et al: Esophageal cancer in Linxian County, China: A possible

etiology and mechanism (initiation and promotion). In E Hecker, NE Fusenig, W Kunz et al (Eds): Carcinogenesis, Vol. 7: Cocarcinogenesis and Biological Effects of Tumor Promoters, pp 167-174, New York: Raven Press 1982
10. Dunham LJ, Bailar JC: World maps of cancer mortality rates and frequency ratios. J. nat. Cancer Inst. 41 (1968) 155-203
11. Eps LW: Esophageal cancer. Paper of Post Graduate Course 1970 Medical Library of the St. Elizabeth Hospital, Curaçao, 1970
12. Gissman L: Papilloma viruses and their association with cancer in animals and in man. Cancer Surv. 3 (1984) 161-181
13. Hecker E: Aktuelle Probleme der Krebsentstehung. Z. Krebsforsch. 78 (1972) 99-122
14. Hecker E: Definitions and terminology in cancer (tumor) etiology - an analysis aiming at proposals for a current internationally standardized terminology. a) Int. J. Cancer 18 (1976) 122-129. b) Z. Krebsforsch. 86 (1976) 219-230. c) Gann 67 (1976) 471-481. d) Bull. Wrld Hlth Org. 54 (1976) 1-10.
15. Hecker E: Structure-activity relationships in diterpene esters irritant and cocarcinogenic to mouse skin. In TJ Slaga, A Sivak, RK Boutwell (Eds): Carcinogenesis, Vol. 2: Mechanisms of Tumor Promotion and Cocarcinogenesis, pp 11-48. New York: Raven Press 1978
16. Hecker E: Diterpene ester type modulators of carcinogenesis - new findings in the mechanisms of chemical carcinogenesis and the etiology of human tumors. In E. C. Miller, J. A. Miller, T. Horono et al (Eds): Naturally Occurring Carcinogens - Mutagens and Modulators of Carcinogenesis, pp 263-286. Tokyo: Japan Sci. Soc. Press 1979
17. Hecker E: Co-carcinogenesis and tumor promoters of the diterpene ester type as possible carcinogenic risk factors. J. Cancer Res. clin. Oncol. 99 (1981) 103-124
18. Hecker E: Prototype processes as experimental models in multifactorial carcinogenesis. J. Cancer Res. clin. Oncol. 99 (1981) A29
19. Hecker E: Co-carcinogens of the tumor promoter type as potential risk factors of cancer in man - a first complete experimental analysis of an etiological model situation and some of its consequences. In M. Börszönyi, N. E. Day, K. Lapis et al (Eds): Models, Mechanisms and Etiology of Tumour Promotion, pp 441-446. Lyon: IARC 1984. (IARC Sci. Publ. No. 56)
20. Hecker E: Concluding remarks and future perspectives. In M. Börszönyi, N. E. Day, K Lapis et al (Eds): Models, Mechanisms and Etiology of Tumour Promotion, pp 509-521. Lyon: IARC 1984. (IARC Sci. Publ. No. 56)
21. Hecker E: Cocarcinogens of the initiation(or-tumor)-promoter type as environmental risk factors of cancer in man - experimental analysis of an etiologic model situation of life style cancer and current problems of assessment of cancer risk in multifactorial carcinogenesis. Acta Pharmacol. Toxicol. 55, Suppl. 2 (1984) 145-164
22. Hecker E: Multifaktorielle und Mehrstufen-Karzinogenese - ätiologische (epidemiologische) und experimentelle Modelle sowie aktuelle Probleme der Bewertung von Krebsrisikofaktoren der Umwelt. In K. E. Appel, A. G. Hildebrandt (Hrsg.): Tumorpromotoren - Erkennung, Wirkungsmechanismen und Bedeutung, S. 14-42. München: MMV Medizin Verlag 1985. (BGA-Schriften Nr. 6)
23. Hecker E, Fusenig NE, Kunz W et al (Eds): Carcinogenesis - A Comprehensive Survey. Vol. 7: Cocarcinogenesis and Biological Effects of Tumor Promoters. New York: Raven Press 1982.
24. Hecker E, Lutz D, Weber J et al: Multistage tumor development in the human esophagus - the first identification of cocarcinogens of the tumor promoter type as principal carcinogenic risk factors in a local life style cancer. In 13th International Cancer Congress, Part B. Biology of Cancer (1), pp 219-238. New York: A. R. Liss 1983
25. Hecker E, Weber J: Cocarcinogens from *Croton flavens* L. and the high incidence of esophageal cancer in Curaçao. In Abstracts of the 7th International Symposium on the Biological Characterization of Human Tumors, Budapest, April 13-15, 1977, p 52; Experientia 34 (1978) 679-682
26. Higginson J: A global perspective of environmental carcinogenesis. In P Emmlot, E Kriek (Eds): Environmental Carcinogenesis, pp 9-22. Amsterdam: Elsevier/North-Holland 1979

27. Hirayama T: Operational epidemiology of cancer. J. Cancer Res. clin. Oncol. 99 (1981) 15-28
28. Hirayama T, Ito Y: A new view of the etology of nasopharyngeal carcinoma. Prev. Med. 10 (1981) 614-622
29. IARC: Approaches to Classifying Chemical Carcinogens According to Mechanism of Action. IARC Techn. Rep. No. 83/001, 1983
30. IARC: Proceedings. Symposium on the Role of Co-carcinogens and Promoters in Human and Environmental Carcinogenesis. Lyon: IARC 1984. (IARC Sci. Publ. No. 56)
31. Ito Y, Ohigashi H, Koshimizu K et al: Epstein-Barr-virus-activating principle in the ether extracts of soils collected from under plants which contain active diterpene esters. Cancer Lett. 19 (1983) 113-117
32. Ito Y, Yamase S, Tokuda H et al: Epstein-Barr virus activation by tung oil, extracts of *Aleurides fordii* and its diterpene ester 12-O-hexadecanoyl-16-hydroxyphorbol-13-acetate. Cancer Lett. 18 (1983) 87-95
33. Kunz HW, Schwarz M, Tennekes H et al: Dose/time response characteristics of chemical carcinogenesis and tumor promotion in liver. Proceedings. Symposium on the Role of Co-carcinogens and Promoters in Human and Experimental Carcinogenesis, May 16-18, 1983, Budapest, Hungary
34. Lutz D, Hecker E: Esophageal cancer on Curaçao - further new tumor promoters from *Croton flavens* L. Book of Abstracts. 8th International Symposium on the Biological Characterization of Human Tumors. May 8-11, 1979, Athens, Greece
35. Marshall E: EPA's high risk carcinogen policy. Science 218 (1982) 975-978
36. Morton JF: A survey of medicinal plants of Curaçao. Econ. Bot. 22 (1968) 87-102
37. Morton JF: Plants associated with esophageal cancer cases in Curaçao. Cancer Res. 28 (1968) 2268-2271
38. Morton JF: Folk remedy plants and esophageal cancer in Coro, Venezuela. Morris Arboretum Bull. 25 (1974) 24-34
39. Morton JF: Plant tannins and esophageal cancer. Proc. 10th International Conference on Toxicology and Occupational Medicine, pp 129-137. Amsterdam: Elsevier/North-Holand 1979
40. Takada K, zur Hausen H: Induction of Epstein-Barr virus antigens by tumor promoters for epidermal and non-epidermal tissues. Int. J. Cancer 33 (1984) 491-496
41. Tuyns AJ, Pequignot G, Abbalucci JS: Oesophageal cancer and alcohol consumption: Importance of type of beverage. Int. J. Cancer 23 (1979) 443-447
42. Todhunter JA: Carcinogen policy at EPA. (Letter). Science 219 (1983) 794
43. Waterhouse J, Muir C, Correa P et al (Eds): Cancer Incidence in Five Continents. Vol. III. Lyon: IARC 1976. (IARC Sci. Publ., No. 15)
44. Weinstein IB: Carcinogen policy at EPA. (Letter). Science 219 (1983) 794-796
45. Wynder EL, Hoffmann DH: Tobacco and health: A societal challenge. New Engl. J Med. 300 (1979) 894-903
46. Wynder EL, Hultberg S, Jacobson F et al: Environmental factors in cancer of the upper alimentary tract. Cancer 10 (1957) 470-487
47. Yamamoto H, Katsuki T, Hinoma Y et al.: Induction of Epstein-Barr virus by a new tumor promoter teleocidin, compared to induction by TPA. Int. J. Cancer 28 (1981) 125-129
48. Yamamoto N: Interaction of viruses with tumor promoters. Rev. Physiol. Biochem. Pharmacol. 101 (1984) 111-159
49. Zeng Y, Zhong JM, Mo YK et al: Epstein-Barr virus early antigen induction in Raji cells by Chinese medicinal herbs. Intervirology 19 (1983) 201-204
50. Zhong SZ: Ancient China's Scientists. Hongkong: Commercial Press 1984
51. Zur Hausen H, O'Neill FB, Freese UK et al: Persisting oncogenic herpesvirus induced by the tumor promoter TPA. Nature 272 (1978) 373-374
52. Zur Hausen H, Bornkamm GW, Schmidt R et al: Tumor initiators and promoters in the induction of Epstein-Barr virus. Proc. nat. Acad. Sci. 76 (1979) 782-785
53. Zur Hausen H, Schulte-Holthausen H, Klein G et al: EBV DNA in biopsies of Burkitt tumors and anaplastic carcinomas of the nasopharynx. Nature 228 (1979) 1076

A Survey of the Familial Aggregation of Esophageal Cancer in Yangcheng County, Shanxi Province

Li Guang-Heng and He Li-Ji

Yangcheng is a mountainous county located at the southern end of the Taihang mountain range in the southeastern part of Shanxi province. It has an area of 1968 km^2, 24 communes, 451 production brigades, 2251 villages, and 81 388 families, with a population of 360 000, mostly peasants. Yangcheng and the other counties nearby are suitable for agricultural production and are very rich in coal resources. The area is also noticeable for its remarkably high incidence of esophageal cancer (EC).

The mortality rate from EC in Yangcheng county is the highest in Shanxi province. In the period 1969–1982, the average total cancer mortality rate was 222.13/100 000, accounting for 22.7% of the total deaths in the population. The crude mortality rate from EC was 149.29/100 000, accounting for 67.2% of all cancer deaths.

The incidence of EC varies widely in different parts of Shanxi province; it is highest in the rural areas along the Taihang mountains and lowest in the north. The mortality rate of EC even within the high incidence area differs widely in different counties and communes. Furthermore, as in Yangcheng, remarkable differences in the EC mortality rate are found in different families in the same villages or brigades where the environment, living conditions, and eating and drinking habits of the people are very much alike. In some of these families, EC occurred in successive generations with obvious familial aggregation, while in many others no EC occurred. Thus, the question arises: does a genetic factor play a role in the causation of EC?

To answer this question, a retrospective survey was conducted in Yangcheng in 1979. Each family was taken as a unit of investigation. Families were visited one by one. A family member, usually a person about 50 years old, was interviewed. The family tree was traced back to the generation of his or her grandparents on the paternal and maternal sides, and all EC patients were recorded. If one or more persons had died of EC, this was taken as a positive family. Families without EC were taken as negative families.

Results

The number of EC deaths in Yangcheng county as well as in its high-risk area, Ciying commune, could be divided into two groups. In one group, there were multiple cases in the families, and in the other, there was only one case of EC per family. The following tables show the results of our investigation.

Cancer of the Liver, Esophagus, and Nasopharynx
Edited by G. Wagner and Zhang You-Hui

Table 1 shows that the EC-positive families accounted for 8.2% of all families in the county, and 9.9% in Ciying commune.

In EC-positive families of Yangcheng county (Table 2), the number of single-case families (3871) was greater than that of multiple-case families (2794). But Table 3 shows that the latter had more deaths from EC (6156) than the former (6290). As for Ciying commune, not only was the number of multiple-case families (254) higher than that of the single-case families (157), but also the percentage of EC deaths (70.4%) was much higher than that of the single-case families (29.6%). Hence the higher the incidence of EC, the more multiple-case families could be found in the commune.

Two-thirds or more of the total male deaths were attributed to EC in the multiple-case families. This was the case in the county as a whole and in the Ciying commune as well. Both showed a very marked difference between the sexes. The sex ratios were much higher in multiple-case families than those observed in single-case families (see Tables 4, 5).

Table 6 shows that in 28.7% of the 2794 multiple-case families, multiple cases of EC appeared in the same generation and in 65.2% in two successive generations. Thus, more than 90% of the multiple EC cases could be found in one and two successive generations. EC cases in three and four successive generations were seldom seen. The rates from Ciying commune were about the same.

Table 1. Number of EC-positive families in Yangcheng county and Ciying commune

Place	Total number of families	EC-positive families	
		Number	%
Yangcheng county	81388	6665	8.2
Ciying commune	4149	411	9.9

Table 2. Percentage of families with single and multiple EC cases

Place	Total number of EC-positive families	Families with a single case of EC		Families with multiple EC cases	
		Number	%	Number	%
Yangcheng	6665	3871	(58.1)	2794	(41.9)
Ciying	411	157	(38.2)	254	(61.8)

Table 3. Percentage of EC deaths from families with a single case and those with multiple cases

Place	Total deaths	EC deaths from families with a single case		EC deaths from families with multiple cases	
		Number	%	Number	%
Yangcheng	11446	5290	(46.7)	6156	(53.8)
Ciying	867	257	(29.6)	610	(70.4)

Table 4. Percentage of male and female EC patients with a positive family history

Place	Males			Females		
	Total No. of deaths	Deaths from families with multiple EC cases		Total No. of deaths	Deaths from families with multiple EC cases	
		Number	%		Number	%
Yangcheng	7868	4964	63.1	3578	1192	33.3
Ciying	635	507	79.8	232	103	44.4

Table 5. Sex ratio of esophageal cancer deaths

Place	Total No. of deaths			Deaths in multiple-case families			Deaths in single-case families		
	M	F	M/F	M	F	M/F	M	F	M/F
Yangcheng	7868	3578	2.20	4964	1192	4.16	2904	2386	1.22
Ciying	635	232	2.37	507	103	4.92	128	129	0.99

Table 6. The distribution of EC patients in multiple-case families

Place	Total No. of multiple EC families	First generation No. of families (%)	Second generation No. of families (%)	Third generation No. of families (%)	Fourth generation No. of families (%)
Yangcheng	2794	803 (28.7)	1821 (65.2)	168 (6.0)	2 (0.1)
Ciying	254	72 (28.4)	163 (64.2)	19 (7.5)	

Table 7. Family history of 475 couples of parents both of whom suffered from EC

Place	Total EC couples in the parental generation	No Ec found on both sides		Ec found only on paternal side		EC found only on maternal side		EC found on both paternal and maternal sides	
		Pairs	%	Pairs	%	Pairs	%	Pairs	%
Yangcheng	475	172	36.2	155	32.6	65	13.7	83	17.5
Ciying	40	10	25.0	18	45.0	4	10.0	8	20.0

Altogether 475 couples in this county died of EC in the parental generation; 36.2% of them had no positive family history on either the paternal or maternal side or both, while 46.3% had a positive family history on the paternal or on the maternal side. The remaining 17.5% had a positive history on both sides. In Ciying commune, 75% of the 40 EC couples presented with a positive history in their ancestors (Table 7).

A comparison was made of the age at death of EC patients in parental and filial generations in Ciying commune (Table 8). The numbers of deaths were 105 in the

Table 8. Comparison of the age of death between parental and filial generations

Age of death in the parental generation (years)	Deaths in parental generation	Death in filial generation at an age older than that of the parental generation	Deaths in filial generation at an age younger than that of the parental generation
30-49	12	14	2
50-54	12	13	4
55-59	16	6	11
60-64	28	3	27
65-69	15	4	16
70-	22	1	25

parental generation and 129 in the filial one. Among the 81 patients in the parental generation, whose age of death was over 55 years, the age of death in 83.2% of their offspring with EC was younger than that of the parents. On the other hand, in the remaining 24 patients in the parental generation who died before 55 years, the age at death in 79.4% of the children was older than that of their parents.

Discussion and Conclusion

1. Yangcheng county is a high incidence area for esophageal cancer, with an average mortality rate of 149.29/100000, which accounts for 67.2% of all cancer deaths. Hundreds of people die of it each year and for a long period its incidence has remained unchanged. Nevertheless, the results of our investigation revealed that among the 81388 families in the whole county, 74723 families, accounting for 91.8%, had no EC patients in more than three successive generations. EC patients were concentrated in only 8.2% of the families.
   In the families with EC patients in Yangcheng county, 58% had only one case per family, and 42% had multiple cases. Of the 11446 EC deaths, 46% were from the former and 54% from the latter families. In the high-risk area of the county, Ciying commune, the proportion of multiple-case families was 62%, and the proportion of EC deaths from the multiple-case families reached 70%.
2. Among families with multiple cases, 65.2% had EC patients in two successive generations, and 6.0% of them in three successive generations. If both parents had developed EC, their descendants often suffered from the same disease. In this series, there were 475 parental couples who died of EC, and in 63.8% of them, EC patients were found on either the paternal or maternal side or both, but mainly on the paternal side (50.1%).
   The age at death of the EC patients in parental and filial generations was variable. We have seen EC at the age of 16 years (female) and 15 years (male) in Ciying commune.
   In view of the facts described above, the high incidence of EC could hardly be explained solely by environmental factors. Most likely, quite a number of people in this county are prone to develop EC due to an inherited susceptibility. Therefore, it is very important to study thoroughly the genetic etiology of this cancer.

3. In the high-risk population, susceptible people must be protected. Measures should be taken, such as reinforcement of medical facilities, setting up networks for cancer control at the grassroot level, conducting thorough investigations in certain communes, popularizing the knowledge of hygiene and sanitation among the people, and persuading them to change some of their bad living habits, such as eating excessively hot food or eating too fast. We should also endeavor to treat the inflammation and epithelial dysplasia of the esophagus if detected. Patients should be diagnosed early and properly treated.

   We have set up family health records and charts of the families with a positive EC history in Yangcheng. Besides, we have tried to find out the susceptible individuals in this county and put them under surveillance, aiming not only at reducing the scale of mass survey but also focusing our limited manpower and material resources on people who are at high risk. Some experimental studies have been carried out in this county, where a cancer hospital has been in existence for nearly 10 years. Although there are a lot of difficulties to be overcome, we are determined to control EC in this high-incidence area, based on a better understanding of its etiology, both genetic and environmental.

Chemical Factors in the Pathogenesis of Esophageal Carcinoma

R. Preußmann

Research into etiological factors of esophageal cancer has increased considerably in the past 1 or 2 decades. There are several reasons for the growing interest in this specific tumor site, one of the more important being the epidemiological identification of defined high-risk areas for this type of cancer [4, 22], such as, for example, the Iranian part of the Caspian Sea and Linxian County in China, both areas belonging to the same belt of high incidence of esophageal cancer. Other important areas to be mentioned here are the Transkai in South Africa or Normandy and Brittany in northwestern France.

The second reason for the increasing interest in esophageal cancer is certainly the fact that experimental cancer research has developed reliable animal models for the induction of this tumor, especially by certain N-nitroso compounds [21]. I will, therefore, concentrate on this specific aspect of nitrosamine carcinogenesis, an area to which our own work in Druckrey's group in Freiburg has contributed considerably [5].

First, I will very briefly mention some important environmental and endogenous factors that have been incriminated as causative or contributing factors in the etiology of esophageal cancer in humans. Excessive exposure to tobacco smoke or chewing tobacco, especially together with alcohol abuse, is very often discussed as a major risk factor also for the esophagus [16, 29]. Tobacco and tobacco smoke contain, among other carcinogens, carcinogenic aromatic hydrocarbons, nitrosamines, and direct alkylating agents as possible initiators of transformation; alcohol being mostly discussed as a promoting agent. Some naturally occurring carcinogens, especially of plant origin, might contribute to the induction of esophageal cancer; the carcinogens in bracken [10] and the tannins, especially in hot teas [4], might be involved in certain geographical areas, while plant irritants like those mentioned by Dr. Hecker might be promotors in other areas.

Pyrolysis products from opium are potent mutagens and might play a role in northern Iran [9].

The role of moldy food and of mycotoxins has been extensively discussed in the Chinese high incidence areas [16], where several fungi have been shown to catalyze the formation of nitrosamines. The typical carcinogenic mycotoxins such as aflatoxins in experimental systems do not, however, usually induce tumors of the esophagus.

Cancer of the Liver, Esophagus, and Nasopharynx
Edited by G. Wagner and Zhang You-Hui

Experimental Induction of Esophageal Cancer

Before concentrating on N-nitroso compounds, I will mention two experiments not involving nitrosamines. Kuratsune and his group [14] in Japan succeeded in inducing a few papillomas and carcinomas in mice by oral administration of benzo[a]pyrene or 4-nitro-quinoline-N-oxide in a 70% or even 95% ethanolic solution. These experiments were based on the assumption that alcohol facilitates the penetration of the carcinogen into the esophageal epithelium during the short passage through the esophagus.

Dihydrosafrole, a natural component of aromatic oils of several spices, induced, at very high doses, some tumors of the esophagus in rats [7], but not in mice, where it is hepatocarcinogenic.

The esophagus, as already mentioned, is a major target organ in carcinogenesis experiments using N-nitroso compounds [21]. Of more than 300 different compounds of this type tested, about 30% (130 different nitrosamines) induced benign and, predominantly, malignant tumors in this organ. The rat is certainly the most sensitive species, and a high proportion of tumor induction with high organ-specificity is very easily possible. Esophageal tumors have also been induced with nitrosamines in mice and guinea pigs, while the hamster (Syrian, Chinese, or European) seems to be resistant with regard to the esophagus but not with regard to other organs. This confirms a general experience in organotropic carcinogenesis with nitroso compounds, namely that an extrapolation of such organ-specific carcinogenic effects to other species is usually not possible.

With regard to structure-activity relationships, it is remarkable that it is especially the group of unsymmetrical nitrosamines that selectively induce esophageal cancer in rats of different strains. The only difference between symmetrical nitrosamines (primarily hepatocarcinogens in the rat) and unsymmetrical nitrosamines is that the latter have two different alkyl residues, while in the former both groups are the same.

This seemingly small difference, however, has a profound influence on organotropy. Thus, all methyl- and ethylalkyl nitrosamines are potent esophageal carcinogens. With symmetrical or cyclic nitrosamines, esophageal tumors can also be induced, but the esophagus usually is not the main tumor site; with symmetrical nitrosamines very often only a low incidence is observed in this organ, other organs being more predominant sites.

The effect on the esophagus is not a direct one, although most of the compounds have been tested by the oral route. Intravenous and subcutaneous injection as well as inhalation have also been investigated, using unsymmetrical nitrosamines, and have confirmed that the action on the esophagus is a systemic effect.

Remarkably enough, the rat forestomach, which is considered to be an extended esophagus morphologically, is only rarely the target for tumors with unsymmetrical nitrosamines. On the other hand, in the mouse certain unsymmetrical nitrosamines induce forestomach tumors, the esophagus being only a minor tumor site.

In the rat again, some directly acting nitroso compounds, not requiring metabolic activation, regularly induce tumors of the forestomach after chronic oral administration without ever inducing tumors in the esophagus [5]. The perplexing problem of organ specificity can be further demonstrated by the following experimental results: In the rat methylalkyl nitrosamines up to methylylhexylnitrosamine are carcinogens for the esophagus, as already discussed; methylalkylnitrosamines with alkyl chains of 7, 9, or 11 carbon atoms are hepatocarcinogenic, while methylalkylnitrosamines with alkyl chains of 8, 10, 12, or 14 C-atoms selectively induce tumors of the urinary bladder [17].

Histopathology [5, 22] has diagnosed nitrosamine-derived esophageal tumors as squamous cell papillomas and, predominantly, carcinomas; the tumors show keratinization and horny pearls. The tumors are sometimes hemorrhagic, but they almost never metastasize. Histogenesis studies have shown that hyperplastic changes and papillomas are precursors of squamous cell carcinomas [3].

For the experimental induction of esophageal tumors with nitrosamines it is not necessary to use the preformed nitrosamines. It is also possible to form the respective nitroso compound endogenously in the organism by simultaneously feeding an unsymmetrical secondary amine together with nitrite [23]. The following amines have been used for this type of experiment: methylbenzylamine, methylaniline, and methylcyclohexylamine. It is well known that endogenous nitrosamine synthesis from precursors can be inhibited as well as catalyzed by commonly occurring compounds such as ascorbic acid and vitamin E (tocopherol) as inhibitors or thiocyanate, tannins, or certain phenols as catalysts.

Endogenous nitrosamine formation might very well be a risk factor in several high-incidence areas and should be further investigated. Without going too far into the complex problems of endogenous nitrosation and the connected nitrate/nitrite problem [20], it should be mentioned here that our own field studies in northern Iran together with IARC [12] have shown that children at the age of 4-12 years had rather high salivary nitrite values without an apparently high nitrate burden, while, in comparison, children of the same age in Heidelberg showed very low to non-detectable nitrite concentrations in the saliva (unpublished results). Unfortunately, the changed political situation in Iran did not allow the necessary confirmation of this line of promising research.

Some data are available on the modifying influence of certain agents on nitrosamine-induced esophageal carcinogenesis. Thus, dietary zinc deficiency increased the tumor incidence and shortened the induction time [6]. On the other hand, alcohol (25%) in a combined administration study did not influence nitrosamine-induced esophageal carcinogenesis [24]. The drug disulfiram, which in high doses influences drug-metabolizing enzymes, increased tumor incidence in combined administration with methylbenzylnitrosamine [26] and, in another experiment, changed the organotropy of the hepatocarcinogen diethylnitrosamine (DENA) on combined administration to the induction of esophageal tumors, not seen with DENA alone [25]. Certain dietary staples like brown rice or potatoes can decrease the incidence of esophageal cancer induced by methylbenzylnitrosamine [28].

Finally, a few words should be said about biochemical and pharmacological studies on the mechanism of action [21]. Using whole-body autoradiography, it was shown that unsymmetrical nitrosamines are concentrated in the rat esophagus, especially in the epithelial layer [13]. In vitro studies using rat esophagus tissue clearly showed that the typical microsomal metabolism does occur, the corresponding aldehydes being formed and detected [8, 18, 19]. Microsomal preparations from the esophagus have a high metabolic activity and specific affinity to unsymmetrical nitrosamine. In vivo and in vitro studies have demonstrated alkylation in the rat esophagus at the typical sites of DNA, O^6-alkylation in the esophagus being predominant with esophagus-specific nitrosamines [11, 15, 27].

Studies by Autrup and his colleagues used cultured human esophaguses to investigate the metabolism of several nitrosamines. By measuring the amount of metabolites bound to DNA, the alkylation pattern, and the quantity of metabolites released into the culture medium, they could show that activation does occur, especially with unsymmetrical nitrosamines [1, 2].

Therefore, the question as to whether the human esophagus may be a target for nitrosamine carcinogenesis can clearly be answered: the answer is yes.

References

1. Autrup H, Grafstrom RC, Brugh M et al.: Comparison of metabolism in bronchus, esophagus, colon and duodenum from the same individual. Cancer Res. 42 (1982) 934-938
2. Autrup H, Stoner GD: Metabolism of N-nitrosamines by cultured human and rat esophagus. Cancer Res. 42 (1982) 1307-1311
3. Cardesa A, Ovelar MY, Mohr U: Experimental esophageal neoplasms in the rat: Histogenetic pathways. In C.J. Pfeiffer (Edit.): Cancer of the Esophagus, pp. 199-213. Boca Raton, Fla.: CRC Press 1982
4. Day NE, Muñoz N: Esophagus. In D. Schottenfeld, I. Fraumeni (Eds): Cancer Epidemiology and Prevention, pp. 596-623. Philadelphia: W. B. Saunders 1982
5. Druckrey H, Preussmann R, Ivankovic S et al.: Organotrope carcinogene Wirkung bei 65 verschiedenen N-Nitroso-Verbindungen an BD-Ratten. Z. Krebsforsch. 69 (1967) 103-201
6. Fong LYY, Sivak A, Newberne PM: Zinc deficiency and Zn methylbenzylnitrosamine induced esophageal cancer in rats. J. nat. Cancer Inst. 61 (1978) 145-151
7. Hagan EC, Jenner PM, Fitzhugh OG et al.: Toxic properties of compounds related to safrole. Toxicol. appl. Pharmacol. 7 (1965) 18-24
8. Hecht SS, Reiss B, Lin D et al.: Metabolism of N′-nitrosonornicotine by cultured rat esophagus. Carcinogenesis 3 (1982) 453-456
9. Hewer T, Rose E, Ghadarian P et al.: Ingested mutagens from opium and tobacco pyrolysis products and cancer of the esophagus. Lancet 1978, II: 494-496
10. Hirayama T: Diet and cancer. Nutr. Cancer 1 (1979) 67-81
11. Hodgson RM, Wiessler M, Kleihues P: Preferential methylation of target organ DNA by the esophageal carcinogen N-nitrosomethylbenzylamine. Carcinogenesis 1 (1980) 861-866
12. Joint Iran-International Agency for Research on Cancer Study Group: Esophageal cancer studies in the Caspian littoral of Iran: Results of population studies. J. nat. Cancer Inst. 59 (1977) 1127-1138
13. Kraft PG, Tannenbaum SR: Distribution of N-nitrosomethylbenzylamine evaluated by whole-body radiography and densitometry. Cancer Res. 40 (1980) 1921-1927
14. Kuratsune M, Kohchi S, Horie A: Carcinogenesis in the esophagus. Gann 56 (1965) 177-187
15. Labuc GE, Archer MC: Comparative tumor initiating activities of N-nitrosomethylbenzylamine and N-nitrosodimethylamine. Carcinogenesis 3 (1982) 519-523
16. Li MX, Cheng SJ: Etiology of carcinoma of the esophagus. In G.J. Huang, W.Y. K'ai (Eds): Carcinoma of the Esophagus and Gastric Cardia, pp. 26-51. Berlin: Springer 1984
17. Lijinsky W, Saavedra JE, Reuber MD: Induction of carcinogenesis in Fischer rats by methylalkylnitrosamines. Cancer Res. 41 (1981) 1288-1292
18. Mehta R, Labuc GE, Urbansky SJ et al.: Organ specificity in the microsomal activation and toxicity of N-nitrosomethylbenzylamine in various species. Cancer Res. 44 (1984) 4017-4022

19. Mirvish SS, Wang MY, Smith JW et al.: β- to ω-hydroxylation of the esophageal carcinogen methyl-n-amylnitrosamine by the rat esophagus and related tissues. Cancer Res. 45 (1985) 577-583
20. Preussmann R: Nitrat in der Nahrung - ein Gesundheitsrisiko? In Nitrat in Gemüsebau und Landwirtschaft, pp. 17-35. Zürich: G. Duttweiler Institut 1981
21. Preussmann R, Stewart B: N-Nitroso compounds. In C. E. Searle (Edit.): Chemical Carcinogens, pp. 643-828. Washington, D.C.: Amer. Chem. Soc. 1984. (Amer. Chem. Soc. Monograph, No. 182)
22. Sales D, Levin B: Incidence epidemiology and predisposing factors. In T. R. de Mesters, B. Levin (Eds): Cancer of the Esophagus, pp. 1-20. Orlando: Grune & Stratton 1985
23. Sander J: Untersuchungen über die Entstehung cancerogener Nitrosoverbindungen im Magen von Versuchstieren und ihre Bedeutung für Menschen. Arzneimittel-Forschung 21 (1971) 1572-1580
24. Schmähl D: Investigations on esophageal carcinogenesis by methylphenylnitrosamine and ethylalcohol in rats. Cancer Lett. 1 (1976) 215-216
25. Schmähl D, Krüger FW, Habs M et al.: Influence of disulfiram on the organotropy of the carcinogenic effect of dimethyl- and diethylnitrosamine in rats. Z. Krebsforsch. 85 (1976) 271-276
26. Schweinsberg F, Bürkle V: Wirkung von Disulfiram auf die Toxizität von N-Methyl-N-nitrosobenzylamine bei Ratten. J. Cancer Res. clin. Oncol. 102 (1981) 43-47
27. Silinskas KC, Zucker PF, Archer MC: Formation of O^6-methylguanine in rat liver DNA by nitrosamines does not predict initiation of preneoplastic foci. Carcinogenesis 6 (1985) 773-775
28. van Rendsburg SJ, Hall JM, du Bruyn DB: Effects of various dietary staples on esophageal carcinogenesis induced in rats by subcutaneously administered N-nitrosomethylbenzylamine. J. nat. Cancer Inst. 75 (1985) 561-566
29. Wynder EL, Bross IJ: A study of etiological factors in cancer of the esophagus. Cancer 14 (1961) 389-413

Vitamin Intervention in Precancerous Lesions of the Esophagus in a High-Risk Population of China

J. Wahrendorf, N. Muñoz, Lu Jian-Bang

Results of a study are presented which, in the meantime, have been published elsewhere [1]. A brief summary is given below.

A randomized double-blind intervention trial was carried out in Huixian, People's Republic of China, in a population with a high incidence of esophageal cancer. The aim of the trial was to determine whether a combined treatment with retinol, riboflavin, and zinc could result, after 1 year, in a lower prevalence of precancerous lesions of the esophagus in the group receiving the active treatment as compared with the group receiving a placebo. A random sample of 610 subjects in the age group 35–64 years and with equal numbers in each sex and age group was drawn from two production brigades. A group of 305 subjects received the active treatment [15 mg (50000 IU) retinol, 200 mg riboflavin, and 50 mg zinc] once a week, and a group of 305 individuals received a placebo. The identical-looking treatment or placebo capsules were given weekly to the study participants by "barefoot doctors." On entry to the study and at the end of the treatment 13.5 months later, the study subjects were interviewed, using a questionnaire on smoking, drinking, and dietary habits; they were examined, especially for signs of vitamin A and riboflavin deficiencies, and blood samples were drawn for a biochemical analysis of riboflavin, retinol, beta-carotene, and zinc. Compliance with the treatment, assessed by inspection of follow-up records kept by the "barefoot doctors" and by changes in the blood levels 2 and 13.5 months after initiation of the treatment, was excellent. The final examination of the 567 (93%) subjects also included esophagoscopy, with at least two biopsies taken. The histological slides were read independently and blindly by three pathologists. After a final diagnosis had been reached by consensus, the code for treatment assignment was opened.

The prevalence of esophagitis with or without atrophy or dysplasia was 45.3% in the placebo group and 48.9% in the vitamin-treated group. Esophagitis was accompanied by atrophy in 12.7% and dysplasia in 2.2% in the placebo group and by atrophy in 12.3% and by dysplasia in 2.5% in the vitamin-treated group.

This is the first strictly controlled nutritional intervention study in cancer epidemiology. The results cannot be explained by bias or by confounding as this was a randomized double-blind study. The failure to demonstrate an effect of the vitamin intervention may be interpreted in several ways:

1. The treatment period was not long enough or the dose was not large enough. As lesions such as angular stomatitis and cheilosis disappeared after 3 weeks with a dose of 50 mg riboflavin, this seems unlikely. The retinol dose could not have been larger without continuous clinical monitoring.

2. Riboflavin and retinol may not induce regression of the esophagitis because of

Cancer of the Liver, Esophagus, and Nasopharynx
Edited by G. Wagner and Zhang You-Hui

the persistence of other factors, but may prevent the induction of precancerous lesions. The natural history of chronic esophagitis may be like that of chronic atrophic gastritis, a precursor of gastric cancer which seems to be irreversible. This hypothesis would be difficult to test in that the lesions in question have been shown to begin early in life.

3. The original hypothesis may have been wrong. However, it would be premature to refute the epidemiological evidence for an involvement of vitamin deficiencies in the development of esophageal cancer by this single study.

Reference

1. Muñoz N, Wahrendorf J, Lu Jian-bang, Crespi M, Thurnham DI, Day NE, Zhang Hong-ji, Grassi A, Li Wen-yan, Liu Gui-lin, Lang Yu-quan, Zhang Cai-yun, Zheng Su-fang, Lu Jun-yao, Correa P, O'Conor GT, Bosch X: No effect of Riboflavin, Retinol, and Zinc on Prevalence of Precancerous Lesions of Oesophagus (Randomised Double-blind Intervention Study in High-risk Population of China) Lancet 1985, II, 111–114

Effect of N-Nitrosamine on Human Esophageal Epithelium Collected from Populations from a High-Risk Area for Esophageal Cancer in Northern China

Lu Shih-Hsin, R. Montesano, Zhang Ming-Shu, Feng Luo, Chui Shao-Xing, D. Umbenhauer, R. Saffhill, and M. F. Rajewsky

Esophageal cancer (EC) is a common disease in some provinces in northern China, and Linxian county of Henan province has the highest age-adjusted mortality rate, with 151/100000 in males and 115/100000 in females. Extensive epidemiological and clinical investigations have been undertaken to identify the causative factors of EC in these areas. Among the suspected etiological factors in the environment, N-nitrosamine and its precursors have received the most attention [9, 10].

Earlier studies demonstrated:

1. The amount of nitrosamines in food collected from Linxian is higher than that from Fanxian which is a low-risk area [3, 6, 8, 15].
2. A positive correlation was found between the average incidence rate of marked epithelial dysplasia or carcinomas of the esophagus and the level of nitrates and nitrites in the well water [14].
3. A positive correlation was noted between the amount of nitrites in the saliva in the Linxian population and the incidence rate of marked epithelial dysplasia or carcinomas of the esophagus [5].
4. The amount and frequency of consumption of pickled vegetables commonly eaten in Linxian were shown to be positively correlated with the mortality rate of EC [4].

A major source of human exposure to N-nitroso compounds is the in vivo formation. With the objective of assessing individual exposure to N-nitroso compounds and their precursors, urine samples were analyzed for nitrate and for several N-nitrosamines such as N-nitrosoproline (NPRO) and N-nitrosothiazolidine-4-carboxylic acid (NTCA) as an exposure index. The results described indicated that subjects living in the high-risk area for EC could be exposed to greater amounts of N-nitroso compounds through both ingestion of preformed compounds in foods and/or endogenous formation than those in the low-risk area [10]. In particular, several nitrosamines were found in the gastric juice from the Linxian population, and the amounts of nitrosamines in gastric juice were shown to be positively correlated with various lesions of the esophagus. These observations suggest that the ingestion of nitrosamines in food and endogenously formed N-nitroso compounds may affect the esophageal epithelium and play an important role in the causation of EC in China. We report here on the inhibition of [^{3}H]thymidine ([^{3}H]TdR) incorporation into DNA of the esophageal epithelium and the induction of hyperplasia on the esophagus by nitrosamine, as well as the detection of O^6-methyl-2′-deoxyguanosine (O^6-medGuo) in the DNA of esophageal tissue samples obtained through surgery from patients in high-incidence areas for esophageal cancer, for whom there is some evidence of exposure to N-nitrosamines.

Inhibition of [^{3}H]TdR Incorporation into DNA of Fetal Esophageal Epithelium by Nitrosamines

The inhibition of [^{3}H]TdR incorporation into DNA by nitrosamines is a useful indicator of carcinogenicity in the esophagus of rodents and may serve as a useful short-term bioassay for detecting carcinogens in the human environment [11]. Seiler also found a good correlation between the carcinogenicity and inhibition of [^{3}H]TdR incorporation into DNA in his mouse test [13]. We studied the effect of N-methyl-N-benzylnitrosamine (NMBzA) found in pickled vegetables and in gastric juice from Linxian on [^{3}H]TdR incorporation into the esophageal epithelium DNA of rat and human fetuses. The esophageal epithelium of the rat or the fetus was incubated for 2 days; then [^{3}H]TdR and NMBzA or diethylnitrosamine (NDEA) were added. After another 40 min incubation, esophageal DNA was extracted, and DNA radioactivity was determined.

The amounts of [^{3}H]TdR incorporation into the epithelial DNA of rat esophaguses untreated with NMBzA or NDEA showed 84 ± 16 cpm/μg DNA and 93 ± 12 cpm/μg DNA, respectively. In the rat esophaguses treated with NMBzA or NDEA, the amount of [^{3}H]TdR incorporation into the epithelium DNA was inhibited. The inhibition of [^{3}H]TdR incorporation into the esophageal epithelium DNA was enhanced along with the increase of nitrosamine doses (Table 1).

In the human fetus untreated esophaguses the amounts of [^{3}H]TdR incorporation into the epithelium DNA were 103 ± 9 cpm/mg DNA. [^{3}H]TdR incorporation into the epithelium DNA of fetal esophaguses was inhibited by NMBzA or NDEA. The inhibition of [^{3}H]TdR incorporation into the esophageal epithelium DNA was also enhanced along with the increase of nitrosamine doses (Table 2).

Table 1. Inhibition of [^{3}H]TdR incorporation into DNA of esophageal epithelium in rats by nitrosamines

Dose (mM)	No. of tests	NMBzA (cpm/μg DNA)	P value	NDEA (cpm/μg DNA)	P value
0	12	84 ± 16		93 ± 12	
0.5	6	67 ± 10	<0.05	95 ± 11	<0.1
1.0	6	59 ± 8	<0.01	90 ± 9	<0.1
2.0	6	46 ± 6	<0.01	81 ± 9	<0.05
5.0	6	31 ± 6	<0.01	53 ± 11	<0.01
10.0	6	14 ± 4	<0.01	43 ± 6	<0.01

Table 2. Inhibition of [^{3}H]TdR incorporation into DNA of esophageal epithelium in human fetus by nitrosamines

Dose (mM)	No. of tests	NMBzA (cpm/μg DNA)	P value	NDEA (cpm/μg DNA)	P value
0	22	103 ± 9		103 ± 9	
0.5	4	95 ± 11	<0.1	105 ± 17	<0.5
1.0	4	89 ± 10	<0.05	101 ± 15	<0.1
2.0	4	60 ± 10	<0.05	78 ± 11	<0.05
5.0	4	50 ± 10	<0.01	67 ± 11	<0.05
10.0	4	16 ± 3	<0.01	31 ± 5	<0.01

The doses causing 50% inhibition were 5.2 mM and 2.5 mM in the human fetus and in the rat, respectively, for NMBzA, which is a specific carcinogen for the rat esophagus, and 8.8 mM and 8.0 mM for the esophageal noncarcinogen NDEA. NMBzA can affect the esophageal epithelium of rat and human fetus, but the sensitivity in rats is higher than in the human fetus.

We also studied the effect of N-3-methylbutyl-N-1-methyl-acentonylnitrosamine (MAMBNA) found in moldy food on the esophageal epithelium DNA of adult populations from Jiao-xian, which is a low-risk area for esophageal cancer. Esophageal biopsies from 70 subjects were obtained during endoscopic examination. These biopsies were cut into 1-mm-thick pieces and divided into two groups: one group was incubated with only [^{3}H]TdR as control group; the other group was incubated with [^{3}H]TdR (5 μCi/ml) and MAMBNA. Incubation was carried out in a medium with 10% fetal calf serum in a shaken bath at 37 °C for 1 h and then fixed in methanol. We found that the labeled cells in the basal layer of the esophageal epithelium treated with MAMBNA were even fewer than in that untreated. These results also demonstrate that MAMBNA inhibited the [^{3}H]TdR incorporation into the human esophageal epithelium DNA.

Action of Nitrosamine on DNA Polymerase in the Fetal Esophageal Epithelium

The existence of molecular weight forms of DNA polymerase in different cellular locations of the mammalian tissue was identified, and these enzyme activities showed quite different properties [1, 2]. There is a relationship between DNA synthesis in vivo and in tissue slices and the activity of these enzymes. In order to study the mechanism of the inhibition of [^{3}H]TdR incorporation into the esophageal epithelial DNA, we studied the level of DNA polymerase in the fetal esophagus. The results showed that the levels of DNA polymerase α and β in the fetal untreated esophagus were 832 ± 123 cpm and 719 ± 102 cpm, respectively, while the levels of DNA polymerase α and β in fetal esophagus treated with NMBzA were 361 ± 62 cpm and 289 ± 59 cpm, respectively. NMBzA significantly suppressed the activity of DNA polymerase α and β (Table 3).

Our results demonstrate that the inhibition by NMBzA of [^{3}H]thymidine incorporation may be due to an inhibition of DNA synthesis and DNA repair.

Table 3. Effect of NMBzA and NDEA on DNA polymerase of esophagus and liver in the human fetus

Group	No. of tests	DNA polymerase in esophagus (cpm/μg protein/h)		DNA polymerase in liver (cpm/μg protein/h)	
		α	β	α	β
Control	4	832 ± 123	719 ± 102	700 ± 200	725 ± 110
NMBzA	4	361 ± 62*	289 ± 59*	–	–
NDEA	4	–	–	340 ± 115*	315 ± 140*

* $P < 0.05$

O^6-Methyldeoxyguanosine (O^6-MedGuo) in Esophageal DNA of Populations from Linxian

O^6-MedGuo has been indicated to be one of the DNA adducts which seem more critical in the induction of tumors by nitroso compounds. In order to identify the high-risk area for EC – Linxian is causally associated with exposure to nitrosamines – a radioimmunoassay using monoclonal antibody against O^6-MedGuo was used to detect the presence of these DNA adducts in the esophageal epithelium of the Linxian population.

A total of 37 human tissue specimens derived from patients who underwent surgery for cancer of the esophagus in Linxian county were analyzed; for comparison, 12 tissue samples obtained from hospitals in Europe were similarly analyzed. The results demonstrated that 17 samples from Linxian county showed a level of O^6-MedGuo ranging from 15 to 50 fmol/mg DNA, 10 showed higher levels up to 160 fmol/mg DNA, and the remaining 10 samples from Europa showed levels of 45 fmol O^6-MedGuo/mg DNA, 7 being below the limit of detection (Fig. 1). Another 38 human esophageal specimens from Linxian and epithelia of 20 fetuses were analyzed using radioimmunoassay. Nineteen samples showed a level O^6-MedGuo ranging from 5 to 10 fmol/mg DNA. Fourteen samples showed a higher level

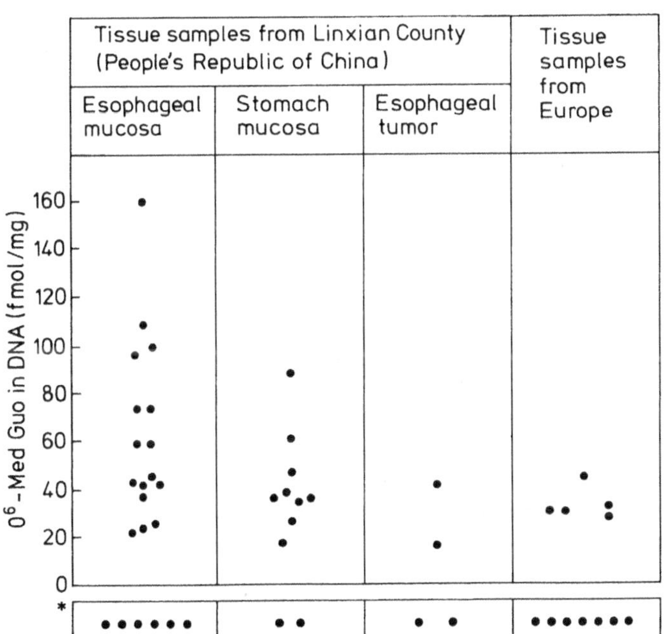

Fig. 1. O^6-Methyl-2′-deoxyguanosine content of DNA in the human esophageal and cardiac stomach mucosa and in samples of esophageal tumor tissue from Linxian County (People's Republic of China). For comparison, the levels observed in various tissue samples, including eosphagus, from Europe are shown. Inhibition values of less than 20% were considered negative and are listed in the *boxes marked with an asterisk*. An additional 6 samples of esophageal mucosa and tumors from Europe with less than 1 mg DNA (0.26–0.92 mg) were also assayed, with negative results

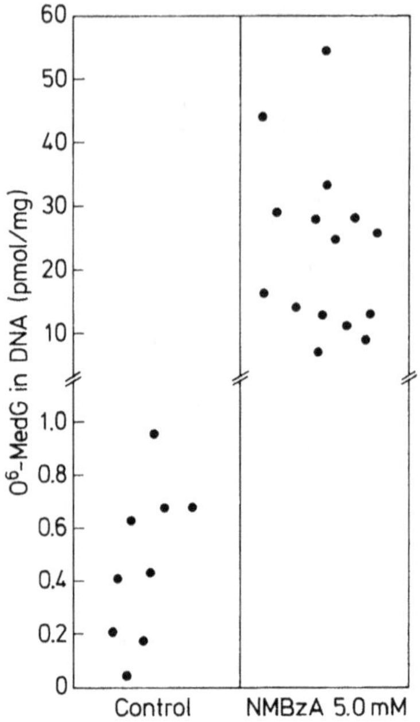

Fig. 2. Levels of O^6-MedG in the NMBzA of human fetal esophageal tissues

up to 43 fmol/mg DNA. The remaining five samples were below 5 fmol/mg DNA. The levels of O^6-MedGuo from all the fetal tissue samples were below 5 fmol/mg DNA, and among these samples seven were zero.

We also carried out in vitro experiments. Fetal esophageal epithelium collected from 14- to 16-week-old water bag-induced abortuses were cultured for 8 h with or without various doses of NMBzA in a medium. The samples cultured without NMBzA showed that the level of O^6-MedGuo was almost zero. The samples cultured with NMBzA at a dose of 0.5 mM showed levels of O^6-MedGuo ranging from 6 to 28 fmol/mg DNA (17.03 ± 8.42), while at a dose of 5.0 mM, the levels of O^6-MedGuo were 27.9–65.19 (44.27 ± 13.57). The level of O^6-MedGuo was raised along with the NMBzA dose, showing the dose response curve of Fig. 2.

The presence of O^6-MedGuo in the esophageal epithelium DNA from Linxian populations must result from a relatively recent exposure to N-nitroso compounds ingested from food or formed endogenously in vivo. The approach and the results obtained appear particularly promising in assessing the role of N-nitroso compounds in the etiology of esophageal cancer in northern China.

Induction of Hyperplasia in Human Esophageal Epithelium by Nitrosamine

In order to observe the possible carcinogenic action of NMBzA on the human esophageal epithelium, we cultured the esophageal epithelium of human fetuses. Esophageal epithelium was organ cultured in a minimum essential medium and cultured up to 3 months in the presence or absence of NMBzA. Explants cultured in the absence of NMBzA for 4 weeks or longer revealed themselves to be normal. Cultured explants treated with NMBzA showed considerable variation with each esophagus in the degree of proliferation. The epithelial layer became thicker, the basal cells were active, the size of the cells was irregular, and the nucleoli were prominent. These phenomena indicated that the cells were proliferation-induced by NMBzA.

References

1. Chang LMS, Bollum FJ: Low molecular weight deoxyribonucleic acid polymerase in mammalian cells. J. biol. Chem. 246 (1971) 5835-5837
2. Chang LMS, Bollum FJ: Variation of deoxyribonucleic acid polymerase activities during rat liver regeneration. J. biol. Chem. 247 (1972) 7948-7950
3. Co-ordinating Group for Research on the Etiology of Esophageal Cancer of North China: The epidemiology of esophageal cancer in North China and preliminary results in the investigation of its etiological factors. Sci. Sin. 18 (1975) 131-148
4. Co-ordinating Group for Research on Etiology of Esophageal Cancer in North China: The preliminary studies on epidemiological factors of esophageal cancer. Res. Cancer Prev. Treatm. 2 (1977) 1-8
5. Department of Chemical Etiology and Carcinogenesis, Chinese Academy of Medical Sciences: Further studies on the etiology of esophageal cancer. Chin. med. J. 58 (1978) 593-597
6. Li MH, Lu SH, Ji C et al.: Formation of carcinogenic N-nitroso compounds in corn-bread inoculated with fungi. Sci. Sin. 22 (1979) 471-477
7. Lu SH, Kuo LP, Li FM et al.: The determination of nitrosamines in gastric juice of subjects in Linxian which is a high incidence area of esophageal cancer. Chin. J. Oncol., Suppl., 1985
8. Lu SH, Li MH, Ji C et al.: A new N-nitroso compound, N-3-methylbutyl-N-methylacetonylnitrosamine in corn-bread inoculated with fungi. Sci. Sin. 22 (1979) 601-608
9. Lu SH, Lin P: Recent research on the etiology of esophageal cancer in China. J. Gastroent. 20 (1982) 361-367
10. Lu SH, Ohshima H, Bartsch H: Recent studies on N-nitroso compounds as possible etiological factors in esophageal cancer. In I. K. O'Neill, R. C. von Borstel, C. T. Miller et al. (Eds): N-Nitroso Compounds: Occurrence, Biological Effects and Relevance to Human Cancer, pp. 947-956. Lyon: IARC 1984. (IARC Scientific Publications, No. 57)
11. Mirvish SS, Chu C, Clayon DB: Inhibition of ^{3}H-Thymidine incorporation into DNA of rat esophageal epithelium and related tissues by carcinogenic N-nitroso compounds. Cancer Res. 38 (1978) 458-466
12. Office of Prevention and Treatment for Cancer: Collection of Mortality Rate for Cancer in China. Beijing Ministry of Public Health, 1978
13. Seiler JP: Inhibition of testicular DNA synthesis by chemical mutagens and carcinogens. Preliminary results in the validation of a novel short-term test. Mut. Res. 46 (1977) 305-310
14. Wang YL, Lu SH, Li MH: Determination of nitrates and nitrite in well water from commune, Lin-Xian County, Henan Province. China J. Oncol. 1 (1979) 201-205
15. Wang GH, Zhang WX, Chai WG: The identification of natural Roussin red methyl ester. Acta Chem. Sin. 38 (1980) 95-102

Papillomavirus Infections in Esophageal Cancer

H. zur Hausen and E.-M. de Villiers

During the past few years one role of papillomavirus infections in human genital cancer became apparent (reviewed in [3]). Cervical dysplasias as precursor lesions of genital cancer can be induced by specific human papillomavirus (HPV) types. Biopsies derived from cervical, vulvar, and penile cancer regularly contain specific types of HPV DNA, in contrast to precursor lesions. In the latter the DNA persists in an episomal state. The malignant tumors preferentially contain viral DNA integrated into chromosomal DNA. The integrational pattern reveals a remarkable specificity on the side of the viral genome. Transcripts of specific open reading frames are produced within the tumor cells and point to an active role of the viral genome in malignant conversion of the cells. Very recently evidence has been obtained suggesting a failing cellular control of viral genome expression as a main factor in malignant conversion of the cells [3].

Since papillomavirus infections and chemical and physical carcinogens interact synergistically in inducing malignant conversion in a number of animal and human systems, it is an interesting problem to analyze human tumors known to be linked to chemical factors for persisting papillomavirus infections. This includes in particular, oral, laryngeal, and lung cancer, which are clearly related to smoking habits. It may also have some bearing on esophageal cancer.

During the past 2 years it has been possible to demonstrate known prototypes of HPV in a small number of oral, tongue, laryngeal, and lung cancers (reviewed in [3]). This led to the working hypothesis that the majority of as yet negative tumors may contain the DNA of unidentified papillomavirus infections that could interact in concert with carcinogens present in tobacco smoke.

A recent analysis of biopsies from esophageal cancer and of cross-hybridization of DNA from cell lines derived from these tumors with 26 known prototypes of HPV yielded negative results (de Villiers and zur Hausen, unpublished data). There are however some hints that specific types of HPV may be involved in the etiology of this tumor. Syrjänen et al. [1] reported the presence of koilocytotic cells in precursor lesions of esophageal cancer. These cells are regarded as indicative of HPV infection. Similarly, Winkler et al. [2] found distinctive histologic evidence of HPV infection in 2 papillomas and in 11 focal epithelial hyperplasias out of a total of 75 lesions tested.

By analyzing one esophageal papilloma, positive hybridization signals were obtained with HPV 18 DNA (de Villiers et al., unpublished data). The low intensity of the signals suggested that the biopsy most likely contains a different yet HPV 18-related type of HPV. The putative viral DNA of this papilloma is presently being cloned and will be further analyzed. Although still very scarce, the available

Cancer of the Liver, Esophagus, and Nasopharynx
Edited by G. Wagner and Zhang You-Hui

results raise the possibility that esophageal cancer may result from a persistent papillomavirus infection which upon interaction with chemical factors develops into a malignant cell clone.

References

1. Syrjänen K, Pyrhönen S, Aukee S, Koskela E: Squamous cell papilloma of the oesophagus: a tumour probably caused by human papilloma virus. Diagn Histopathol 5 (1982) 291-296
2. Winkler B, Capo V, Neumann W, Ma A, La Porta R, Reilly S, Green PM, Richart RM, Crum CP: Human papillomavirus infection of the oesophagus. A clinicopathologic study with demonstration of papillomavirus antigen by the immunoperoxidase technique. Cancer 55 (1985) 149-155
3. Zur Hausen H: Human papillomaviruses: why are some types carcinogenic? In Oldstone M, Notkins A (Eds): Concepts in Viral Pathogenesis. Berlin - Heidelberg - New York: Springer (to be published)

Experience with Combined Preoperative Irradiation and Surgery for Squamous-Cell Carcinoma of the Esophagus

Huang Guo-Jun and Gu Xiang-Zhi

Results of the treatment of carcinoma of the esophagus by either radiotherapy or surgery alone have not been satisfactory. With the aim of improving such a situation, clinical studies with combined preoperative irradiation and surgery were carried out in 408 selective cases (1959–1976) and in 83 randomized cases (1977–1982) with squamous cell carcinoma of the esophagus. In the first study, the majority of patients had tumors of poor or questionable resectability as clinically evaluated before treatment. The primary tumors were located in the upper and middle thirds of the esophagus in 79.9% and were ypTNM stages III and IV in 81.6% of the cases. In this study, the resectability rate was 81.9%, the operative mortality 3.4%, and the 5-, 10-, and 15-year survival rates 33.8%, 23.0%, and 17.9%, respectively. During the same period, 736 patients with tumors more distally located and of better resectability were treated by surgery alone. In 43.8% of these the tumor was located in the lower third of the esophagus. The operative mortality was 3.0% and the 5-year survival rate 29.8% in this group of cases.

In the randomized study 160 patients, all with midthoracic esophageal carcinoma averaging 5.2 cm in length, were eligible for analysis, of which 83 were treated by combined therapy and 77 by surgery alone. The results, both early and late, as obtained by combined therapy versus those obtained by surgery alone, were as follows: resectability rates 95.2% vs. 89.6%, 30-day resection mortality rates 3.8% vs. 4.3%, incidence rates of intrathoracic anastomotic leakage 0% vs. 1.7%, incidence rates of lymph node metastasis 21.5% vs. 30.4%, incidences of residual tumor at the esophageal stump 0% vs. 2.9%, and 5-year survival rates 45.5% vs. 25.0%.

The fact that the incidence of anastomotic leak in the combined therapy group was not higher, if not lower, than that of the group treated by surgery alone may serve to indicate that preoperative irradiation at the recommended dosage had no untoward effects on esophageal healing, as in about half of the cases of the combined therapy group the esophageal anastomotic site was within the field of preoperative irradiation. The lower incidences of residual tumor at the esophageal stump and of lymph node metastasis in the cases treated by combined therapy, as compared with those in the group treated by surgery alone, may also serve to indicate the good tumoricidal effects of preoperative irradiation.

Based on the experience with the two clinical studies, it was concluded that the combination of preoperative irradiation and surgery in the treatment of squamous cell carcinoma of the esophagus has merits in promoting resectability and long-term survivals over single modality by surgery alone. With the recommended dosage and rest intervals, preoperative irradiation has no untoward effects on the healing power of the irradiated esophagus and poses no additional difficulty on surgical manipulation. This combined modality is especially indicated in cases of midthoracic esophageal carcinoma with borderline resectability.

Cancer of the Liver, Esophagus, and Nasopharynx
Edited by G. Wagner and Zhang You-Hui

A Study of Tumor-Associated Antigens

Dong Zhi-Wei, Wei Shu-Min, Li Zhen-Pu, Wan Wen-Hui, and Xu Xin-Lai

Introduction

The development of the hybridoma technique [8] has provided a powerful new tool for studies of tumor-associated antigens. Since 1978 Koprowski [9] and other investigators have prepared monoclonal antibodies (McAbs) to human melanoma, leukemia, lymphoma, colon cancer, breast cancer, lung cancer, and others. And some new tumor-associated antigens have been identified [4, 11]. However, there are only a few studies on antigens of gastric cancer. The mortality rate of gastric cancer is the highest one in China. Therefore, it is very interesting and necessary to investigate the antigens of gastric cancer in order to develop new approaches to the diagnosis and therapy of gastric cancer.

In the present study, we prepared and characterized three McAbs against gastric cancer and identified the corresponding antigens.

Materials and Methods

Cells. Gastric cancer cell line MGC803 was established in the Department of Biology, Shan-Dong Normal University, from a surgical specimen of a patient with low-differentiated gastric cancer and was cultured in RPM1 1640 medium supplemented with 20% serum from newborn calves. Murine myeloma cell line NS-1 was kindly provided by Dr. Pen in the Cancer Research Institute of the Chinese Academy of Medical Sciences. Pooled lymphocytes and AB0 red blood cells from blood donors were separated by Ficoll-Hypaque gradient centrifugation. Normal bone marrow cells were contributed by patients with chest diseases and were confirmed by histopathological examination.

Reagents. Horseradish peroxidase (HRP, Sigma), fluorescence isothiocyanate (FITC, Merck), propidium iodide (PI, Sigma), 3,3′-diaminobenzidine tetrahydrochloride (DAB, Sigma), 1,2-phenylenediamine (OPD, Merck), Sepharose-CL-4B (Pharmacia), RNase (Sigma), pronase (Merck), trypsin (Sigma), and specific rabbit anti-mouse Ig heavy and light chain antibodies (Bionetics) were purchased. The conjugate of affinity-purified rabbit anti-mouse IgG (cross-reacted with IgM) with HRP (HRP-R α MuIgG) and conjugate of rabbit anti-mouse IgG with FITC (FITC-R α MuIgG) were prepared in our lab.

Cancer of the Liver, Esophagus, and Nasopharynx
Edited by G. Wagner and Zhang You-Hui

The Production of McAb

Balb/c mice were immunized with MGC803 cells twice (i.p., 5×10^6 cells/each time) at weekly intervals and boosted 2 weeks later (i.p., 5×10^6 cells). Three days after the last immunization, the spleen cells from the immunized mice were fused with myeloma cell lines NS-1 using polyethylene glycol (PEG, mol. wt. 1000, Baker) as described [6]. Fusions were carried out at a spleen cell to myeloma cell ratio of 10:1. The cells were resuspended in HAT medium and planted in 24 or 96 well plates (Costar), then cultured at 37 °C, in an atmosphere of 5% CO_2 in the air. Two weeks later, the hybridoma supernatants from visible colonies were screened with an enzyme-linked immunofiltration assay. Only the hybridomas, which reacted with MGC803 cells, but did not react with pooled lymphocytes, were chosen and subcloned with limiting dilution. The subcloned hybridoma secreting McAb against MGC803 cells was then injected into mineral oil primed Balb/c mice, and the ascites were collected from the mice 7–10 days later.

Enzyme-Linked Immunofiltration Assay (ELFA) [5]

Target cells were immobilized on the filter which had been placed at the bottom of wells with a tiny drain hole linked to a vacuum system. After washing three times with vacuum system, hybridoma supernatants were added and incubated for 1 h at room temperature. After washing thoroughly, HRP-R α MuIgG (1:2000) and a substrate solution containing OPD and H_2O_2 were added sequentially with 30 min incubation and washing between two additions. The reaction was terminated by the addition of 12.5% sulfuric acid, and the color intensity was measured at 492 nm with an enzyme-linked immunoadsorbent assay (ELISA) reader. NS-1 cell culture supernant containing normal mouse serum diluted to 1:1000 was run in parallel as a negative control.

Indirect Immunofluorescence Staining (IF)

Target cells were washed with PBS and resuspended at 10^7 cells/ml in 1% BSA-PBS. Fifty microliters of cells were incubated with an equal volume of hybridoma supernatant of 1:400 diluted ascites for 1 h at 4 °C. The cells were washed three times with 0.1% BSA-PBS; then 100 µl FITC-R α MuIgG in a 1:20 dilution was added. After 60-min incubation at 4 °C, the cell pellet was washed with 0.1% BSA-PBS, and a drop of cell suspension on a slide was observed with an epifluorescence microscope (Nikon). A similar observation with pooled lymphocytes was used as a negative control.

Analysis of Cells with Flow Cytometry [2]

As above 2×10^6 target cells were stained with IF, then resuspended and fixed in 50% ethanol for 4 h at 4 °C. The target cells were further treated with RNase (500 u/ml) for 30 min at 37 °C. After washing, the cells were stained with PI (50 µg/ml) for 30 min at 4 °C. Following washing and resuspending, the cells were passed through a 40-µm pore size nylon mesh and analyzed with FACS III which was equipped with a 50-μm-diameter nozzle and an argon ion laser. The excitation wavelength was 488 nm, and a 520-nm bandpass filter and 620-nm pass filter were used for detecting green and red fluorescence, respectively. The measured data were stored and processed by computer.

Biochemical and Immunochemical Analysis of Antigens

A quantity of 10^7 target cells were frozen and thawed twice until 95% of the cells were broken with intact nuclei. The intact cells and nuclei were eliminated by 600-g centrifugation for 20 min, and a crude cell membrane pellet was obtained after centrifugation at 100000 g for 1 h (4 °C); 200 μl lysate buffer (0.5% NP-40, 0.5% DOC, 50 mM NaCl, 10 mM PMSF, 1 mM EDTA in 20 mM Tris-HCl buffer, pH 8.2) was added into the pellet, and the mixture was shaken (40 times/min) for 15 min at 4 °C. Following centrifugation at 100000 g for 1 h, the supernatant was collected as an antigen extract.

Ten microliters of antigen extract was added on the nitrocellulose membrane as spots and dried at room temperature. Spots on the membrane were treated with trypsin (5 mg/ml), pronase (0.6 mg/ml) for 1 h at 37 °C, and sodium periodate (1 mg/ml) for 1 h at 4 °C, respectively. After washing, the spots were blocked with 5% BSA-PBS. Then McAb, HRP-R α MuIgG (1:1000) substrate solution containing DAB and H_2O_2 were added sequentially, thoroughly washing between additions.

A parallel experiment omitting treatment with enzymes or sodium periodate was run as a control.

The antigen extract was run on a SDS-polyacrylamide gel [10] (12.5%, reduced and nonreduced condition). After electrophoresis, the gel was immersed into a buffer solution (20% methanol, 20 mM Tris, and 150 mM glycine, pH 8.0) for 10 min. The antigens in the gel were electroblotted onto a nitrocellulose membrane [3] (6-8 V/cm, 16-18 h, 4 °C). The blotted membrane was blocked with 5% BSA (containing 150 mM NaCl, 10 mM Tris-HCl, pH 8.0) for 15 min, then incubated with McAb (supernatant or 1:500 dilution ascites) for 60 min at room temperature. The antigen bands were visualized by adding HRP-R α MuIgG and substrate solution as described above.

Results

McAbs Against Gastric Cancer Cell Line MGC803

Three McAbs were obtained in different fusions and designated as PCl, PD4, and PC6, respectively. Their Ig subclasses were IgM and IgG2b (Table 1).

Binding Capacities of McAbs with Various Cells

The specificities of McAbs were characterized with ELFA. Table 2 shows the binding capacities of McAbs with various cells. It is obvious that McAbs had high binding capacities with gastric cancer cells in different patterns and low reactions with

Table 1. Monoclonal antibodies against gastric cancer cell lines

Designation	Immunogen	Subcloning (times)	Ig Subclasses[a]
PCl	MGC803	7	IgM
PD4	MGC803	7	IgG2b
PC6	MGC803	7	IgG2b

[a] Ig subclasses were tested with the Ouchterlony method

lung cancer cells. With the exception of McAb PCl reacting with one of the hepatoma cell lines, the McAbs did not react with other tested tumor cells and lymphocytes, AB0 red blood cells, fibroblasts, or normal bone marrow cells. The binding capacities of McAbs with target cells could be eliminated by the absorption of MGC803 cells, but not irrelevant cells (for example, pooled lymphocytes).

Localization of Correspondent Antigens with IF

Immunofluorescence stain of target cells with McAbs showed a typical membrane fluorescence in fixed or unfixed condition. Moreover, only a given percentage of cells could be stained as positive, and the fluorescence intensity of cells varied from one to the other (Fig. 1).

Analysis of Antigen Expression by Using Flow Cytometry

The membrane PCl antigen of target cells was stained with IF, and nuclear DNA was labeled with PI. By a two-parameter analysis of flow cytometry it was shown that there was a high level of PCl antigen expression in the G_1 phase of the cell cycle for MGC803 cells as well as in the G_1 and G_2-M phases for SGC7901 (Fig. 2).

Sensitivity of Antigens to Treatment of Heating, Sodium Periodate, and Enzymatic Digestion

MGC803 cells were boiled for 20 min and the antigen activity was evaluated with IF stain. Table 3 showed that PCl and PD4 antigens were quite sensitive to heat, whereas the PC6 antigen was resistant. The treatment with sodium periodate did not affect the activity of the antigens, but treatment with trypsin and pronase destroyed the antigens.

Immunochemical Analysis of the Antigens

By using Western blotting, it was shown that the PCl antigen has a band with a 42-kd molecular weight and the PD4 antigen had a band with a 40-kd molecular weight. There was no band for the PC6 antigen and negative control (Fig. 3). The PCl and PD4 antigen bands could be abolished by the absorption of conjugates of Sepharose-CL-4B with correspondent McAbs PCl and PD4, respectively. However, the absorption of the conjugate of Sepharose-CL-4B with McAb PCl did not affect the PD4 antigen band, and vice versa. In addition, the antigen bands were not

Table 2. Binding capacities of McAbs with various cells

Cells	Binding capacities		
	PC1	PD4	PC6
Gastric cancer			
MGC803	+++	+++	+++
SGC7901	+++	+++	−
BGC823	+	++	−
Kato III	+++	−	++
Esophageal cancer			
109	−	−	−
Hepatoma			
7402	+++	−	−
7703	−	−	−
Colon cancer			
B77	−	−	−
B80	−	−	−
Breast cancer			
BCP037	−	−	−
Lung cancer			
L-a-1	+	+	+
L-a-2	+	+	+
L-a-3	+	+	+
L-s	+	+	−
Tongue cancer			
TCA	−	−	−
Bladder cancer			
5637	−	−	−
Osteosarcoma			
OS-732	−	−	−
Lymphoma			
Raji	−	−	−
Leukemia			
Molt-3	−	−	−
Molt-4	−	−	−
Lymphoblasts			
UC-729-6	−	−	−
Lymphocytes			
Autologous	−	ND	ND
Allogenic	−	−	−
Red blood cells			
A type	−	−	−
B type	−	−	−
0 type	−	−	−
Normal bone marrow	−	−	−
Fibroblasts			
2BS	−	−	−

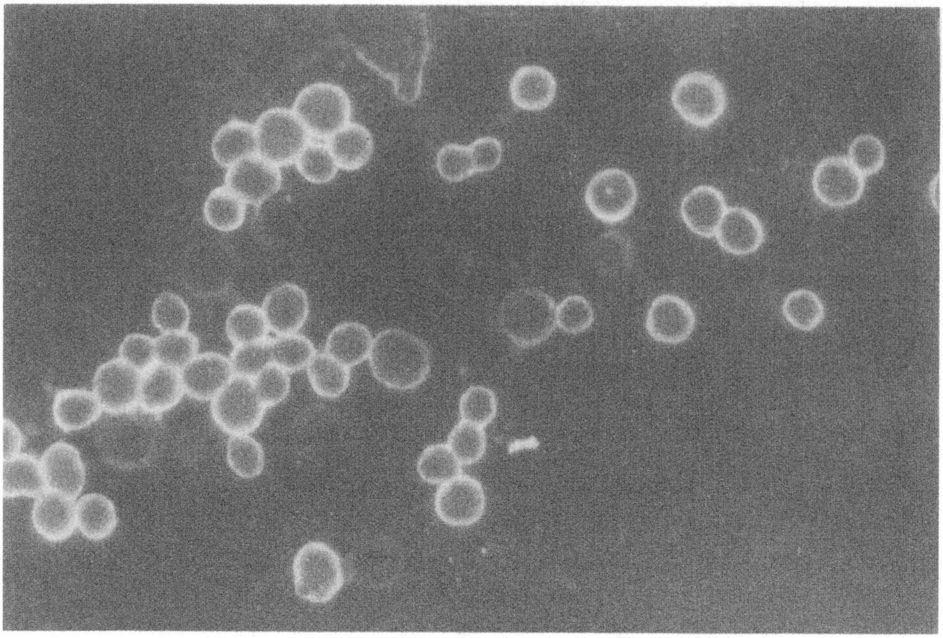

Fig. 1. Immunofluorescence stain of gastric cancer cells MGC803 with McAb PCl, ×200

affected by blocking of human IgG. Moreover, the PCl and PD4 antigen bands were visualized by Western blotting for target cells MGC803 and SGC7901, but only negative results were obtained, for example, for colon cancer cells B-80 and leukemia cells Molt-4, as well as for lymphocytes.

Discussion

Up to the present, the nature of the majority of tumor-associated antigens has not been clarified. Among a few defined antigens, the 19-9 antigen identified by Koprowski et al. [1] is a gastrointestinal cancer antigen, being a monosialoganglioside related to Lewis A substance. It is obvious that the antigens reported here are different.

The McAbs PCl, PD4, and PC6 were obtained by a fusion of myeloma cells with spleen cells immunized with gastric cancer cell line MGC803. The binding capacities of these McAbs were restricted to gastric cancer cells and lung cancer cells. The antigens PCl and PD4 were sensitive to heat and digestion of proteases and resistant to treatment with sodium periodate, indicating the nature of proteins. This point of view was confirmed by Western blotting analysis, and the molecular weights for PCl and PD4 antigens were 42 kd and 40 kd, respectively, whereas PC6 antigen was resistant to heat and treatment with sodium periodate, but sensitive to protease digestion, probably being a glycoprotein, although this was not confirmed by Western blotting. These antigens are mainly located on the membrane of target

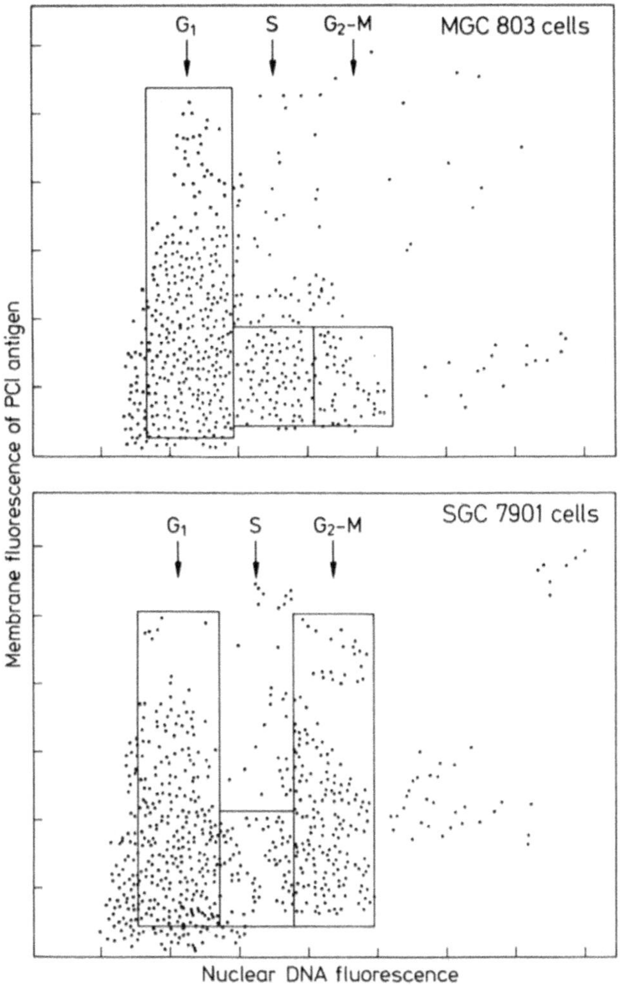

Fig. 2. Two-parameter analysis of gastric cancer cells with flow cytometry. The membrane PCl antigen of target cells was stained with IF (green fluorescence) and nuclear DNA was labeled with PI (red fluorescence). *Upper,* MGC803 cells; *lower,* SGC7901 cells. *Longitude,* membrane fluorescence of PCl antigen; *Latitude,* nuclear DNA fluorescence

Table 3. Sensitivity of antigens to treatment of heat, sodium periodate and enzymatic digestion

	Antigens		
	PCl	PD4	PC6
Nontreatment	+++	+++	+++
Treatment			
Heat (100 °C, 20′)	–	–	+++
Sodium periodate	+++	+++	+++
Trypsin	–	–	+
Pronase	–	–	–

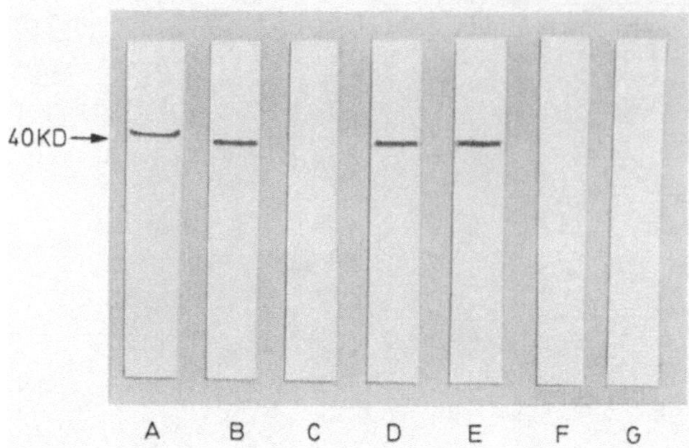

Fig. 3. Immunochemical analysis of the antigens with Western blotting. *A*, reacted with McAb PCl; *B*, reacted with McAb PD4; *C*, reacted with McAb PC6; *D*, blocked with human IgG, then reacted with McAb PD4; *E*, absorbed with conjugate of Sepharose-CL-4B with McAb PCl, then reacted with McAb PD4; *F*, absorbed with conjugate of Sepharose-CL-4B with McAb PD4, then reacted with McAb PD4; *G*, reacted with normal mouse serum (1:1000)

cells. However, the levels of antigen expression were quite heterogeneous in the cell population. By using two-dimensional flow cytometry, it was demonstrated that the heterogeneity of PCl antigen expression was partially dependent cell on cycle, and a high level of PCl antigen expression was found in the G_1 phase of MGC803 as well as the G_1 and G_2-M phase of SGC7901.

For their restricted distribution and identified molecular weight, PCl and PD4 antigens were not related to AB0, HLA, AFP, CEA, and Fc receptor as well as other gastric cancer-associated antigens reported [7].

The relationship between these novel antigens and cancerous development is not clear. The distribution of these antigens in human normal and tumor tissues and the potential use of these McAbs in the diagnosis and treatment of cancer are under investigation.

References

1. Atkins BF, Ernst CS, Herlyn M, Steplewski Z, Sears HF, Koprowski H: Gastrointestinal Cancer-associated Antigen in Immunoperoxidase Assay. Cancer Res. 43 (1982) 4820-4823
2. Braylan RC, Benson NA, Nourse V, Kruth HS: Correlated Analysis of Cellular DNA, Membrane Antigens and Light Scatter of Human Lymphoid Cells. Cytometry 2 (1982) 337-343
3. Burnette WN: "Western Blotting": Electrophoretic Transfer of Proteins from Sodium Dodecyl Sulfate-Polyacrylamide Gels to Unmodified Nitrocellulose and Radiographic Detection with Antibody and Radioiodinated Protein. A. Anal. Biochem. 112 (1981) 195-203
4. Dippold WG, Lloyd KO, Li LTC, Ikeda H, Oettgen HF, Old LJ: Cell Surface Antigens of Human Malignant Melanoma: Definition of Six Antigenic Systems with Mouse Monoclonal Antibodies. Proc. nat. Acad. Sci 77 (1980) 6114-6118
5. Dong ZW, Li ZP, Wan WH, Xu XL: Application of enzyme-linked immunofiltration to

screening and characterization of monoclonal antibodies. Chin. J. Microbiol. Immunol. 5 (1985) 33-36
6. Galfré G, Milstein C: Preparation of Monoclonal Antibodies: Strategies and Procedures. In J.J. Langone, H. van Vunakis (Eds): Immunochemical Techniques, Part B, pp. 3-46. New York: Academic Press 1981. (Methods in Enzymology, Vol. 73)
7. Hirohashi S, Watanabe M, Shimosato Y, Sekine T: Monoclonal Antibody Reactive with the Sialyl-Sugar Residue of a High Molecular Weight Glycoprotein in Sera of Cancer Patients. Gann 75 (1984) 485-488
8. Köhler G, Milstein C: Continuous Cultures of Fused Cells Secreting Antibody of Predefined Specificity. Nature 256 (1975) 495-497
9. Koprowski H, Steplewski Z, Herlyn D, Herlyn M: Study of Antibodies against Human Melanoma Produced by Somatic Cell Hybrids. Proc. nat. Acad. Sci 75 (1978) 3405-3409
10. Laemmli UK: Cleavage of Structural Proteins during the Assembly of the Head of Bacteriophage T4. Nature 227 (1970) 680-685
11. Magnani JL, Nilsson B, Brockhaus M, Zopf D, Steplewski Z, Koprowski H, Ginsburg V: A Monoclonal Antibody-defined Antigen Associated with Gastrointestinal Cancer is a Ganglioside Containing Sialylated Lacto-N-Fucopentaose II. J. Biol. Chem. 257 (1982) 14365-14369

IV Cancer of the Nasopharynx

Epidemiology of Nasopharyngeal Carcinoma with Special Reference to Early Detection and Pre-NPC Conditions

G. de Thé and Zeng Yi

The relationships between the Epstein-Barr virus (EBV) and nasopharyngeal carcinoma (NPC) are very strong and probably of a causal nature, but yet poorly understood in their molecular mechanisms. While the EBV may or may not infect the epithelial cells of the nasopharynx during primary infection, its presence in the epithelial tumor cells is constant in the undifferentiated carcinoma of the nasopharynx. Furthermore, reactivation of EBV latency in the nasopharynx represents a late step prior to clinical onset. Such a reactivation is accompanied by the synthesis of specific IgA, which was found to be most instrumental for early detection of NPC.

That NPC patients had a high level of IgA antibody was first observed by Wara et al. in 1975 [7]. Soon after, Henle and Henle [5] and Desgranges and de Thé [2] showed that such IgA antibodies were directed against EBV/VCA and EA. The regular presence of such antibodies in patients with nasopharyngeal carcinoma originating from different geographical areas and their absence in patients with other ENT tumors suggested that such an antibody could represent a useful marker for the diagnosis of the disease.

Population Screening and Early Detection of NPC

Soon after the observations mentioned above, Zeng et al. [10] initiated a major population survey in a rural area of the eastern part of the Guang-Xi Autonomous Region of the People's Republic of China. The county of Zang-Wu, with a population of 450000, was selected, and individuals aged 30 years and over were registered and asked to give blood to search for IgA/VCA antibodies. As seen in Table 1,

Table 1. IgA/VCA serological population surveys in rural and urban population of the Guang-Xi autonomous region

	No. persons surveyed	No. with IgA/VCA	% IGA/VCA+ in surveyed population	No. NPCs detected	Ca In situ	Clinical stages I	II	III	IV	NPC detection in population	NPC among IgA/VCA+ individuals
Rural Zangwu	148029	3533	2.38%	55	1	12 (22%)	19 (34%)	17 (31%)	6 (11%)	37/100000	1.55%
						56% (I+II)					
Urban Wuzhou	20726	1136	5.50%	35		15 (43%)	17 (48.5%)	3 (9.5%)	0	168/100000	2.70%
						91.5% (I+II)					

Cancer of the Liver, Esophagus, and Nasopharynx
Edited by G. Wagner and Zhang You-Hui

2.38% of the 148029 persons screened were found to have IgA/VCA antibodies [9, 12]. The 460 individuals found to have IgA/VCA antibodies at a titer equal or superior to 1:80 were clinically examined, and 55 cases of nasopharyngeal carcinoma were diagnosed at different clinical stages.

The city of Wu-Zhou, with a population of 170000, was chosen for both cancer registration and further seroepidemiological studies. The NPC annual incidence was found to be 20 per 100000 individuals. The survey of 20726 workers aged 40 years and over showed that 1136 individuals had IgA/VCA antibodies [11, 13]. Clinical examination of these persons led to the detection of 35 cases of NPC, the clinical stages being given in Table 1. The prevalence rate of NPC as detected in Wu-Zhou reached 150/100000 in the 40- to 69-year-old age group, a high figure if one considers that the hospitalized patients were not included in that figure. When one compares the results of the serological surveys among rural and urban populations, one sees that the proportion of the IgA-positive individuals was lower in Zang-Wu (2.38%) than in Wu-Zhou (5.5%). This may reflect differences in the immunoenzymatic test used. The detection rate of NPC and the proportion of NPC at early clinical stages was, however, greater in the city of Wu-Zhou than in the rural area of Zang-Wu. This might be related to a better awareness of NPC and better health delivery systems in towns than in rural areas.

The use of IgA/EA antibodies instead of IgA/VCA antibodies to detect early NPC allowed us to decrease substantially the number of screened persons to be clinically examined, since only 0.05% of the general population exhibited IgA/EA antibodies, 43% of those already having clinical NPC.

Follow-up of IgA/VCA-Positive Individuals

In Zangwu county, 1138 individuals with IgA/VCA antibodies were followed up yearly for 3 years, from both serological and clinical viewpoints. It can be observed in Table 2 that two groups were at high risk for developing NPC: (a) individuals who increased their IgA/VCA titers fourfold or more had an 18.5% chance of developing NPC within 3 years; (b) individuals who had stable IgA/VCA antibody

Table 2. Stability and fluctuations of IgA/VCA antibody titers over 3 years in relation to risk of developing NPC in Zangwu county

No. persons IgA/VCA+	Stability (no change in IgA/VCA)	Loss of IgA/VCA (retroversion)	Increase[a]	Decline[a]	Up and down
1138 (100%)	455 (40%)	398 (35%)	81 (7.1%)	162 (14.2%)	42 (3.7%)
NPC patients detected Total = 21 cases	6[b]	0	15[c]	0	0

[a] By fourfold in titers

[b] These 6 cases represent 1.32% of the 455 individuals with stable titers and 28% of the 21 NPCs detected

[c] These 15 cases represent 18% of the 81 subjects with increasing IgA/VCA titers and 71% of the 21 NPCs detected

titers had a 1.32% chance of developing NPC within this period. The first group was of great interest, since it represented only 7.1% of the total IgA/VCA-positive population but led to 71.5% of the detected NPC. Therefore, if interventions are to be contemplated to prevent NPC, they should be performed on individuals with increasing IgA/VCA antibody titers, since one out of five will eventually develop the disease within 3 years.

If one tries to evaluate the time which elapsed between the first bleeding and subsequent tumor diagnosis in this series, one sees that, for stage I, such intervals varied from 8 to 30 months, for stage II between 10 and 48 months, and for stage III between 9 and 34 months. These surprising results may reflect important individual variations in the rate of NPC development. The survey of IgA-positive individuals in the town of Wu-Zhou is being pursued in order to better characterize the yearly rate of seroconversion (from IgA/VCA negative to positive) and of retroversion (from IgA/VCA positive to negative) and the conditions of increasing titers.

Pre-NPC Conditions

In parallel with these population surveys, we were interested in investigating what the presence of IgA antibodies to VCA and EA meant from an immunovirological viewpoint in the nasopharyngeal mucosa. In order to see whether the presence of IgA/VCA antibodies reflected a specific viral activity in the NP mucosa, 56 individuals exhibiting IgA/VCA antibodies for more than 18 months were biopsied. Four NPC cases were detected among these 56 individuals (two at an early stage of the disease and two at stage III). A further 14 individuals without detectable abnormalities in their nasopharynx exhibited EBV-DNA sequences and/or EBNA in their nasopharyngeal mucosa [1]. In a further study, exfoliated cells from the nasopharynx of both IgA-positive and IgA-negative individuals (obtained with a negative pressure apparatus developed by Zhanjiang Medical College in 1976 [14]) were investigated comparatively for the presence of EBNA and EBV-DNA sequences by spot followed by blot hybridizations. As seen in Table 3 [3, 6], both groups differed, but less than expected. One-third to one-fifth of IgA/VCA-positive individuals had detectable EBNA or EBV-DNA, respectively, in their exfoliated cells, as compared with one-fifth and one-seventh of the IgA/VCA-negative individuals. The EBNA test was regularly found to be a more sensitive test than blot hybridization. Forty-six of these IgA-positive and -negative individuals were again studied a year later, and it was noted that four out of seven individuals, who a year previously had detectable EBV-DNA sequences in their nasopharyngeal cells, failed to do so a year later. Conversely, 2 out of 15 individuals lacking detectable EBV-DNA in their exfoliated

Table 3. Comparative detection of EBV/DNA and EBNA in exfoliated nasopharyngeal cells of IgA/VCA-positive and -negative individuals

	No. tested	EBV/DNA positive [3]	No. tested	EBNA positive [6]
IgA/VCA+ individuals	62	13 (21%)	26	9 (34%)
IgA/VCA− individuals	39	6 (15%)	46	9 (20%)

cells were positive a year later. Thus, the presence of EBV-DNA sequences in the nasopharyngeal mucosa appears not to be directly related to the presence of antibodies to IgA/VCA. This observation was surprising to us, and we are in the process of investigating whether the presence of viral DNA in nasopharyngeal cells among both groups of IgA-positive and IgA-negative individuals might not reflect the difference in the cell population involved (lymphoid cells in IgA-negative and epithelial cells in IgA-positive individuals).

From an immunovirological viewpoint, the development of IgA/VCA and IgA/EA antibodies together with IgG/EA antibodies reflects a reactivation of the EBV latency and characterizes pre-NPC conditions [4]. What is happening in the virus-cell relationship in the nasopharyngeal mucosa just prior to tumor development remains unknown. Further investigation of these events is critical from both the fundamental and applied viewpoints.

Prospect of Better Control of NPC

Table 4 gives the comparative distribution of clinical staging of 1066 NPC cases from the outpatient clinics of hospitals outside the surveyed area and of the 35 cases detected during the serological screening in Wu-Zhou city (see also Table 1 and [8, 13]). Although the two groups were different by the number involved, the differences are striking: early stages (I + II) represent 30% of the cases in outpatient clinics, whereas they represent more than 90% when systematic screening is implemented. If one considers the tumorous process limited to the nasopharyngeal mucosa (stage I), the difference is even more striking: 1.7% versus 43%. Such a shift has a tremendous impact on NPC control, since NPC patients at stage I exhibit a 90% five years disease-free survival as compared with less than 30% in patients at stage III. Today, most patients in NPC-endemic areas arrive so late that 70% of them die within 1 year following diagnosis (at stages IV, V). If early diagnosis is implemented, the situation can be completely reversed, with an 80% cure rate at 5 years for the early stages (I, II). Such an effect can be achieved before the mode of action of the EBV in the molecular pathogenesis of NPC is understood.

Table 4. Comparative distribution of clinical stages of NPC cases diagnosed in outpatient clinics or detected by serological screening

	No. cases	Stages			
		I	II	III	IV
Outpatient clinic	1066 (100%)	18 (1.7%)	312 (29.2%)	556 (52.2%)	180 (16.9%)
		(30.9%)			
Serological screening	35 (100%)	15 (43%)	17 (48.5%)	3 (8.5%)	
		(91.5%)			

References

1. Desgranges C, Bornkamm GW, Zeng Y et al.: Detection of Epstein-Barr viral DNA in the nasopharyngeal mucosa of Chinese with IgA/EBV-specific antibodies. Int. J. Cancer 29 (1982) 187-191
2. Desgranges C, de Thé G: IgA and nasopharyngeal carcinoma. In G. de Thé, Y. Ito, F. Rapp (Eds): Oncogenesis and Herpes-viruses III, pp. 883-891. Lyon: IARC 1978. (IARC Scientific Publications No. 25)
3. Desgranges C, Pi GH, Bornkamm G et al.: Presence of EBV-DNA sequences in nasopharyngeal cells of individuals without IgA/VCA antibodies. Int. J. Cancer 32 (1983) 543-545
4. de Thé G, Zeng Y, Desgranges C et al.: The existence of pre-nasopharyngeal carcinoma conditions should allow preventive interventions. In Prasad et al. (Eds): Nasopharyngeal Carcinoma: Current Concepts, pp. 365-374. Kuala Lumpur: University of Malaya 1983
5. Henle G, Henle W: Epstein-Barr virus-specific IgA serum antibodies as an outstanding feature of nasopharyngeal carcinoma. Int. J. Cancer 17 (1976) 1-7
6. Shen SJ, Chen CP, Ma JL et al.: Further study on detection of EBNA from nasopharyngeal exfoliated cells of patients with nasopharyngeal carcinoma. Acta Zhanjiang med. Coll. 1 (1983) 34-37
7. Wara WM, Wara DW, Phillips TL et al.: Elevated IgA in carcinoma of the nasopharynx. Cancer 35 (1975) 1313-1315
8. Zeng Y, Gi ZW, Wang PC et al.: Induction of Epstein-Barr virus antigen in Raji cells and P3HR-1 cells by culture fluids of anaerobes from nasopharynx of patients with nasopharyngeal carcinoma and with other ear-nose-throat diseases. Cancer Letters (in press)
9. Zeng Y, Liu YX, Liu ZR et al.: Application of an immunoenzymatic method and an immunoauroradiographic method for a mass survey of nasopharyngeal carcinoma. Intervirology 13 (1980) 162-168
10. Zeng Y, Liu YX, Wei JN et al.: Serological mass survey of nasopharyngeal carcinoma. Acta Acad. Med. Sin. 1 (1979) 123-126
11. Zeng Y, Zhang LG, Li HY et al.: Serological mass survey for early detection of nasopharyngeal carcinoma in Wuzhou City, China. Int. J. Cancer 29 (1982) 139-141
12. Zeng Y, Zhong JM, Li LY et al.: Follow-up studies on Epstein-Barr virus IgA/VCA antibody positive persons in Zangwu County, China. Intervirology 20 (1983) 190-194
13. Zeng Y, Zhang LG, Wu YC et al.: Follow-up studies on NPC in EB virus IgA/VCA antibody positive persons in Wuzhou City, China. Chin. J. Virol. 1 (1985) 7-11
14. Zhanjiang Medical College: Diagnosis of nasopharyngeal carcinoma by cytological examination of exfoliated cells by negative pressure suction. Chin. med. J. 1 (1976) 45-47

Histopathological Aspects of Nasopharyngeal Carcinoma

K. Shanmugaratnam

The development and structure of the normal nasopharynx have an important bearing on the histogenesis and histomorphology of cancers that may arise in this area. Approximately 60% of the nasopharyngeal surface in adults is lined by stratified squamous epithelium which shows little or no keratinization [1]. Patches of ciliated epithelium and transitional or intermediate-type epithelium occur throughout the nasopharyngeal surface.

The nasopharyngeal mucosa has a total surface area of 50 cm^2 [1]; the lateral walls, which contain the pharyngeal recesses or fossae of Rosenmueller, have the largest surface area. The nasopharyngeal epithelium, endodermal and branchiogenic in origin, is largely derived from the third brachial arch and, to a lesser extent, from the endodermal aspect of the dorsal part of the mandibular arch [26, 54]. During fetal life, it is essentially a columnar ciliated epithelium of the respiratory type with foci of presquamous change; true squamous metaplasia occurs only after birth [19].

The nasopharyngeal mucosa is "lymphoepithelial" inasmuch as it contains abundant lymphoid tissue; the lymphocytes are present not only in the lamina propria but also in the epithelial layer. Electron microscopic studies have demonstrated an intimate relationship between lymphocytes and nasopharyngeal epithelial cells with occasional cell membrane discontinuity and cytoplasmic bridging [14].

The nasopharyngeal wall also contains seromucous glands, soft tissue, and other specific tissue elements. Consequently, a variety of malignant tumors may arise in the nasopharynx:

1. Nasopharyngeal carcinoma (NPC) – a malignant tumor of the epithelium lining the surfaces and crypts of the nasopharynx (ICD 147)
2. Malignant tumors of glandular epithelium – adenocarcinoma, adenocystic carcinoma, and other tumors of the salivary gland type (ICD 147)
3. Malignant tumors of soft tissues (ICD 147)
4. Malignant tumors of other tissue elements, e.g., melanoma (ICD 147)
5. Malignant tumors of bone and cartilage (ICD 170)
6. Malignant lymphomas (ICD 200–203)

Nasopharyngeal carcinoma (NPC) is the most common form of nasopharyngeal malignancy in all human populations. The ratio of NPC to other cancers arising in the nasopharynx is highest in populations with a high incidence of nasopharyngeal cancer. Geographical variations in the incidence of cancer of the nasopharynx (ICD 147) are essentially due to variations in the incidence of NPC.

Cancer of the Liver, Esophagus, and Nasopharynx
Edited by G. Wagner and Zhang You-Hui

Histogenesis

The epithelial origin of NPC is obvious from the light microscopic, immunohistochemical, and ultrastructural features of the neoplasm. A cohesive or carcinomatous growth pattern of the tumor cells is evident by light microscopy, the presence of keratin proteins is invariably demonstrable by immunocytological staining [9, 15, 30, 43], and the presence of keratin fibrils, tonofilaments and desmosomes is invariably demonstrable by electron microscopy [14, 29, 51]. Tissue cultures from NPC biopsies have shown a transient growth of epithelial sheets, fibroblasts, and lymphoid cells [10, 14], but growth of NPC explants in nude mice has revealed that only epithelial cells are malignant [22].

Histological studies have also provided convincing evidence that NPC arises from the surface epithelium of the nasopharynx. This epithelium may be demonstrably continuous with the tumor and may show malignant in-situ changes [28, 47]. It has been reported that the development of NPC may be preceded by reserve cell hyperplasia [35], atypical metaplasia, and atypical hyperplasia [27] of the surface epithelium. The tumor cells do not show mucin secretion or glandular differentiation, and there is no evidence to support glandular origin.

The question of which type of epithelium lining the nasopharyngeal surface is the source of NPC is not settled. Some authors have expressed the view that NPC arises exclusively from stratified squamous epithelium [23, 52]; this view is supported by the demonstration of squamous differentiation in all tumors by immunohistochemistry and electron microscopy. Others have favored an origin from transitional epithelium [13] or ciliated columnar respiratory epithelium [11, 28, 29, 47, 49]. This view has derived some support from ultrastructural studies showing common cellular organelles in normal respiratory epithelium and some NPC tumor cells which contain a cytoplasmic vacuolar system with a well-defined Golgi complex and endoplasmic reticulum as well as cytoplasmic tonofilaments [29]; it is not contradicted by the presence of keratin proteins in the tumor cells since these may also be found in respiratory epithelium [49].

It has also been proposed that the nonkeratinizing and undifferentiated types of NPC arise from primitive stem cells or intermediate cells which are capable of differentiating into mature squamous or respiratory epithelium [4]. Such stem cells are present in the basal layer of all types of epithelium in the nasopharynx. It is, therefore, reasonable to postulate that NPC may arise from any of the types of epithelium that line the nasopharyngeal surface [28, 47, 49].

Histopathological Classification

The classification of NPC into various histological types is based on light microscopy. Several schemes have been proposed. Some authors have favored the subdivision of NPC into two main types - squamous cell carcinoma and undifferentiated carcinoma [32, 33, 47]. Others have divided NPC into a multiplicity of types on the basis of cytological, structural, and stromal variations [28, 58].

According to the classification proposed by WHO [48], three histological types are recognized on the basis of their light microscopic appearances:

1. Squamous cell carcinoma (SCC). This type shows definite evidence of squamous differentiation with intercellular bridges and/or keratinization over most of its extent; it may be subdivided into three grades: (a) well differentiated, (b) moderately differentiated, and (c) poorly differentiated.
2. Nonkeratinizing carcinoma (NKC). This type shows no evidence of squamous differentiation but the tumor cells have well-defined cell margins and exhibit a stratified or pavemented arrangement; a plexiform growth pattern is seen in some cases.
3. Undifferentiated carcinoma (UC). The tumor cells in this type generally have pale or vesicular nuclei and prominent nucleoli. They have indistinct cell margins and exhibit a syncytial rather than pavemented appearance. Spindle-shaped tumor cells, some with hyperchromatic nuclei, may be present. The tumor cells are arranged in irregular but moderately well defined masses - the so-called Régaud type [38] - or in strands of loosely connected cells in a lymphoid stroma - the so-called Schmincke type [42].

The term "lymphoepithelial carcinoma" is used in the WHO scheme to describe nonkeratinizing and undifferentiated types of NPC (NKC and UC) in which numerous lymphocytes are found among the tumor cells. It has been proposed that these types of NPC (WHO types 2 and 3) should each be formally subdivided into two subtypes - with and without lymphoid stroma [23-25]. Lymphocytic infiltration of varying degree may be seen in most NPCs, even in SCC [36, 46], although this is seldom as striking as in NKC and UC. Some of the lymphocytes seen in tumor biopsies, especially those in the stroma, may represent residual nasopharyngeal lymphoid tissue, but a substantial proportion of those intimately admixed with tumor cells probably represent reactive lymphocytic infiltration. This view is supported by a significant accumulation of T-lymphocytes [18] and IgA-containing B-lymphocytes [57] in the tumor. Localized amyloid deposits may be found in a small proportion of tumor biopsies [36].

Problems in Diagnosis

The diagnosis of NPC is based on the site of origin of the tumor and its histological features. In the majority of cases a definitive diagnosis may be made with little difficulty by biopsy. Indeed, the histological features of the most common undifferentiated type are sufficiently characteristic to enable a presumptive diagnosis of NPC even when the biopsy samples are taken from metastatic or secondary sites.

False-negative diagnoses result from biopsy samples that are inadequate - either because they do not include tumor tissue or because the histological features are obscured by traumatic distortion or tumor necrosis. False-positive diagnoses are exceptionally rare and may not be expected from experienced pathologists. Some of the follicular cells of reactive lymphoid hyperplasia may resemble NPC cells, and invaginations of surface or crypt epithelium in the lamina propria may simulate invasion when sectioned tangentially; the true nature of these cellular aggregates may be established by serial sectioning and careful microscopy.

Among other malignancies that occur in the nasopharynx, lymphomas are the most likely to be confused with NPC. Some types of lymphoma, especially the large cell immunoblastic types, may resemble NPC and some undifferentiated NPCs, especially those with poor cell cohesion, may simulate lymphoma. These diagnostic difficulties are readily resolved by the use of electron microscopy or immunohistochemical techniques. By immunohistological staining, keratin is the most reliable epithelial marker for identifying NPC and excluding lymphoma [9, 15, 30, 43, 49]; some markers of lymphoid cells are equally reliable for identifying lymphoma and excluding NPC [6]. Other nasopharyngeal malignancies seldom cause diagnostic difficulties.

Problems of Classification

The histological classification of NPC has been the subject of long-standing debate. Some standardization of histological criteria and terminology has followed the publication of the WHO classification [48] but the controversy remains. It is important to recognize that the validity and merits of any classification depend on its objectives and on whether the criteria for the definition of histological types are sufficiently distinctive to allow a fair measure of reproducibility among observers.

One of the objectives of classification is to assist histological diagnosis of the tumor by categorizing and describing its morphological variants; some of the schemes with many subtypes have this objective in view. A more important objective is to subdivide the tumor into histomorphological types that share important biological characteristics in clinical behavior, response to therapy, epidemiology, and etiology.

The main practical difficulty in classification lies in the fact that the differences between histological types of NPC, whatever the scheme adopted, are not sharp. The prototypes are easily distinguished but many tumors, especially in high-risk populations, exhibit intermediate or mixed features [44, 45]. NKC and UC have been defined in the WHO scheme [48] as tumors in which squamous differentiation is not evident by light microscopy, but it is more realistic to describe them as tumors with little or no evidence of squamous differentiation [56]. Lymphocytic infiltration may be present in all types of NPC [36, 46] but is more marked in NKC and UC. The differences with respect to squamous differentiation and lymphocytic admixture, which are the bases of classification, are not qualitative but quantitative.

Correlations Between Histological Type and Biological Characteristics

Despite the problems in classification mentioned previously, significant differences have been observed in the biological attributes of the major histological types of NPC.

Geography and Race. Undifferentiated carcinoma comprises a significantly higher proportion of tumors among Chinese [46, 50], who have the highest incidence of NPC, and among United States Blacks [12] and Ugandans [41], who have relatively low or intermediate risks for the disease.

Age. Undifferentiated carcinoma comprises a significantly higher proportion of tumors occurring among children and adolescents [7, 8, 16, 31]; conversely, SCC is more common among older patients [39].

Epstein-Barr Virus. Patients with poorly differentiated and undifferentiated types of NPC have higher mean titers of antibodies against various EBV-related antigens [33, 34, 50, 53, 55], and it has been reported that the presence of EBV genomes and EBV nuclear antigen in the tumor cells is restricted to these types [2, 3, 17, 21]. NPC-EBV relationships are strong and almost invariably demonstrable in undifferentiated NPCs (UC). NPCs of intermediate differentiation (NKC) also exhibit EBV relationships, although they are not as strong and consistent as in UC; NKCs with lymphocytic infiltration have stronger EBV relationships than those without [23, 25]. NPC-EBV relationships are rarely demonstrable in well-differentiated SCCs [20, 25, 33]. The differences between histological types of NPC in their EBV-related serological reactivities have been less marked in high-risk populations [46, 50]. It is also relevant to note that EBV serological reactivities may vary in strength during the course of the disease and with the extent of tumor growth [5].

Survival Rates. The 5-year survivals are approximately 20%–30% for all NPCs and 60%–70% in cases where the tumor is confined to the nasopharynx [46]. The survival rates for the undifferentiated and poorly differentiated NPCs are generally better [16, 37, 40, 46], probably because they are more responsive to radiotherapy. Better 3-year survivals, with no significant difference in the 5-year survival rates, were observed in NPCs with marked lymphocytic infiltration [46].

Comment

The histological types of NPC are not sharply distinct and some observer variations may be expected whatever scheme of classification is adopted. Despite these variations, histological classification has achieved a measure of success in predicting EBV associations and response to radiotherapy. The question arises as to how the classification can be modified or the definitions of tumor types sharpened to achieve a greater measure of comparability and biological correlation.

Ultrastructural [51] and immunocytochemical [15] studies have not established any difference between the tumor types. It has been suggested that NKC and UC may have close similarities in their monoclonal keratin antibody-staining properties and that immunocytological studies, using standard tumor-specific antibodies and well-evaluated monoclonal antibodies against various classes of cytokeratins, may help to elucidate the histogenesis of the tumors [49]; it remains to be seen whether such investigations will reveal differences between the tumor types that are sharper or more relevant than those provided by light microscopy.

The classical types of SCC and UC may be recognized fairly easily with a high degree of comparability between observers. NKC was introduced into the WHO classification [48] by consensus among the participating pathologists to categorize an intermediate type of NPC that is essentially nonkeratinizing but not quite undifferentiated and to promote investigations on this group of tumors. Subsequent studies have shown that NKC has close biological similarities with UC and that the similarities are more marked in tumors with lymphocytic infiltration [23, 25]. It is also probable that these characteristics are shared by poorly differentiated SCC in which evidence of squamous differentiation is only focal or barely discernible and which often coexists with NKC or UC in high-risk populations [46]. It is the well-differentiated and moderately differentiated SCC with more obvious and extensive evidence of keratinization that appears to be biologically different. It is therefore recommended that further correlative studies using the WHO classification should include a subdivision of SCC according to the grade of differentiation and a further subdivision of all tumor types according to the degree of lymphocytic infiltration.

References

1. Ali MY: Histology of the human nasopharyngeal mucosa. J. Anat. 99 (1965) 657-672
2. Andersson-Anvert M, Forsby N, Klein G et al.: Relationship between the Epstein-Barr virus and undifferentiated nasopharyngeal carcinoma: Correlated nucleic acid hybridization and histopathological examination. Int. J. Cancer 20 (1977) 486-494
3. Andersson-Anvert M, Forsby N, Klein G et al.: Relationship between the Epstein-Barr virus genome and nasopharyngeal carcinoma in Caucasian patients. Int. J. Cancer 23 (1979) 762-767
4. Batsakis JG, Solomon AR, Rice DH: The pathology of head and neck tumors: Carcinoma of the nasopharynx, Part II. Head Neck Surg. 3 (1981) 511-524
5. Bertram G, Pearson GR, Faggioni A et al.: Long-term survey of EBV-serology and non-EBV related tests in correlation to the clinical course. In U. Prasad, D. V. Ablashi, P. H. Levine et al. (Eds): Nasopharyngeal Carcinoma: Current Concepts, pp. 115-124. Kuala Lumpur: University of Malaya Press 1983
6. Borowitz MJ, Stevanovic G, Gottfried M: Differential diagnosis of undifferentiated malignant tumors with monoclonal antibody T29/33. Hum. Path. 15 (1984) 928-934
7. Brugere J, Point D, Sancho-Garnier H et al.: Epidemiology of malignant tumors of the nasopharynx in France: Retrospective and prospective studies. In de Thé G, Ito Y (Eds): Nasopharyngeal Carcinoma: Etiology and Control, pp. 241-249. Lyon: IARC 1978. (IARC Sci. Publ., No. 20)
8. Cammoun M, Ellouz R, Behi et al.: Histological types of nasopharyngeal carcinoma in an intermediate risk area. In de Thé G, Ito Y (Eds): Nasopharyngeal Carcinoma: Etiology and Control, pp. 13-16. Lyon: IARC 1978. (IARC Sci. Publ., No. 20)
9. Costa J: The histopathological diagnosis of nasopharyngeal carcinoma. In Grundmann E, Krueger GRF, Ablashi DV (Eds): Nasopharyngeal Carcinoma, pp. 7-10. Stuttgart: Fischer 1981. (Cancer Campaign, Vol. 5)
10. De Thé G, Ho JHC, Kwan HC et al.: Nasopharyngeal carcinoma I. Types of cultures derived from tumour biopsies and non-tumorous tissues of Chinese patients with special reference to lymphoblastoid transformation. Int. J. Cancer 6 (1970) 189-206
11. Digby KH: Nasopharyngeal carcinoma. Ann. roy. Coll. Surg. Engl. 9 (1951) 253-265
12. Easton JE, Levine PH, Hyams VJ: Nasopharyngeal carcinoma in the United States: A pathological study of 177 U.S. and 30 foreign cases. Arch. Otolaryng. 106 (1980) 88-91
13. Ewing J: Lymphoepithelioma. Amer. J. Path. 5 (1929) 99-107
14. Gazzolo L, de Thé G, Vuillaume M et al.: Nasopharyngeal carcinoma II. Ultra-structure of normal mucosa, tumour biopsies and subsequent epithelial growth in vitro. J. nat. Cancer Inst. 48 (1972) 73-86
15. Gusterson BA, Mitchell DP, Warburton MJ et al.: Epithelial markers in the diagnosis of nasopharyngeal carcinoma: An immunocytochemical study. J. clin. Path. 36 (1983) 628-631
16. Hoppe RT, Williams J, Warnke R et al.: Carcinoma of the nasopharynx - the significance of histology. Int. J. Radiat. Oncol. Biol. Phys. 4 (1978) 199-205

17. Huang DP, Ho HC, Henle W et al.: Presence of EBNA in nasopharyngeal carcinoma and control patient tissue related to EBV serology. Int. J. Cancer 22 (1978) 266-274
18. Jondal M, Klein G: Classification of lymphocytes in nasopharyngeal carcinoma (NPC) biopsies. Biomedicine 23 (1975) 163-165
19. Kangasuntheram R, Ramsbotham M: Development of the human nasopharyngeal epithelium. Acta Anat. 70 (1968) 1-13
20. Karpinski A, Krueger GRF, Wustrow J et al.: Epstein-Barr virus antibody titers in various histological types of carcinoma of the nasopharynx. In Grundmann E, Krueger GRF, Ablashi DV (Eds): Nasopharyngeal Carcinoma, pp. 95-99. Stuttgart: Fischer 1981. (Cancer Campaign, Vol. 5)
21. Klein G: The Epstein-Barr virus and neoplasia. New Engl. J. Med. 293 (1975) 1353-1357
22. Klein G, Giovanella BC, Lindahl T et al.: Direct evidence for the present of Epstein-Barr virus DNA and nuclear antigen in malignant epithelial cells from patients with poorly differentiated carcinoma of the nasopharynx. Proc. nat. Acad. Sci. 71 (1974) 4737-4741
23. Krueger GRF: Nasopharyngeal carcinoma. In Purtilo DT (Edit.): Immune Deficiency and Cancer, pp. 37-68. New York: Plenum Publ. Corp. 1984
24. Krueger GRF, Wustrow J: Current histological classification of nasopharyngeal carcinoma (NPC) at Cologne University. In Grundmann E, Krueger GRF, Ablashi DV (Eds): Nasopharyngeal Carcinoma, pp. 11-15. Stuttgart: Fischer 1981. (Cancer Campaign, Vol. 5)
25. Krueger GRF, Kottaridis SD, Wolf H et al.: Histological types of nasopharyngeal carcinoma as compared to EBV serology. Anticancer Res. 1 (1981) 187-194
26. Langebartel DA: The Anatomical Primer. An Embryological Explanation of Human Gross Morphology. Baltimore: University Park Press 1977
27. Li ZQ, Chen JJ, Li WJ: Early detection of nasopharyngeal carcinoma (NPC) and nasopharyngeal mucosal hyperplastic lesions (NPHL) with its relationship to carcinomatous change. In Prasad U, Ablashi DV, Levine PH et al. (Eds): Nasopharyngeal Carcinoma - Current Concepts, pp. 17-23. Kuala Lumpur: University of Malaya Press 1983
28. Liang PC, Chen CC, Chu CC et al.: The histological classification, biological characteristics and histogenesis of nasopharyngeal carcinoma. Chin. med. J. 81 (1962) 629-658
29. Lin HS, Lin CS, Yeh S et al.: Fine structure of nasopharyngeal carcinoma with special reference to the anaplastic type. Cancer 23 (1969) 390-405
30. Madri JA, Barwick KW: An immunohistochemical study of nasopharyngeal neoplasms using keratin antibodies. Amer. J. surg. Path. 6 (1982) 143-149
31. McConnell EM: Nasopharyngeal carcinoma in children and young adults. Brit. J. Cancer 12 (1958) 195-201
32. Micheau C: Anatomie pathologique et essai de classification des épithéliomas du nasopharynx. Bull. Cancer (Paris) 62 (1975) 277-286
33. Micheau C, de Thé G, Orofiamma B et al.: Practical value of classifying NPC into two major microscopic types. In Grundmann E, Krueger GRF, Ablashi DV (Eds): Nasopharyngeal Carcinoma, pp. 51 57. Stuttgart: Fischer 1981. (Cancer Campaign, Vol. 5)
34. Miller D, Goldmann JM, Goodman ML: Etiologic study of nasopharyngeal cancer. Arch. Otolaryng. 94 (1971) 104-108
35. Prasad U: Significance of metaplastic transformation in the pathogenesis of nasopharyngeal carcinoma. In Grundmann E, Krueger GRF, Ablashi DV (Eds): Nasopharyngeal Carcinoma, pp. 31-39. Stuttgart: Fischer 1981. (Cancer Campaign, Vol. 5)
36. Prathap K, Looi LM, Prasad U: Localized amyloidosis in nasopharyngeal carcinoma. Histopathology 8 (1984) 27-34
37. Pearson GR, Neel HB, Weiland LH et al.: Antibody dependent cellular cytotoxicity and disease course in North American patients with nasopharyngeal carcinoma: A prospective study. Int. J. Cancer 33 (1984) 777-778
38. Regaud C, Reverchon L: Sur un cas d'épithélioma épidérmoïde developpé dans le massif maxillaire supérieur, étendu aux téguments de la face, aux cavités buccale, nasale et orbitaire, ainsi qu'aux ganglions du cou, guéri par la curiethérapie. Rév. Laryng. 42 (1921) 369-378
39. Resta L, Rocco R, Santangelo A: Morphologic and classificatory considerations about 140 cases of carcinoma of the nasopharynx. Tumori 31 (1983) 313-321

40. Scanlon PW, Rhodes RE, Woolner LB et al.: Cancer of the nasopharynx: 142 patients treated in the 11 year period 1950-1960. Amer. J. Roentgenol. 99 (1967) 313-325
41. Schmauz R, Templeton AC: Nasopharyngeal carcinoma in Uganda. Cancer 29 (1972) 610-621
42. Schmincke A: Über lympho-epitheliale Geschwülste. Beitr. Path. Anat. 58 (1921) 161-170
43. Sesterhenn J, Sesterhenn K, Hyams V et al.: Demonstration of keratin antigens in undifferentiated carcinoma of the nasopharyngeal type and malignant lymphomas - a contribution of practical differential diagnoses. In Prasad U, Ablashi DV, Levine PH et al. (Eds): Nasopharyngeal Carcinoma - Current Concepts, pp. 47-54. Kuala Lumpur: University of Malaya Press 1983
44. Shanmugaratnam K: The pathology of nasopharyngeal carcinoma. In Biggs PM, de Thé G, Payne LN (Eds): Oncogenesis and Herpes Viruses, pp. 239-248. Lyon: IARC 1972. (IARC Sci. Publ., No. 2)
45. Shanmugaratnam K: Histological typing of nasopharyngeal carcinoma. In de Thé G, Ito Y (Eds): Nasopharyngeal Carcinoma: Etiology and Control, pp. 3-12. Lyon: IARC 1978. (IARC Sci. Publ., No. 20)
46. Shanmugaratnam K, Chan SH, de Thé G et al.: Histopathology of nasopharyngeal carcinoma: Correlation with epidemiology, survival rates and other biological characteristics. Cancer 44 (1979) 1029-1044
47. Shanmugaratnam K, Muir CS: Nasopharyngeal carcinoma: Origin and structure. In Muir CS, Shanmugaratnam K (Eds): Cancer of the Nasopharynx, pp. 153-162. Copenhagen: Munksgaard 1967. (UICC Monograph Series, 1)
48. Shanmugaratnam K, Sobin L (Eds): Histological Typing of Upper Respiratory Tract Tumours. Geneva: WHO 1978. (Int. Histological Typing of Tumours, No. 19)
49. Shi S-R, Goodman ML, Bhan AK et al.: Immunohistochemical study of nasopharyngeal carcinoma using monoclonal keratin antibodies. Amer. J. Pathol. 117 (1984) 53-63
50. Sugano H, Sakamoto G, Sawaki S et al.: Histopathological types of nasopharyngeal carcinoma in a low-risk area: Japan. In de Thé G, Ito Y (Eds): Nasopharyngeal Carcinoma: Etiology and Control, pp. 27-39. Lyon: IARC 1978. (IARC Sci. Publ., No. 20)
51. Svoboda DJ, Kirchner FR, Shanmugaratnam K: Ultrastructure of nasopharyngeal carcinomas in American and Chinese patients. An application of electron microscopy to geographic pathology. Exp. mol. Path. 4 (1965) 189-204
52. Teoh TB: Epidermoid carcinoma of the nasopharynx among Chinese, a study of 31 necropsies. J. Path. Bact. 73 (1957) 451-465
53. Uhlmann C, Krueger GRF, Sesterhenn K et al.: Nasopharyngeal and adjacent neoplasms: A clinico-pathologic and immunologic study. Arch. Otorhinolaryng. 218 (1978) 163-177
54. Williams PL, Warwick R (Eds): Grays Anatomy. 36th Ed. Edinburgh: Churchill Livingston 1980
55. Wilmes E, Wolf H, Deinhardt F et al.: EBV serology in NPC and related malignancies. In Grundmann E, Krueger GRF, Ablashi DV (Eds): Nasopharyngeal Carcinoma, pp. 145-150. Stuttgart: Fischer 1981. (Cancer Campaign, Vol. 5)
56. Weiland LH: Clinical pathology of nasopharyngeal carcinoma: Current Studies. In Prasad U, Ablashi DV, Levine PH et al. (Eds): Nasopharyngeal Carcinoma - Current Concepts, pp. 35-38. Kuala Lumpur: University of Malaya Press 1983
57. Wustrow J, Karpinski A, Haas W et al.: Correlation of histological NPC tumor types with local and peripheral T- and B-cell values. In Grundmann E, Krueger GRF, Ablashi DV (Eds): Nasopharyngeal Carcinoma, pp. 193-199. Stuttgart: Fischer 1981. (Cancer Campaign, Vol. 5)
58. Yeh S: A histological classification of carcinomas of the nasopharynx with a critical review as to the existence of lymphoepitheliomas. Cancer 15 (1962) 895-920

Prospective Study of Serum VCA-IGA Antibody in the Normal Population in Guangdong Province of China

Li Chen-Chuan, Chen Ai-Mei, and Liang Yi-Ren

Nasopharyngeal carcinoma (NPC) is one of the most common malignancies in the Guangdong province of China. It represents 31.5% of all malignant tumors based on the hospital registry in this province [1]. A number of studies have demonstrated the higher serological reactivity to EBV-associated antigens among NPC patients compared with controls, independent of race and geography. Over 90% of NPC patients were positive for IgA antibodies to VCA at 1:10 dilution, as opposed to 0.6–6.0 in the control groups. GMTs of VCA-IgA were approximately 25-fold higher in NPC patients than in the various control groups [2]. But how about the EBV serology reactivity for normal individuals? There is very little information on this aspect.

During the year of 1983, a mass screening by serum VCA-IgA antibody detection was carried out on a series of 12273 persons from the normal population in Guangdong province. The purpose of this serological study was to investigate the presence of antibodies to the EBV-VCA antigen and the prospective follow-up of individuals with positive reactivity to the VCA antigen in order to find out early NPC cases.

Materials and Methods

A minimal amount of blood was taken from the fingertip of each of 12273 persons and tested by immunoenzymatic assay in which the kit was prepared by the Shanghai Bioproduct Institute. The assay method was the same as the routine indirect immunoenzymatic method [3].

Results and Analysis

1. Table 1 shows the results of serum VCA-IgA antibody detection for 12273 members of the normal population in Guangdong Province. The positive detection rate for males was 5.62% and for females 7.20%; the average was 6.25%. There was no significant difference ($P > 0.05$).
2. The results of serum VCA-IgA antibody detection for the normal population by sex, age, and titer distribution are shown in Table 2. Among 767 persons with positive results, 80% had titers of antibody $\leq 1:10$ and $20\% \leq 1:20$.
3. Nasopharyngeal carcinoma detection rate among those with positive serum VCA-IgA antibody: among 12273 blood samples, 767 showed positive results; and a re-checkup for serum VCA-IgA antibody and a clinical examination were

Cancer of the Liver, Esophagus, and Nasopharynx
Edited by G. Wagner and Zhang You-Hui

Table 1. The result of serum VCA-IgA antibody detection in 12273 persons from the normal population in Guangdong province

	No.	%	No. of Positives	% of Positives
Male	7414	60.4	417	5.62
Female	4859	39.6	350	7.20
M+F	12273	100.0	767	6.25

Table 2. Results of serum VCA-IgA antibody detection by sex, age, and titer distribution

Age groups	Males								Females						M+F
	(−)	1:5	1:10	1:20	1:40	1:80	1:160	1:320	(−)	1:5	1:10	1:20	1:40	1:80	
0-									1						1
5-	4		1						2						7
10-	9	1		1					8						19
15-	175	3	1	1					178	6	5				369
20-	767	10	7	2					663	37	17	6		1	1510
25-	859	18	11	2					688	16	19	7	1	1	1622
30-	953	24	15	3			1		825	27	22	9	2		1881
35-	736	16	18	7					608	23	8	5	1		1422
40-	919	26	18	8[a]	2	1	1		553	16	15	6			1565
45-	986	32	27	5		1			579	31	14	10	3	1	1689
50-	835	29	30	9	2	7[b]		1[a]	272	15	3	9			1212
55-	480	19	14	11	2	1			79	7	4				617
60-	193	7	5	5	2				34	1	1				248
65-	51	1	3	4				1[a]	10						70
70-	30	1							9		1				41
M+F	6997	187	150	58	8	10	2	2	4509	179	109	52	7	3	12273

[a] NPC patient detected
[b] Two NPC patients

Table 3. Comparison of VCA-IgA antibody detection among three main dialect groups in Guangdong province

	No. of cases	No. of positives	% of positives	No. of NPC cases	Detection rate of NPC/100000
Cantonese group	9205	587	6.38	5	54.3
Hakka group	809	64	7.91	0	0
Southern Fukeinese group	579	23	3.97	0	0
Other provinces	1680	93	5.54	0	0
Total	12273	767	6.25	5	40.7

conducted for these serum VCA-IgA-positive persons. A nasopharyngeal biopsy was carried out for those persons with high titer of VCA antibody (≤1:20) and suspicious lesions. Up to December 1983, five NPC patients were confirmed by pathological examination. The distribution of VCA antibodies ranged from 1:20 to 1:320, GMT 104.71. All five persons were males. Thus, the detection rate for the normal population by serum VCA-IgA antibody detection was 40.7/100000 (5/12273) (Table 3). The detection rate of NPC for males was 67.4/100000 (5/7414).

All these five NPC patients detected in our series were males above 40 years of age and Cantonese dialect-speaking people. Thus the NPC detection rate for males above 40 years of age was 143.1/100000 (5/3494) (Table 4); for Cantonese dialect-speaking males aged above 40 years it was 179.7/100000 (5/2783) (Table 5). Thus, it seems that the high-risk people for NPC were the Cantonese dialect-speaking males aged above 40 years. We plan to follow up these 767 persons with positive results, especially those with titers higher than 1:20, in order to facilitate the early diagnosis of NPC. Up to December 1983, we reexamined these persons by the serum VCA-IgA method; another two persons with high titers (1:160) of VCA-IgA antibody and EA-IgA antibody-positive were discovered (Table 2). These two persons are highly suspect of having NPC, and close observation of these persons is needed. These two persons are also 40 years of age and Cantonese dialect-speaking males, but a nasopharyngeal biopsy has not been taken because no suspicious lesion has been found.

Table 4. Serum VCA-IgA-positive and NPC cases detected among different dialect groups above 40 years of age

	No. of detections	No. of (+)	%	NPC cases	Detection rate (/100000)
Male	3494	275	7.87	5	143.1
Female	1536	137	8.92	0	0
M+F	5442	412	7.57	5	91.0

Table 5. Positivity (%) of serum VCA-IgA-positive and NPC cases detected among Cantonese people

	No. of detections	No. of (+)	%	NPC cases	Detection rate (/100000)
Male	2783	207	7.44	5	179.1
Female	1777	99	8.41	0	0
M+F	3960	306	7.73	5	126.3

4. Concerning the different dialect groups in a series of 12273 persons in the normal population, no NPC patient was detected except in Cantonese dialect-speaking people.

In summary, the results of EBV-VCA-IgA antibody detection among 12273 Chinese in Guangdong province are that five NPC patients were found among 767 persons with positive results. These five patients were males above 40 years of age, all speaking Cantonese dialect. These results suggest that Cantonese-speaking males above 40 years of age should be considered at high risk for NPC. This finding will be beneficial for the discovery and early diagnosis of NPC.

References

1. Li C-C: NPC Epidemiology, Risk Factors and Screening for Early Detection, in Marks PA (Edit.): New York: Grune & Stratton 1980
2. Li W-J et al.: Report on the Results of Serum VCA-IgA Detection by Using Immune Enzymatic Method for 1006 Cases of Pretreated Nasopharyngeal Carcinoma and 2114 Controls. WHO/WPRO Report of the Symposium on NPC, Guangzhou, China, Dec. 7-10, 1981. Manila 1982
3. Liu Y-X: Detection of EB Virus-Specific IgA Antibody from Patients with Nasopharyngeal Carcinoma by Immunoenzymic Method. J. Chinese Oncology 1 (1979) 8

Prospective Studies on Nasopharyngeal Carcinoma and Epstein-Barr Virus Inducers

Zeng Yi

Nasopharyngeal carcinoma (NPC) is common in southern China. The purpose of our studies was first to find simple and sensitive techniques that can be conveniently applied in the high-risk NPC areas for the early detection of NPC, and second to clarify the role of Epstein-Barr (EB) virus, environmental, and genetic factors in the development of NPC.

Prospective Studies

Serological mass surveys of NPC and follow-up studies on the EB virus IgA/VCA antibody-positive persons were carried out in Zangwu county of Guangxi Autonomous Region by an immunoenzymatic test [1, 2, 3]. NPC patients could be detected in their early stage, but it is rather difficult to carry out follow-up studies because many IgA/VCA antibody-positive persons live in remote areas, and clinical examinations are not carried out periodically for some persons. Therefore, another serological mass survey has been carried out in Wuzhou city since 1980 [4, 5]. Altogether 20726 persons aged 40 years and older were examined and the antibody-positive persons were followed up for 4 years. As shown in Table 1, among 20726 persons examined 1136 persons had the IgA/VCA antibody; the positive rate was 5.5%. From them 18 NPC patients were diagnosed clinically and histologically. Ten were at stage I, 6 at stage II, and 2 at stage III. The IgA/VCA antibody-positive persons were reexamined clinically and histologically once a year for 4 years; during this period 17 additional NPC cases were diagnosed, 5 at stage I, 11 at stage II, and 1 at stage III. Thus 16 of the 17 cases (94.1%) were in the early stages. The only stage III case had an antibody titer of 1:40 in the first bleeding, and some suspected lesions were found in the nasopharyngeal mucosa, but this patient refused to have a biopsy

Table 1. Clinical stage of NPC patients found in a mass survey and in the outpatient clinic

		Clinical stages				Total
		I	II	III	IV	
Screening action	Number of cases	15	17	3	0	35
	%	43.0	48.5	8.5	–	100.0
Outpatient clinic	Number of cases	18	312	526	180	1036
	%	1.7	30.1	50.8	17.4	100.0

Cancer of the Liver, Esophagus, and Nasopharynx
Edited by G. Wagner and Zhang You-Hui

taken, and the NPC developed into stage III 2 years and 8 months later. Altogether 35 NPC patients were detected, among them 15 cases (43%) at stage I and 17 (48.5%) at stage II; the early cases (I + II) amounted to 91.5%. The detection rate of early cases is 2.9 times higher than that of the outpatient clinic. IgA/VCA antibodies could be detected 16-41 months prior to the clinical diagnosis of NPC patients (Table 1). No NPC patients were found among 19590 persons without IgA/VCA antibody for a period of 4 years. If IgA/VCA-positive persons are examined routinely once a year, NPC patients can be detected at an early stage.

The detection rate of NPC in IgA/VCA antibody-positive persons is 61.6 times the annual incidence of NPC in the general population of the same age group. These results further indicate that the EB virus plays an important role in the development of NPC and that serological screening and follow-up studies are valuable for the early detection of NPC.

Epstein-Barr Virus Inducers

Our previous data showed that the geometric mean titer of complement-fixing antibodies to EB virus in sera from persons aged 20 years and older in high-risk areas for nasopharyngeal carcinoma (NPC) was significantly higher than that from persons of the same age group in NPC low-risk areas [6] and that the positive rate of IgA/VCA antibody to EBV from normal individuals in NPC high-risk areas increased with increasing age [1]. The detection rate of NPC from persons examined serologically and from IgA antibody-positive persons in some factories was much higher than that from the general population of the same age group in Wuzhou city [5]. Therefore, it is necessary to determine whether factors (inducers) causing an activation of the EB virus are present in foods, Chinese medical herbs, and other plant products.

Epstein-Barr Virus Early Antigen Induction in Raji Cells by Extracts from Plants

Ether extracts from more than 1693 plants including Chinese medicinal herbs were studied for the induction of EB virus EA in the Raji cell system. Fifty-three herbs were found to have inducing activity [7, 8].

Many such plants such as *Aleurites fordii, Sapium sebiferum, Wikstroemia indica,* and *Euphorbia antiquorum* grow in the NPC high-risk areas (Table 2).

Epstein-Barr Virus Activation in Raji Cells with Ether Extracts of Soil

The EB virus inducers were found in samples collected from the soil under tung oil trees *(Aleurites fordii), Wikstroemia indica, Sapium sebiferum, Euphorbia antiquorum,* and other plants growing in southern China where NPC is prevalent [9] (Table 3). Some vegetables grown on these soils also contained EB virus inducers [10].

Table 2. Effect of extracts from plants on EB virus induction in Raji cells. Four millimolar n-butyrate alone gave a 0.4%-1% positive rate

Extract from plants (1-12.5 r/ml)	EA-positive cells (%)
Euphorbia humifusa	40
Euphorbia helioscopia	36.4
Euphorbia antiquorum	36
Sapium sebiferum	24.8
Croton lachnocarpus	22.4
Euphorbia lunulata	17.2
Aleurites fordii (tung oil tree)	42
Daphne genkwa	46
Stellera chamaejasme	46
Wikstroemia chamaedaphne	53
Wikstroemia indica	50
Edgeworthia chrysantha	43
Caesalpinia sappan	8
Desmodium styracifolium	6
Premna fulva	42
Sparganium stoloniferum	16
Daturamonium	50
Tinospora sp.	7
Aleuritopleris argentea	17
Clematis intricata	3
Belamcanda chinesis	36
Ixeris debilis	9.2

Enhancement of Lymphocyte Transformation In Vitro

The enhancing effect of extracts from plants on the transformation of lymphocytes by EB virus was tested in a soft agar system. *Daphne genkwa, W. chamaedaphne, W. indica, Stellera chamaejasme,* and *Sparganium stoloniferum* were found to induce EA of EB virus in Raji cells and also to enhance the transformation of lymphocytes by EB virus; but some plants such as *Abrus fruticulosus* and *Bulbophyllum inconspicuum* had no inducing activity of EA and also no enhancing effect on transformation (Table 4) [11].

Enhancement of the Growth of Chicken Sarcoma and Papilloma by Extracts from Some Plants

The enhancing effect of extracts of *W. chamaedaphne* and *W. indica* on the growth of sarcoma was studied in chicken [12]. The weight of tumors in these two groups is 2.5-3.0 and 2.6-4.1 times higher than that in virus control groups, respectively (Table 5). The effect of the extracts on tumor promotion was also studied in mice [13]. There was no papilloma in the control group (DMBA), but the percentage of papilloma in mice in the croton oil, *W. chamaedaphne,* and *W. indica* groups was 77%, 35%, and 27%, respectively (Fig. 1). These results indicate that both *W. chamaedaphne* and *W. indica* act as croton oil (TPA) and are considered to be promotors.

Table 3. Induction of EB virus EA in Raji cells by extracts of soil samples from Wuzhou city and Zangwu county. Controls: B (n-butyrate) + C (croton oil) = 45.7%; B only = 0.4%; C only = 0.8%; untreated Raji cells = 0%; NT, not tested

Soil samples	Positive sample No.	EBV EA-positive cells (%) Ether extract (γ/ml)		
		10	2	0.4
Under tung oil trees	15	25.0	14.0	2.6
along the road and	3	14.0	11.4	0.6
the Western River	5	10.6	0.0	0.0
(11/19+)	8	4.0	3.0	2.0
	11	2.6	0.6	6.0
	2	1.4	2.2	1.4
	1	2.0	0.6	1.0
	14	0.0	1.8	1.0
	17	0.8	1.2	1.6
	18	1.4	0.6	0.8
	4	1.0	0.0	0.0
Under tung oil trees	35	6.6	9.6	4.6
along the road and	21	8.0	2.8	2.0
the Kui River	31	2.0	8.0	1.0
(8/20+)	22	0.0	4.0	0.0
	23	8.0	1.6	0.4
	36	2.0	1.0	2.0
	29	2.0	0.4	0.8
	39	0.6	0.8	1.4
From the dock of Western River (1/4+)	41	2.0	0.6	0.8
Under				
Codiacum variegatus	76	2.8	8.0	6.0
Codiacum variegatus	77	8.0	6.0	1.6
Codiacum variegatus	78	2.0	8.0	12.0
Euphorbia milli	80	NT	4.0	30.0
(4/4+)				

Table 4. Enhancing effect of extracts from some plants on the transformation of human lymphocytes by EB virus. TPA (5 ng/ml), 186; $P < 0.05$–0.01

Plant extract	Concentration (r/ml)			
	0	0.2	2	20
Stellera chamaejasme	68	131 (1.9)[a]	187 (2.8)	254 (3.7)
Wikstroemia chamaedaphne	68	158 (2.3)	210 (3.1)	190 (2.9)
Daphne genkwa	68	160 (2.4)	210 (3.1)	229 (3.4)
Wikstroemia indica	68	111 (1.6)	200 (2.9)	280 (4.1)
Sparganium stoloniferum	63	137 (2.2)	161 (2.6)	284 (4.5)
Bulbophyllum inconspicuum	55	40 (0.7)	40 (0.7)	42 (0.7)
Abrus fruticulosus	55	44 (0.8)	42 (0.7)	48 (0.8)

[a] Ratio of colonies in experimental group to colonies in control group

Table 5. Enhancing effect of extracts of *Wikstroemia chamaedaphne* and *W. indica* on the growth of chicken sarcoma by Rous sarcoma virus. Virus control, 346 mg; ratio = experimental group / virus control group

	Control (ethyl alcohol)	*Wikstroemia chamaedaphne* (mg)		*Wikstroemia indica* (mg)	
Concentration	10%	0.5	2.5	0.02	0.1
Weight of tumor (mg)	458	850	1050	900	1444
Ratio	1	2.5	3.0	2.6	4.1

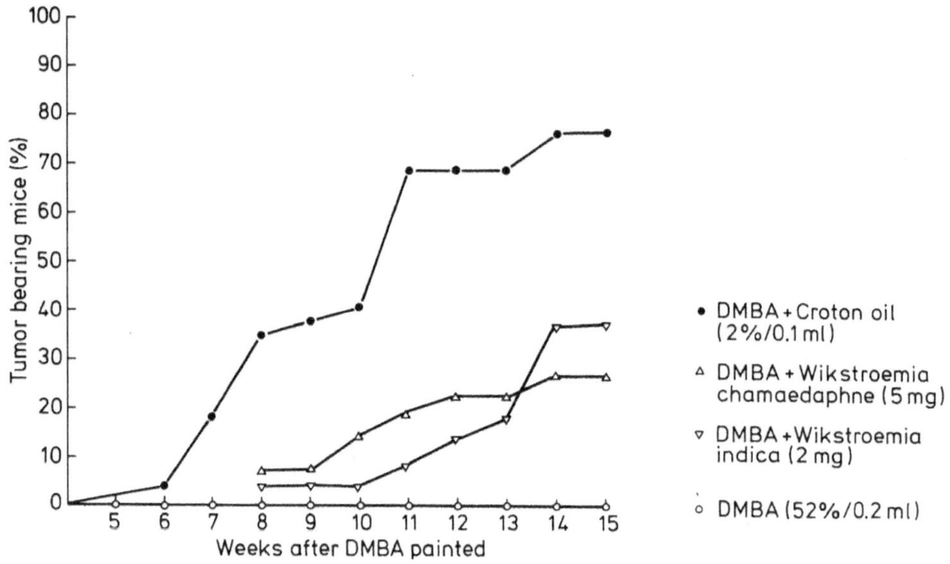

Fig. 1. Effect of plant extracts on tumor promotion

Table 6. Enhancement of cervical cancer in mice by *Wikstroemia chamaedaphne* (WC) and HHPA. Comparing data from groups C, D, and E, the difference is significant ($P < 0.05$)

Groups	No. of mice	Total cancer	%	Invasive cancer	%
WC	38	0	0	0	0
HHPA	36	0	0	0	0
MCA	23	13	56.5	4	30.7
WC + MCA	29	24	82.8	21	87.5
HHPA + MCA	45	38	84.4	30	78.5

Enhancement of Cervical Carcinoma in Mice by *Wikstroemia chamaedaphne* and HHPA

The enhancing effect of *W. chamaedaphne* (WC) and of HHPA on cervical cancer induced by methylcholanthrene (MCA) was studied in mice (Table 6). The ratio of cancer induced by WC extract and HHPA with MCA was 82.5% and 84.4%, and the rate for invasive cancer (later stage) was 87.5% and 78.5% respectively. The incidence of cancer in the control groups (MCA alone) was significantly lower, with a ratio of 56.5% (noninvasive) and 30.7% (invasive). These data indicate that WC extracts and HHPA enhance the development of cervical carcinoma in mice [14].

Some extracts from plants including Chinese medicinal herbs were found to have an inducing activity of early antigen in Raji cells, to enhance the transformation of lymphocytes by EB virus in vitro, and to enhance tumor growth by Rous sarcoma virus, DMBA, and MCA in vivo. These data indicate that some extracts from plants acting as TPA could activate EB virus and were considered to be tumor promotors. There might be a relationship between the activation of EB virus by certain environmental factors and the development of NPC, but this requires confirmation.

References

1. Zeng Y, Liu YX, Liu CR et al.: Application of Immunoenzymatic Test and Immunoautoradiographic Method for the Mass Survey of Nasopharyngeal Carcinoma. Chin. J. Oncol. 1 (1979) 2-7 and Intervirology 13 (1980) 162-168
2. Zeng Y, Liu YX, Wei JN et al.: Serological Screening of Nasopharyngeal Carcinoma. Acta Acad. Med. Sin. 1 (1979) 123-126
3. Zeng Y, Zhong JM, Li LY: Follow-up Studies on Epstein-Barr Virus IgA/VCA Antibody-positive Persons in Zangwu County, China. Intervirology 20 (1983) 190-194
4. Zeng Y, Zhang LG, Li HY et al.: Serological Mass Survey for Early Detection of Nasopharyngeal Carcinoma in Wuzhou City, China. Int. J. Cancer 29 (1982) 139-141
5. Zeng Y, Zhang LG, Wu YC, et al: Prospective studies on nasopharyngeal carcinoma in Epstein-Barr Virus IgA/VCA Antibodies-Positive Persons in Wuzhon city, China Int. J. Cancer 36 (1985) 545-547
6. Tumor Control Team, Zhonshan County; Department of Microbiology, Zhongshan Medical College; Laboratory of Tumor Viruses, Institute of Cancer, Institute of Epidemiology, Chinese Academy of Medical Sciences: A Study on the Complement Fixing Antibody to EB Virus from Normal Individuals in Guangdong Province and Beijing. Chin. J. ENT 1 (1978) 23-25
7. Zeng Y, Zhong TM, Mo YK et al.: Epstein-Barr Virus Early Antigen Induction in Raji Cells by Chinese Medicinal Herbs. Intervirology 19 (1983) 201-204
8. Zeng Y, Ni HY, Ye SC et al.: Epstein-Barr Inducers in Plants and Chinese Medicinal Herbs. (Unpublished Data)
9. Zeng Y, Miao XC, Jiao B et al.: Epstein-Barr Virus Activation in Raji Cells with Ether Extracts of Soil from Different Areas in China. Cancer Lett. 23 (1984) 53-59
10. Zhong JM, Zeng Y: Epstein-Barr Virus Inducers in Vegetable Grown from the Soil Containing Inducers. (Unpublished Data)
11. Hu YL, Zeng Y: The Extract from some Chinese Herbs Enhanced the Transformation of Human Lymphocytes by EB Virus. Chinese J. Oncol 1 (1985) 417-419
12. Hu YL, Zeng Y: Wikstroemia chamaedaphne and Wikstroemia indica Enhanced the Tumor Growth by Rous Sarcoma Virus. (Unpublished Data)
13. Hu YL, Zeng Y: Wikstroemia chamaedaphne and Wikstroemia indica Enhanced the Tumor Growth by Methylcholanthrene in mice (Unpublished Data)
14. Sun Y, Chen MH, Zeng Y et al.: Tumor-promoting Effect of Diterpene Ester HHPA and Extract of Wikstroemia chamaedaphne on Cervical Cancer in Mice. (Unpublished Data)

Control of Epstein-Barr Virus-Related Disease

H. Wolf

Introduction

The Epstein-Barr virus (EBV) is the causative agent of infectious mononucleosis and has been linked as an etiological factor with nasopharyngeal carcinoma and possibly African Burkitt's lymphoma and B-cell lymphomas in immunologically deprived persons. Whereas infectious mononucleosis is the clinical manifestation of primary infection, which affects - with or without clinical symptoms - more than 90% of the population, the EBV-related neoplasias have to be considered as secondary diseases. The incidence of nasopharyngeal carcinoma (NPC) ranges from very low (0.1/100000/year) in most Western countries to very high (above 30/100000/year) in some areas of southeast Asia. It is the most frequent neoplasia of man in several areas of south China [22]. The diagnosis of EBV-related infections and neoplastic diseases is complicated by the fact that, following primary infection in the earlier years of life, the virus persists lifelong in the parotid gland of very probably all healthy individuals [26]. From epithelial cells of the parotid gland and possibly other sites of the oropharynx the virus is released into the saliva and can more or less continuously infect new lymphocytes in the oral cavity [15]. In the EBV-primed host, production of EBV in the peripheral lymphocytes seems to be inhibited by suppression or very early elimination of cells entering a lytic cycle of virus replication. Therefore, antibody titers to viral antigens, e.g., to virus capsid antigen (VCA) decline and may even become undetectable in case of antibodies to early antigens (EA) and the lymphocyte-detected membrane antigen ("LYDMA"). At any time there is about 1 in 10000 lymphocytes in the immune host, harboring latent EBV genomes and possessing the potential for indefinite growth when transplanted into tissue culture [7].

Whereas in most cells of those human tumors which are possibly virus-associated like primary liver carcinoma or cervical carcinoma viral sequences seem to be integrated into the host genome. This event seems to be rare and dispensable for the immortalizing activity of EBV. It has been shown that EBV DNA is able to persist over extended periods in an episomal form [23], although a low level of integration has been demonstrated [13]. The origin of replication of these episomes has been mapped in the *Bam*C fragment of EBV-DNA [31]. For the activity of this origin, a further EBV gene encoding EBNA 1 has to be present in *cis* or *trans*. The gene product binds tightly to the origin of replication and to an area in the *Bam*Q fragment [18]. Within the origin, an enhancer-like activity has been reported [11, 19] which may activate the transcription of a common 5′ end for the mRNAs encoding EBNA 1 and EBNA 2 and probably EBNA 3. Although the mechanisms of cell

Cancer of the Liver, Esophagus, and Nasopharynx
Edited by G. Wagner and Zhang You-Hui

interaction are not yet clear, further studies on the role of the transactive EBNA 1 gene and its likely cellular homologue [2, 10, 29] may be of importance. One of the interesting features of the EBNA 1 is that it is presumably ineffective in rodent cells, which may be a hint to the known tissue specificity of EBV. It is frequently quoted that B-lymphocytes are the primary site of viral latency, and apparently specific cells in the oropharynx [26] are responsible for a persistence of lytically infected cells. The significance of the observations on the biology of EBV is not understood. Neither do we know the exact routes of infection apart from the identification of a complement component, the C3d receptor as the cellular receptor for EBV [5], nor do we understand the maintainance of the apparently rather steady population of EBV genome-containing lymphocytes in the peripheral blood. For a recent discussion of the problems involved in viral persistence see [28].

Methods of Controlling EBV-related Diseases

Early Diagnosis and Subsequent Therapy

Due to the lifelong persistence of EBV and the frequent early infection it is difficult to control EBV-related diseases and particularly the condition of NPC. The regular presence of EBV-DNA in the epithelial tumor cells of NPC [30] suggests the diagnostic utilization of this finding.

Zeng and coworkers have used a simple aspirator to collect cells from the nasopharynx in order to detect viral nucleic acid [1]. The desire for a better cell yield and the possibility of cytological examination on aliquots of the collected material led to the development of specialized and improved equipment by our group [20], which is now also used for other problems such as screening for papilloma viral DNA in aspirates from the cervix [6]. The finding that EBV is produced in specific sites of the oropharynx has, however, made the results of earlier reports using cell aspirates [1] questionable as it is not clear by the techniques used whether early cancer cells, passively absorbed EBV, EBV-producing lymphocytes, or other lytically EBV-producing cells were the cause of the positive signals observed. In situ hybridization and characterization of the positive cells are the necessary next steps unless further help can be expected from this approach.

Chromosomal abnormalities, as they have been described for EBV-containing and EBV-free Burkitt type lymphomas, have not been reported for NPC. This is largely due to the fact that the attempts to grow this tumor in vitro have failed. The successful cultivation of several tumor biopsies in nude mice [3], however, and the development of efficient methods to prepare chromosomal smears directly from such xenografts seem to initiate new developments. This model can be used to study chromosomal modifications precisely. Preliminary data [24] did not show any gross abnormalities or any euploidies and, therefore, did not confirm earlier reports [4].

Development of Serological Test Systems

Based on the pioneering work of Henle et al. [8], serological tests became feasible which led the way to a mass application of serological tests for the early detection of NPC. Especially IgA antibodies to EBV-related antigens were found to be very use-

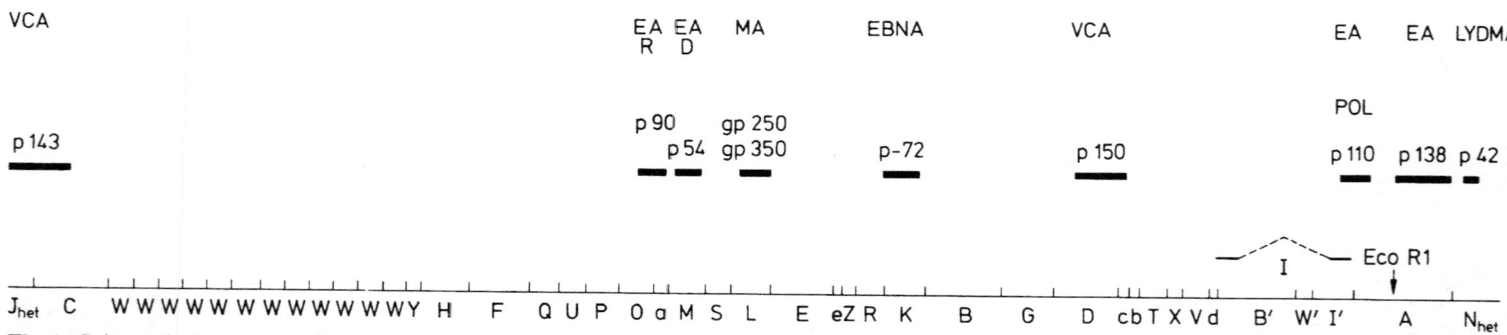

Fig. 1. Schematic drawing of the Epstein-Barr viral genome with *BamH1* restriction endonuclease sites and the location of diagnostically relevant antigens

ful for early diagnosis (for VCA and EA [25]; for MA [33]) and have already been used in a large field trial to assess the impact on the control of NPC [32]. The results are very encouraging (see [28]). Serological prescreening resulted in the detection of NPC in 86% of the NPC patients as compared with 29% in the noncontrolled population and thus allowed an increase of 57% in the fraction of patients with survival rates of almost 80% to over 90%.

Immunofluorescence tests or enzymatic tests derived therefrom [32] are, however, not acceptable in the long run for several reasons. The production of antigen is expensive and the quality of antigen is variable. The tests are laborious, are time consuming, and require expensive microscopes and experienced readers. Still, those sera cross-reacting with cellular antigens cannot be evaluated. Recombinant DNA technology has been used with good results to develop new test systems based on purer antigens. Series of immune precipitations using many separate sera collected from various donors and precipitating radioactively labeled proteins of EBV-producing superinfected Raji cells have been used to define viral gene products as antigens of value for diagnostic tests [27]. In vitro translation of viral mRNA hybrid selected with fragments of EBV-DNA has been used to map viral proteins on the genome [21]. Figure 1 shows the localization and designation of viral genes identified as being useful for diagnostic purposes.

Some of these genes could be expressed in *Escherichia coli* cells after subcloning into expression vectors. Table 1 gives an overview of the *E. coli*-derived EBV-related expression products which could be used for diagnostic purposes. We obtained the expression products of two early antigens, p138 and p54, of EBNA 1, of a virus capsid antigen (p150) and of the major membrane protein (gp350/250). Whenever it was possible, we tried to express the entire coding region (p54). It not, we

Table 1. Expressed EBV-specific proteins in *E. coli* and the host plasmids used.
pUC plasmid-derived proteins are products with only a small heterologous fusion partner; the transcription starts from a lac promotor; pUR plasmids generate large fusion proteins containing the bacterial β-galactosidase

EBV protein	Classification	Expression plasmid	Expressed amino acids of the total EBV protein (%)	Fused foreign amino acids (aa) or β-gal (116 kD)	
				C-terminal	N-terminal
p138	Early protein major DNA-binding protein	pUCARG 1140	375/1128 (33.2%)	6 aa	5 aa
EBNA I	Nuclear antigen, latently expressed in infected cells	pUC8KSH 1.2	191/641 (29.7%)	6 aa	-
p54	Early protein	pUC9MBcE 3.2	404/404 (100%)	14 aa	-
p150	Virus capsid antigen	pUR290CX-H580	185/1381 (13.4%)	β-gal + 14 aa	17 aa
gp250/350	Major membrane antigen	pURLP1.9	634/907 (69.9%)	β-gal + 4 aa	10 aa
gp250/350	Major membrane antigen	pUC19LP1.9	634/907 (69.9%)	9 aa	23 aa

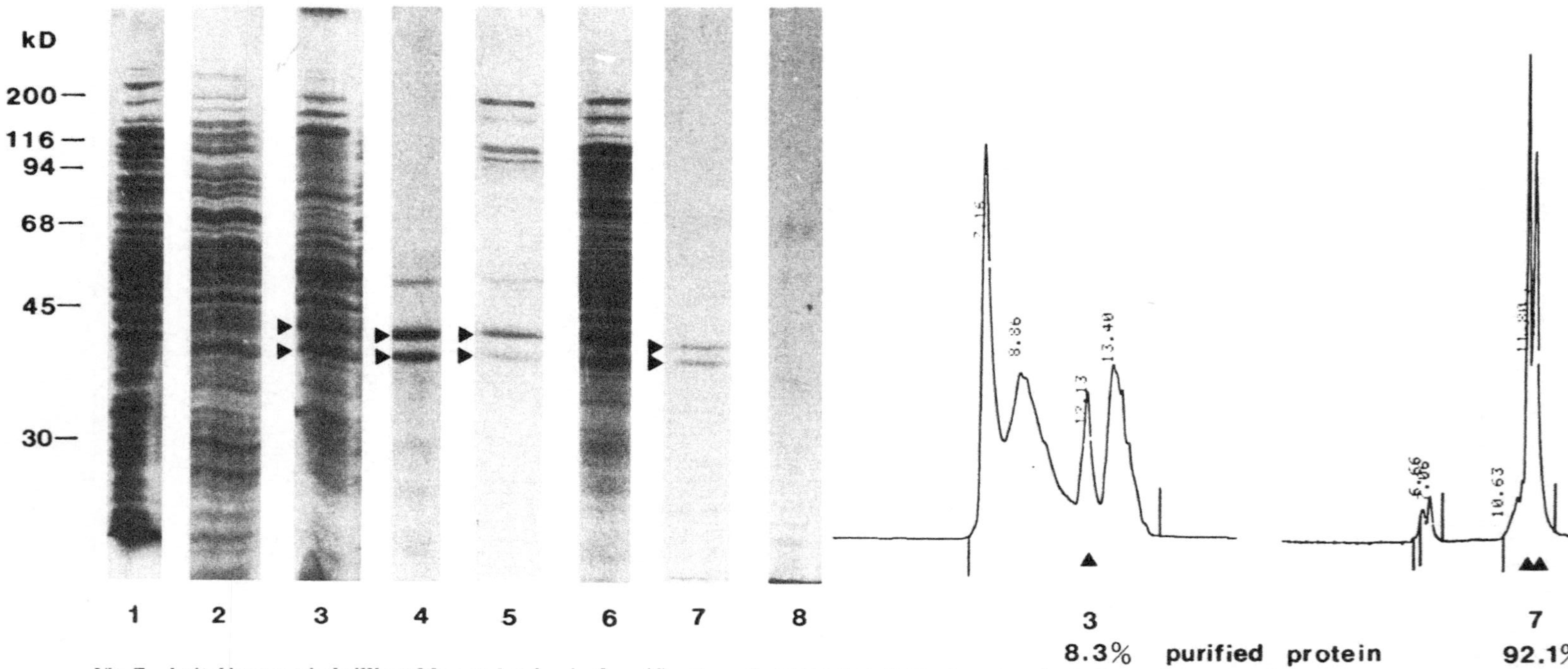

Fig. 2. *Left.* Coomassie brilliant blue stained gel of purification of pUC ARG 1140; the *triangles* indicate the antigenic bands. *1*, pUC 8 (negative control); *2*, bacterial lysate in 4 *M* urea/20 m*M* Tris pH 7.5; *3*, pellet from 2 in 8 *M* urea/20 m*M* Tris pH 7.5/0.1% SDS; *4*, gel filtration fractions 28–30; *5*, gel filtration fractions 73–75; *6*, gel filtration fractions 81–82; *7*, phosphocellulose (after gel filtration) unbound; *8*, phosphocellulose (after gel filtration) bound. *Right.* High-performance liquid chromatography with gel filtration chromatogram shows fractions 3 and 7 of the Coomassie brilliant blue stained gel. Mobile phase: 25 m*M* phosphate buffer pH 7.0 with 150 m*M* sodium chloride; flow rate, 1 ml/min; detector, UV (280 nm)

searched for antigenic parts using computer-aided predictions of antigenic epitopes. The antigenic parts were then expressed as β-galactoside fusion proteins (membrane antigen and capsid antigen) or, if possible, as protein parts with only a few foreign amino acids (EBNA 1 and p 138).

In the case of p 138, which besides p54 is of the highest specific significance for the detection of NPC as judged from the initial immune precipitations, the intact gene was not stably produced in sufficient quantities in *E. coli.* Computer-aided predictions of antigenic epitopes helped to identify two antigenic epitopes. These results were experimentally verified with fusion proteins containing various segments of the p 138 gene. The two antigens were found to be both necessary for detection of antibodies against p 138 in all NPC patients and were fused together into an autologous fusion protein, p 1140, which now has only a few fused bacterial sequences.

The use of the expression products allow the diagnosis and staging of EBV-associated disease [28]. Whereas IgM antibodies to the early antigens and structure proteins indicate a fresh infection, the appearance of IgG antibodies to EBNA and the membrane protein is a sign of past infection. IgA titers to early proteins give a very strong support for the diagnosis of NPC.

An effective application of this antigen set is given only in fast and cheap ELISA tests which are suitable for mass screenings of high-risk collectives. For this purpose it is necessary to purify the expression products from contaminating bacterial proteins which show background reactions as it can be seen in some blots of Fig. 2. An example for the purification is given for the pUC ARG 1140 encoded of the p 138 early protein (Fig. 2).

Figure 3 shows expression products derived from the various vectors after transfer to nitrocellulose, immunostaining with various sera, and antibody-class specific detection reaction. The high specificity of IgA antibodies for NPC diagnostics is clearly visible; in sera from persons without NPC no EBV-specific IgA antibodies are present.

Prevention or Delay of Infection

From the epidemiological work on HBV and its relation to primary liver cell carcinoma it may be concluded that delay of viral infection drastically reduces the cancer risk. It seems not unreasonable to draw similar conclusions for EBV and nasopharyngeal carcinoma. The major membrane antigen of EBV has been found to raise neutralizing antibodies in humans and test animals [15]. This gene has been mapped on the viral genome [9, 17]. Attempts to express this entire gene in bacteria in acceptable amounts failed, although segments of the gene were stably expressed as fusion proteins and some also as nonfusion proteins (Fig. 3). These virus-specific gene products gave rise to antibodies in immunized rabbits which recognized the native MA in virus-producing cells and exercized a neutralizing activity. The requirements for a potential vaccine to be a highly purified pyrogen-free product and the desire to use a product reflecting as authentically as possible the natural antigen were the reasons for expressing this gene in eukaryotic cells. The expression plasmid used as a selective marker the gene for dihydrofolate reductase (DHFR) and thus allows the amplification of the plasmid after transfection into DHFR-neg-

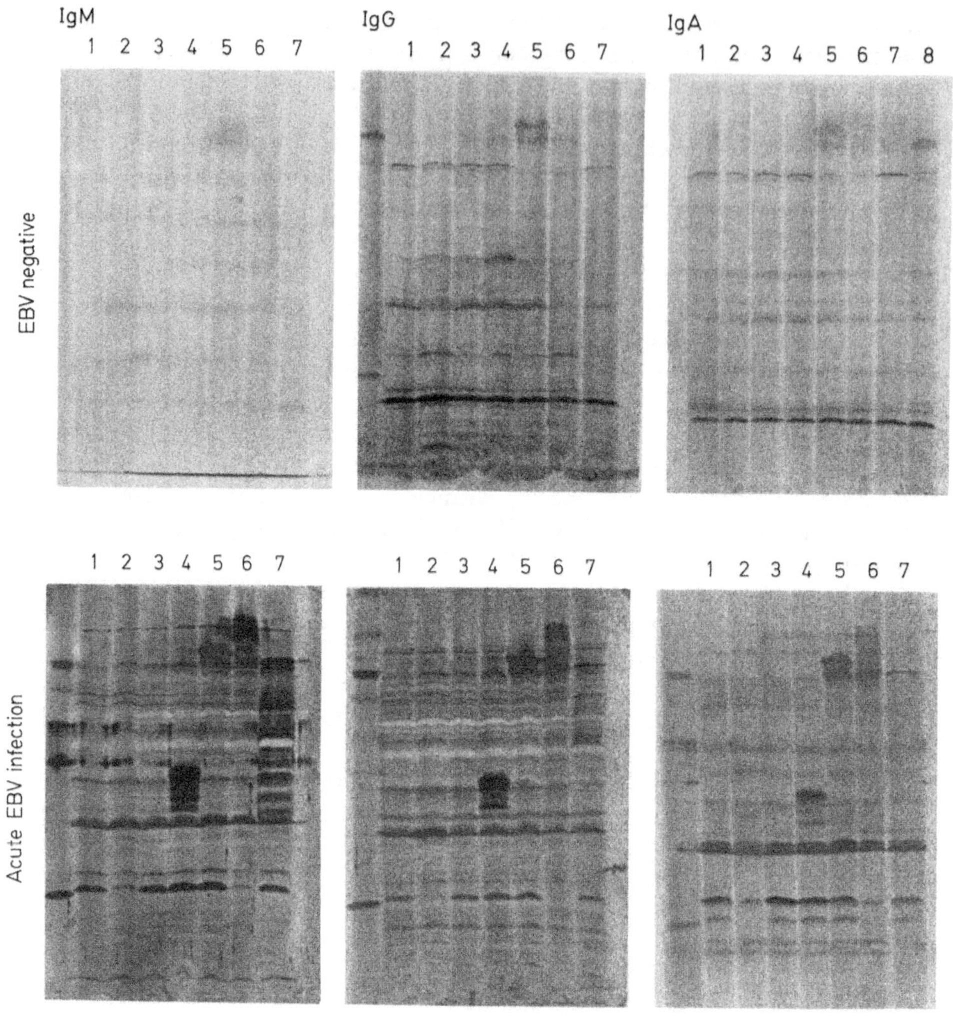

Fig. 3. Western blots of IPTG-induced *E. coli* carrying expression plasmids with the indicated EBV-specific proteins. For size and bacterial fusion parts see Table 1. pUC 8 and pUR 288 (β-galactosidase expression) were applied as negative controls. The bacterial lysates were separated on SDS-PAGE (17.5%), transferred to nitrocellulose, and immunostained with various sera pools (from EBV-negative persons, freshly infected, after infection, NPC patients) and antibody-class-specific second antibodies conjugated with peroxidase. The figure shows the significance and specificity of antibodies to virus proteins dependent on the state of EBV. The EBV-negative serum pool (first row) shows only background reaction.

After primary infection (infectious mononucleosis) a very strong IgM reaction can be observed, especially against the early protein p54 and the membrane protein. But there are no antobodies against the EBNA1 which is significant for latent EBV carriers (row 3 sera of persons with past EBV infection). For these individuals, antibodies of the IgG class to VCA and the membrane protein indicate a status of protection. No antibody titers against the early proteins can be seen.

If patients develop NPC, there is a clear change in antibody distribution and titer. No IgM-specific reaction can be observed in the IgG class; however, nearly all EBV-related expression products were recognized. The relevant diagnostic limit for this disease is the appearance of IgA antibodies to the early proteins p138 and p54

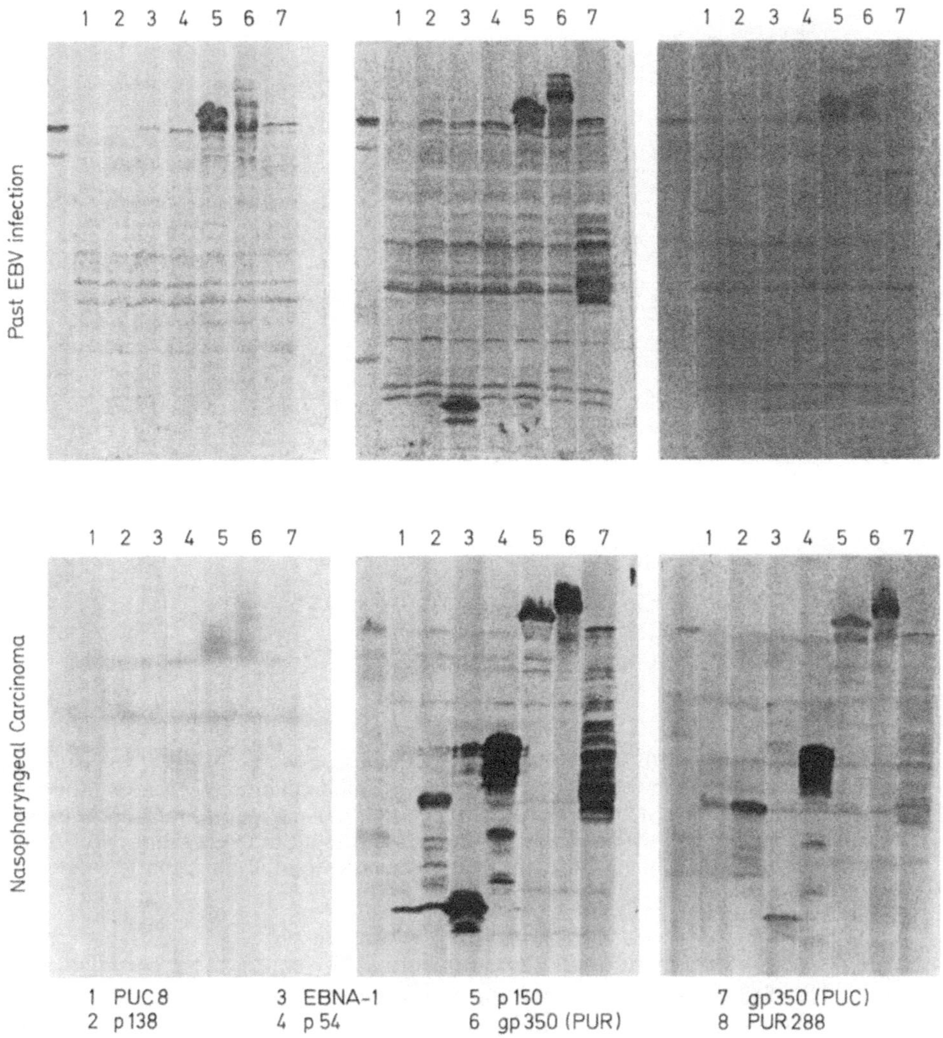

Fig. 3. (continued)

ative cells and the addition of selective pressure by increasing concentrations of methothrexate. Figure 4 shows the identification of MA reaction in a clone with monoclonal antibodies directed to gp350/250, showing that the gene is present in a spliced and unspliced form, reflecting the situation in EBV-producing cells. This product should be usable after appropriate purification as an antigen for immunization.

Because immunization with proteins may not achieve sufficient protection under the conditions of general application due to the lack of compliance with revaccination programs and furthermore due to the cost factors involved in the vaccine production, we [12, 16] have also inserted this gene into the thymidine kinase gene of vaccinia virus. This strategy should permit sufficient protection to control EBV-

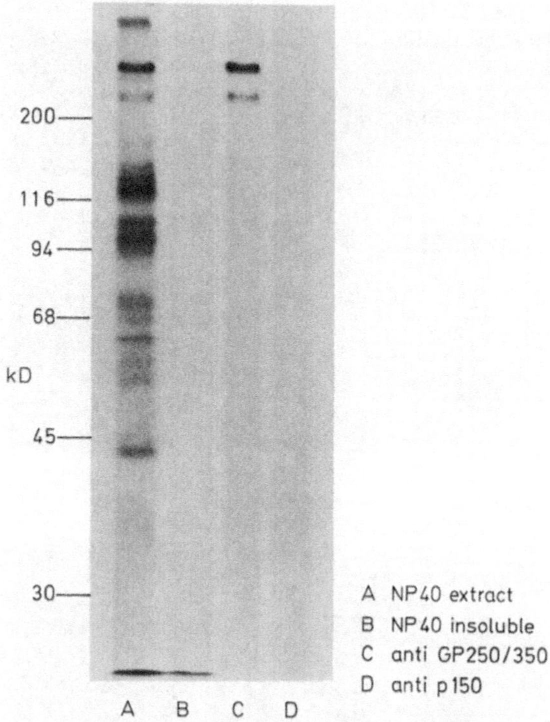

Fig. 4. Expression of gp250/350 in eukaryotic Chinese hamster ovary cells. The cells of a clone, which were found to be gp250/350-positive in an immunoluorescence test, were surface labeled with ^{125}iodine. *A*, NP40 extract of the labeled cells; *B*, pellet of the NP40 extract; *C*, immunoprecipitation of the NP40 extract with a monoclonal antibody against gp250/350; *D*, immunoprecipitation of the NP40 extract with antibodies to p150 (virus capsid antigen)

related diseases with a maximum of two injections. The enormous accumulated risk of up to 1% of the population developing NPC in the high-risk areas of southeast Asia and particularly China may outweigh a relatively small risk of complications following the application of vaccinia viruses. This risk can be further reduced if strains with stable lower or even undetectable neurotropism are used, such as the MVA strain [14].

Although prevention is clearly the idealistic goal for controlling EBV-related diseases, early detection is of immense importance, as most NPC patients in the coming 50 years will be already infected with EBV and are best protected by a continuous monitoring of EBV-related antibodies.

References

1. Desgranges C, de Thé G, Wolf H et al.: Further studies on the detection of the Epstein-Barr virus DNA in nasopharyngeal carcinoma biopsies from different parts of the world. In de Thé G, Epstein MA, zur Hausen H (Eds): Oncogenesis and Herpesviruses II, Part 2, pp. 191-193. Lyon: IARC 1975. (IARC Sci. Publ., No. 11)

2. Dillner J, Sternas L, Kallin B et al.: Antibodies against a synthetic peptide identify the Epstein-Barr virus determined nuclear antigen. Proc. nat. Acad. Sci. 81 (1984) 4652-4656
3. Ebbers J, Lindenberger J, Meyer zum Gottesberge-Orsulakova A et al.: Xenografting of nasopharyngeal carcinoma into athymic mice. (Submitted 1985)
4. Finerty S, Jarvis JE, Epstein MA et al.: Cytogenetics of malignant epithelial cells and lymphoplastoid cell lines from nasopharyngeal carcinoma. Brit. J. Cancer 37 (1978) 231-239
5. Fingeroth J, Weir J, Tedder T et al.: Epstein-Barr virus receptor of human B lymphocytes is the C3d receptor CR2. Proc. nat. Acad. Sci. 81 (1984) 4510-4514
6. Gissmann L, Wolnik L, Ikenberg H et al.: Human papillomavirus types 6 and 11 DNA sequences in genital and laryngeal papillomas and in some cervical cancers. Proc. nat. Acad. Sci. 80 (1983) 560-563
7. Henle W, Diehl V, Hohn G et al.: Herpes-type virus and chromosome marker in normal leukocytes after growth with irradiated Burkitt cells. Science 157 (1967) 1064-1065
8. Henle W, Henle G: Seroepidemiology of the virus. In Epstein MA, Achong B (Eds): The Epstein-Barr-Virus, pp. 61-78. Berlin: Springer 1979
9. Hummel M, Thorley-Lawson D, Kieff E: An Epstein-Barr virus DNA fragment encodes messages for the two major envelope glycoproteins (gp 350/300 and gp 220/200). J. Virol. 49 (1984) 413-417
10. Luka J, Kreofsky T, Pearson GR et al.: Identification and characterization of a cellular protein that cross-reacts with the Epstein-Barr virus nuclear antigen. J. Virol. 52 (1984) 833-838
11. Lupton S, Levine AJ: Mapping genetic elements of Epstein-Barr virus that facilitate extrachromosomal persistence of Epstein-Barr virus-derived plasmids in human cells. Mol. cell. Biol. 5 (1985) 2533-2542
12. Mackett M, Smith GL, Moss B: Vaccinia virus: a selectable eukaryotic cloning and expression vector. Proc. nat. Acad. Sci. 79 (1982) 7415-7419
13. Matsuo T, Heller M, Petti L et al.: Persistence of the entire Epstein-Barr virus genome integrated into human lymphocyte DNA. Science 226 (1984) 1322-1324
14. Mayr A, Stickl H, Müller HK et al.: The smallpox vaccination strain MVA: marker, genetic structure, experience gained with the parenteral vaccination and behavior in organisms with a debilitated defence mechanism. Zbl. Bakt. Mikrobiol. Hyg., 1. Abt. Orig. B 167 (1978) 375-390
15. Morgan DG, Miller G, Niedermann JC et al.: Site of Epstein-Barr virus replication in the oropharynx. Lancet 1979, II: 1154-1157
16. Motz M, Gu SY, Hou YT et al.: (In preparation)
17. Motz M, Seibl R, Wolf H: (In preparation)
18. Rawlins D, Milman G, Hayward SD et al.: Sequence specific DNA binding of the Epstein-Barr virus nuclear antigen (EBNA-1). 10th Int. Herpesvirus Workshop. Ann Arbor, MI 1985
19. Reisman D, Yates J, Sugden B: A putative origin of replication of plasmids derived from Epstein-Barr virus is composed of two *cis*-acting components. Mol. cell. Biol. 5 (1985) 1822-1832
20. Richter W, Gu SY, Seibl R et al.: A new method for examination of carcinomas of the nasopharynx. In Prasad U, Ablashi DV, Levine PH et al. (Eds): Nasopharyngeal Carcinoma - Current Concepts, pp. 25-32. Kuala Lumpur: University of Malaysia Press 1983
21. Seibl R, Wolf H: Mapping of Epstein-Barr virus proteins on the genome by translation of hybrid-selected RNA from induced P3HR-1 cells and induced Raji cells. Virology 141 (1985) 1-13
22. Simon MJ, Shanmugaratnam K (Eds): The Biology of Nasopharyngeal Carcinoma. Geneva: UICC 1982. (UICC Techn. Report Ser., Vol. 71)
23. Tanaka A, Nomoyama M, Hamper B: Partial elimination of latent Epstein-Barr virus genomes from virus-producing cells by cycloheximide. Virology 70 (1976) 167-170
24. Wienberg, Ebbers J, Wolf H: Unpublished
25. Wilmes E, Wolf H, Deinhardt F et al.: EBV-serology in NPC and related malignancies. In Grundmann E, Krueger GRF, Ablashi DV (Eds): Nasopharyngeal Carcinoma, pp. 145-150. Stuttgart: Fischer 1981. (Cancer Campaign, Vol. 5)

26. Wolf H, Haus M, Wilmes E: Persistence of Epstein-Barr virus in the parotid gland. J. Virol. 51 (1984) 795–798
27. Wolf H, Motz M, Kühbeck R et al.: Strategies to the economic preparation of Epstein-Barr virus proteins of diagnostic and protective value by genetic engineering: a new approach based on segments of virus-encoded gene products. In Williams et al. (Eds): Virus-associated Cancers, pp. 525–539. New York: Oxford University Press 1984
28. Wolf H, Motz M, Modrow S et al.: Epstein-Barr virus and nasopharyngeal carcinoma. In Viruses in Human Tumors. Basel: Karger (in press)
29. Wolf H, Seibl R: Benign and malignant disease caused by EBV. J. invest. Derm. 83 (1984) 88 s–95 s
30. Wolf H, zur Hausen H, Becker V: EB viral genomes in epithelial nasopharyngeal carcinoma cells. Nature, New Biol. 244 (1973) 245–247
31. Yates J, Warren N, Reisman D et al.: A *cis*-acting element from the Epstein Barr viral genome that permits stable replication of recombinant plasmids in latently infected cells. Proc. nat. Acad. Sci. 81 (1984) 3806–3810
32. Zeng Y, Zhang LG, Li HY et al.: Serological mass survey for early detection of nasopharyngeal carcinoma in Wuzhow City, China. Int. J. Cancer 29 (1982) 139–141
33. Zhu XX, Zeng Y, Wolf H: Detection of IgG and IgA antibodies to Epstein Barr virus membrane antigen in the sera from patients with nasopharyngeal carcinoma and normal individuals. Int. J. Cancer (in press)

The Role of Epstein-Barr Virus in Nasopharyngeal Carcinoma

G. W. Bornkamm

Introduction

Shortly after the discovery of the Epstein-Barr virus (EBV) in cultured Burkitt's lymphoma (BL) cells, the association of the virus with another human malignant disease became apparent. Old et al. [21] noted first that patients with nasopharyngeal carcinoma (NPC) have unusually high antibody titers against viral antigens. This finding has since been widely confirmed and extended (for review, see [7, 10]). NPC is characterized by particular epidemiological features. It is the most frequent cancer in adult males in some parts of south China, with an age peak between 45 and 55 years. It occurs, however, with a lesser frequency all over the world. The Mediterranean countries are known as areas with an intermediate risk. Remarkably, there is a second peak at the age of 10–20 years for the occurrence of NPC outside China.

The epithelial tumor cells harbor multiple copies of the viral genome and express the viral nuclear antigen EBNA [13, 23, 29, 33]. The viral DNA in the tumor cells is predominantly present in an episomal state [14].

The association of NPC with EBV is of practical importance for the diagnosis of the disease. The IgA antibodies against viral capsid antigen (VCA) and, less consistently, against early antigens (EA) are readily detectable in the serum of patients with NPC [9]. They provide, moreover, a useful tool for early diagnosis, since they are usually present before the clinical onset of NPC [12, 32] and also help to monitor the course of the disease [11].

The aspect of early diagnosis of NPC by the aid of EBV serology is the subject of Zeng's chapter and will not be treated here. I will review briefly what is known or, rather, what is not known about the role of EBV in the development of NPC. I will discuss in particular the physiological virus-host interaction and will try to relate the development of NPC to the physiology of a natural infection with the virus. Since so little is known about NPC, more questions will be raised than answers can be provided.

Is EBV Consistently Associated with NPC?

To answer this question, it is necessary to consider the histopathological classification of carcinomas located in the nasopharynx. The WHO classification discriminates between three types of tumors:

Cancer of the Liver, Esophagus, and Nasopharynx
Edited by G. Wagner and Zhang You-Hui

1. Keratinizing squamous cell carcinoma
2. Nonkeratinizing squamous cell carcinoma
3. Undifferentiated nasopharyngeal carcinoma

The first type, the keratinizing squamous cell carcinoma, is not associated with EBV. The third type, the undifferentiated tumor, is the type which is frequently observed in south China and which is invariably linked to EBV. The second group, the nonkeratinizing differentiated tumors, is not homogeneous with regard to the presence of EBV DNA. The subclassification into tumors with or without lymphoid infiltration has turned out to be useful in the sense that tumors with lymphoid infiltration are associated with EBV, whereas tumors without lymphoid infiltration are not related to the virus [15]. So far, there is no exception from the rule that the undifferentiated tumor following the characteristic epidemiological pattern is invariably linked to EBV.

Do Disease-Specific Subtypes of EBV Exist?

To study this question, we have characterized in detail the virus isolate M-ABA, which is derived from the tumor cells of a nasopharyngeal carcinoma transplanted into a nude mouse [6]. The restriction pattern of M-ABA EBV was compared with that of several other isolates from BL and other diseases and revealed no evidence of disease-specific subtypes [3]. Moreover, three distinct regions of M-ABA EBV encompassing about 7 kbp were sequenced and differed from those of B95-8 virus only at very few positions [17, Barrell, personal communication]. From the frequency of restriction fragment length polymorphisms we can conclude that the NPC-derived virus is as closely related to BL-derived isolates as any two isolates originating from other sources. Thus, we have to assume that a subtype of EBV which could account for the development of NPC does not exist.

Natural Infection and the Sites Suspected of Virus Production

Infection by EBV is mediated by close salivary contact. The primary infection is either asymptomatic or leads to the clinical picture of infectious mononucleosis (IM). This disease is characterized by the polyclonal proliferative response of the B-lymphocytes infected with the virus and the defense mechanisms of the immune system against this B-cell proliferation. Similarly to the infection of human B cells in vitro, the infection is nonproductive, giving rise to EBNA, but not VCA and EA expression in the infected cells. The white blood picture is dominated by the T-lymphocytes limiting the proliferative B-cell response. During the early phase of IM, virus-induced natural killer cells are dominant [28]. Later during the course of IM a specific T-cell response develops. The immune T-cells are able to eliminate the virus-infected cells in an HLA-restricted fashion. The antigen on the virus-infected cells is operationally defined as lymphocyte-detected membrane antigen (LYDMA) and is believed to be encoded by the virus [19, 24]. During the course of infectious mononucleosis and possibly lifelong thereafter, virus is excreted in the oropharynx and shed in the saliva, pointing to the oropharynx as the site of virus production.

Virus excretion is enhanced in immunosuppressed individuals, suggesting that the production of virus is modulated by the immune system [27, 31]. Even though the target cell for virus production has long been debated, there is general consent that epithelial cells in the oropharynx, rather than the nonproductively infected B-lymphocytes, replicate and shed the virus. The glandular epithelial cells of the salivary glands [20, 30] as well as the surface epithelial cells of the oropharynx [26] have been suspected as sites of virus production. Recently, by studying oral lesions called hairy leukoplakias in patients with AIDS, evidence has been provided by Greenspan et al. [8] that EBV is produced in epithelial cells of the lateral part of the tongue. It appears most likely that this is also a site of virus production in individuals not suffering from AIDS. The data suggest that EBV is latently maintained in the basal epithelial layer and is being produced when terminal differentiation of the epithelial cells is initiated. In this respect, EBV appears to mirror the behavior of papilloma viruses.

With the dual tropism, productive infection of epithelial cells and nonproductive infection of lymphocytes, EBV closely resembles Marek's disease virus (MDV), which replicates in the epithelial cells of feather follicles and which infects T-lymphocytes in a nonproductive fashion, giving rise to the development of T-cell lymphomas in chicken.

A number of questions remain unresolved. How does the virus enter the epithelial cells? Three different mechanisms may be considered. First, EBV only might infect a specific subclass of epithelial cells which carry a receptor for the virus. Secondly, EBV might replicate in the presence of a helper virus, giving rise to the formation of pseudotypes which can infect epithelial cells. Thirdly, fusion with EBV-infected lymphocytes might be an alternative way for the virus to enter the epithelial cells [2].

Another unresolved problem is how the production of the virus in the epithelial cells can be modulated by the immune system. Is the production of the virus related to the turnover of epithelial cells? And, if so, is the turnover of epithelial cells modulated by the immune system?

The urgent question with respect to the role of EBV in NPC is whether the target cell for virus production is related to the target cell of NPC. NPC might thus be considered as an "accident" where terminal differentiation and virus production is blocked and the cells continue to proliferate. In this context, it might be interesting to study other tumors, namely carcinomas of the tongue, for the presence of EBV DNA. It is noteworthy that a number of tumors other than NPC were reported to be associated with EBV, i.e., undifferentiated carcinomas of the parotid gland [16, 25], undifferentiated carcinomas of the thymus [18], poorly differentiated supraglottic laryngeal carcinomas [4], and undifferentiated or poorly differentiated carcinomas of the palatine tonsil [5].

This could point to a common developmental origin of the target cells of EBV-associated undifferentiated or poorly differentiated carcinomas in the primitive pharynx.

The characterization of the tumor cells of NPC by monoclonal antibodies, the search for the corresponding cells during embryonic development, and the elucidation of the possible relationship of this cell type to the lytic cycle of the virus remains an urgent and challenging task.

Are Viral Gene Functions Involved in the Malignant Growth of NPC Cells?

As stated earlier, NPC cells stain positive for EBNA. Up to now, no studies have been reported looking for an expression of distinct antigens in NPC cells by the use of monospecific antisera against EBNA 1, EBNA 2, the membrane antigen expressed in immortalized lymphocytes, or other antigens expressed during the abortive or lytic virus cycle. The only information we have about the transcriptional activity of the viral genome in NPC cells stems from the work of Raab-Traub et al. [22]. These data support the view that the genes transcribed in EBV-infected proliferating B-lymphocytes are also transcriptionally active in NPC cells and suggest a possible role of these genes for cell proliferation in this case, too.

Similarly to EBV-positive Burkitt's lymphoma, the question remains why the EBV genome-carrying tumor cells are not eliminated by the immune T-cells which recognize and kill the LYDMA-positive cells in an HLA-restricted fashion. The question whether LYDMA is expressed in NPC cells in concert with HLA class I genes and whether the tumor cells are accessible to the action of cytotoxic T-cells in vitro has not yet been addressed experimentally.

In some tumors transplanted into nude mice, RNA species were also detected which are transcribed only during the abortive or lytic cycle of the virus. It is not known whether an induction of an abortive or lytic cycle is also observed in human tumors in vivo.

Do Viral Genes Cooperate with Cellular Oncogenes in NPC?

Even though this is a very obvious question, nothing is known about oncogene activation in NPC. I do not know of any studies in which NPC DNA has been transfected into target cells to look for focus formation or growth in platelet-poor plasma. Moreover, I do not know of any recent cytogenetic studies in which the modern high-resolution banding technique has been used to look for chromosomal aberrations. This is obviously a gap which will have to be filled within the next few years.

Perspectives

Even though the association of EBV with NPC is very well documented, our understanding of the role of the virus in this malignancy is still at its very beginning. I have raised only some of the obvious open questions.

Besides the cytogenetic analysis with improved banding techniques and the search for activated oncogenes, the characterization of the target cell of NPC and the elucidation of its relationship to the target cell of virus production will be of primary importance for a better understanding of this tumor.

References

1. Andersson-Anvret M, Forsby N, Klein G, Henle W: Relationship between the Epstein-Barr virus and undifferentiated nasopharyngeal carcinoma: correlated nucleic acid hybridization and histopathological examination. Int. J. Cancer 20 (1977) 486-494
2. Bayliss GJ, Wolf H: An Epstein-Barr virus early protein induces cell fusion. Proc. Natl. Acad. Sci. USA 78 (1981) 7162-7165
3. Bornkamm GW, Delius H, Zimber U, Hudewentz J, Epstein MA: Comparison of Epstein-Barr virus strains of different origin by analysis of viral DNAs. J. Virol. 35 (1980) 603-618
4. Brichacek B, Hirsch I, Sibl O, Vilikusova E, Vonka V: Association of some supraglottic laryngeal carcinomas with EB virus. Int. J. Cancer 32 (1983) 193-197
5. Brichacek B, Hirsch I, Sibl O, Vilikusova E, Vonka V: Presence of Epstein-Barr virus DNA in carcinoma of the palatine tonsil. J. Natl. Cancer Inst. 72 (1984) 809-811
6. Crawford DH, Epstein MA, Bornkamm GW, Achong BG, Finerty S, Thompson JL: Biological and biochemical properties of isolates of Epstein-Barr virus from the malignant epithelial cells of two nasopharyngeal carcinomas. Int. J. Cancer 24 (1979) 294-302
7. Epstein MA, Achong BG (eds): The Epstein-Barr virus. Springer Verlag, Berlin-Heidelberg-New York 1979
8. Greenspan JS, Greenspan D, Lennette ET, Abrams DI, Conant MA, Petersen V, Freese UK: Replication of Epstein-Barr virus within the epithelial cells of oral "hairy" leukoplakia, an AIDS-associated lesion. N. Engl. J. Med. 313 (1985) 1564-1571
9. Henle G, Henle W: Epstein-Barr virus-specific IgA serum antibodies as an outstanding feature of nasopharyngeal carcinoma. Int. J. Cancer 17 (1976) 1-17
10. Henle W, Henle G: Epstein-Barr virus and human malignancies. In: Advances in Viral Oncology, Vol. 5, Klein G (ed), Raven Press, New York (1985) 201-238
11. Henle W, Ho JHC, Henle G, Chan JCW, Kwan HC: Nasopharyngeal carcinoma: significance of changes in Epstein-Barr virus-related antibody patterns following therapy. Int. J. Cancer 20 (1977) 663-672
12. Ho JHC, Kwan HC, Ng MN, de Thé G: Serum IgA antibodies to Epstein-Barr virus capsid antigen preceding symptoms of nasopharyngeal carcinoma cells. Lancet I (1978) 436
13. Huang DP, Ho JHC, Henle W, Henle G: Demonstration of Epstein-Barr virus-associated nuclear antigen in nasopharyngeal carcinoma cells from fresh biopsies. Int. J. Cancer 14 (1974) 580-588
14. Kaschka-Dierich C, Adams A, Lindahl T, Bornkamm GW, Bjursell G, Klein G: Intracellular forms of Epstein-Barr virus DNA in human tumour cells in vivo. Nature 260 (1976) 302-306
15. Krueger GRF, Wustrow J: Current histological classification of nasopharyngeal carcinoma (NPC) at Cologne University. In: Cancer Campaign, Vol. 5, Nasopharyngeal Carcinoma, Grundmann E, Krueger GRF, Ablashi DV (eds), Gustav Fischer Verlag, Stuttgart-New York (1981) pp. 11-16
16. Lanier AP, Bornkamm GW, Henle W, Henle G, Bender TR, Talbot ML, Dohan PH: Association of Epstein-Barr virus with nasopharyngeal carcinoma in Alaskan native patients: serum antibodies and tissue EBNA and DNA. Int. J. Cancer 28 (1981) 301-305
17. Laux G, Freese UK, Bornkamm GW: Structure and evolution of two related transcription units of Epstein-Barr virus carrying small tandem repeats. J. Virol. 56 (1985) 987-995
18. Leyvraz S, Henle W, Chaninian AP, Perlmann C, Klein G, Gordon RE, Rosenblum M, Holland JF: Association of Epstein-Barr virus with thymic carcinoma. New Engl. J. Med. 312 (1985) 1296-1299
19. Misko IS, Moss DJ, Pope JH: HLA antigen-related restriction of T lymphocyte cytotoxicity to Epstein-Barr virus. Proc. Natl. Acad. Sci. USA 77 (1980) 4247-4250
20. Morgan DG, Miller G, Niederman JC, Smith HW, Dowaliby JM: Site of Epstein-Barr virus replication in the oropharynx. Lancet II (1979) 1154-1157
21. Old LJ, Boyse EA, Oettgen HF, de Herven E, Geering G, Williams B, Clifford P: Precipitating antibody in human serums to an antigen present in cultured Burkitt's lymphoma cells. Proc. Natl. Acad. Sci. USA 56 (1966) 1691-1704

22. Raab-Traub N, Hood R, Yang C-S, Henry II B, Pagano JS: Epstein-Barr virus transcription in nasopharyngeal carcinoma. J. Virol. 48 (1983) 580-590
23. Reedman B, Klein G: Cellular localization of an Epstein-Barr virus (EBV)-associated complement-fixing antigen in producer and non-producer lymphoblastoid cell lines. Int. J. Cancer 11 (1973) 499-520
24. Rickinson AB, Wallace LE, Epstein MA: HLA-restricted T cell recognition of Epstein-Barr virus infected B cells. Nature 283 (1980) 865-867
25. Semundsen AK, Albeck H, Hansen JPH: Epstein-Barr virus in nasopharyngeal and salivary gland carcinomas in Greenland Eskimoes. Br. J. Cancer 46 (1982) 721-728
26. Sixbey JW, Nedrud JG, Raab-Traub N, Hanes RA, Pagano JS: Epstein-Barr virus replication in oropharyngeal epithelial cells. New Engl. J. Med. 310 (1984) 1225-1230
27. Strauch B, Andrews LL, Siegel N, Miller G: Oropharyngeal excretion of Epstein-Barr virus by renal transplant patients and other patients treated with immunosuppressive drugs. Lancet I (1974) 234-237
28. Svedmyr E, Jondal M: Cytotoxic effector cells specific for B cell lines transformed by Epstein-Barr virus are present in patients with infectous mononucleosis. Proc. Natl. Acad. Sci. USA 72 (1975) 1622-1626
29. Wolf H, zur Hausen H, Becker V: EB-viral genomes in epithelial nasopharyngeal carcinoma cells. Nature New Biol. 244 (1973) 245-247
30. Wolf H, Haus M, Wilmes E: Persistence of Epstein-Barr virus in the parotid gland. J. Virol. 51 (1984) 795-798
31. Yao QY, Rickinson AB, Gaston JSH, Epstein MA: In vitro analysis of the Epstein-Barr virus - host balance in longterm renal allograft recipients. Int. J. Cancer 35 (1985) 43-49
32. Zeng Y, Yuxi L, Chunren L, Sanwen C, Jihneng W, Jisong Z, Huijong Z: Application of an immunoenzymatic method and an immunoautoradiographic method for a mass survey of nasopharyngeal carcinoma. Intervirology 13 (1980) 162-168
33. zur Hausen H, Schulte-Holthausen H, Klein G, Henle W, Henle G, Clifford P, Santesson L: EBV DNA in biopsies of Burkitt tumours and anaplastic carcinomas of the nasopharynx. Nature 228 (1970) 1056-1058

The Role of Promotion in the Carcinogenesis of Nasopharyngeal Carcinoma

Yao Kai-Tai, Wu Peng-Nian, and Jiang Ji-Wen

It is well known that evidence for the chemical promotion of cocarcinogenesis was first provided by Berenblum. Subsequently, Mottram, Boutwell, Van Duren, and Hecker were responsible for defining many important aspects of the initiation and promotion of two-stage carcinogenesis. Recently, the concept of two-stage carcinogenesis has been extended to the carcinogenesis of the liver, urinary bladder, kidney, lung, and mammary gland [11]. As for nasopharyngeal carcinoma (NPC) carcinogenesis, the role of promotion largely remains to be explored.

Environmental Factors in the Pathogenesis of NPC

The association of Epstein-Barr (EB) virus with poorly differentiated or undifferentiated carcinoma of the nasopharynx is well known. But crucial evidence for supporting an etiological role of the EB virus in NPC is still lacking. Most probably some environmental factors are also important for the development of NPC.

In 1976, a general survey of cancer mortality was conducted in Hunan Province. The mortality rate of NPC in Hunan Province was lower than that in Guangdong, Guangxi, and Fujian, but higher than that of other provinces in China. The geographical distribution of NPC in Hunan has its peculiarities. There is a high-risk area in the west of Hunan, a mountain area, separated from Guangdong and Guangxi geographically (Fig. 1). The mortality rate of NPC in the south of Hunan is comparable to that in the west of Hunan, the high-risk center being located in Guangdong and Guangxi, as suggested by the trend surface analysis [14].

This distribution was confirmed by a survey of the NPC mortality rate which was conducted in 1980 [12]. Furthermore, a case-control study including 270 pairs was carried out [13]. The results of both studies indicated that the average exposure rate to firewood as a fuel showed a significant difference between NPC and controls (Table 1). The relative risk for firewood exposure was also high (Table 2). Moreover, 3,4-benzpyrene (3,4-BP) contents in smoke samples collected from a high-risk area were higher than those from a low-risk area [9]. But the preliminary study demonstrated that there was no difference in 3,4-BP contents between smoke samples from NPC patients and non-NPC inhabitants in the same area (Tables 3, 4). The data implied that some other factors were needed for the development of NPC.

Ho et al. [4] in Hongkong suggested that consumption of salted fish, especially when starting in early childhood, might be an important risk factor for NPC. Huang et al. [5] also reported that tumors in the nasal fossa of rats could be induced by feeding salted fish, which might contain a certain amount of nitrosamines [3]. Actu-

Cancer of the Liver, Esophagus, and Nasopharynx
Edited by G. Wagner and Zhang You-Hui

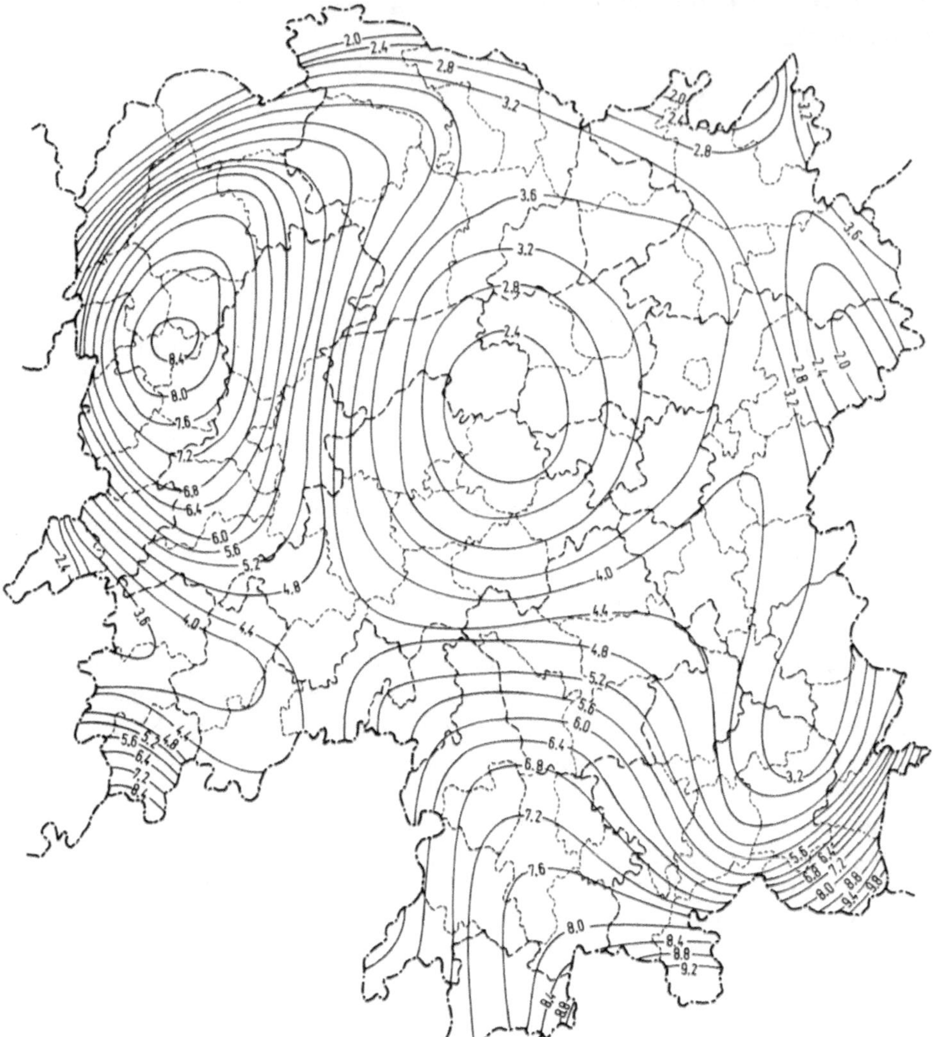

Fig. 1. Nasopharyngeal carcinoma mortality rates in Hunan Province; goodness of fit $C = 100\ (1 - P/Q = 18.047)$

ally, the fact that nasopharyngeal carcinoma of rats could be induced by nitrosamines had already been reported in the early 1970s [1]. Later [15], it was found that subcutaneous injection of N-dinitrosopiperazine took priority for inducing NPC in rats in respect to tissue specificity (Figs 2, 3). The significance of this animal model in the etiology of human NPC remains to be explored. The relationship of chemicals in the environment with the development of human cancer is very complicated, even if chemical factors in the environment play a major role in the development of a given cancer in different geographical areas. The intake of salted fish might play an important role in the pathogenesis of NPC in Hongkong, but it does not seem to

Table 1. Average exposure rate of housing, fuel, drinking water, and cereals in NPC patients and controls

Factor	No. of pairs	Average exposure rate (%)		Mean of difference	t	P
		NPC	Controls			
Housing						
Tile-roofed house	269	91.28	90.05	−0.28	−0.304	0.701
Thatched cottage	269	4.83	4.73	0.10	0.100	0.911
Old house	244	80.03	79.85	0.18	0.175	0.933
House without chimney	270	80.15	74.63	0.22	0.221	0.003
Fuel						
Hard coal	270	13.14	16.64	−3.70	−3.170	0.002
Soft coal	270	6.88	7.34	−0.47	−0.611	0.541
Firewood	270	63.33	59.02	4.32	2.673	0.008
Hay	270	13.31	13.48	−0.11	−0.100	0.920
Sources of drinking water						
Tap water	270	5.69	4.62	1.07	1.230	0.219
Well	270	51.07	55.51	−4.44	−2.107	0.035
River	270	13.73	12.84	0.89	0.524	0.600
Mountain brook	270	5.44	3.78	1.67	1.836	0.066
Pond	270	1.58	0.71	0.87	1.583	0.113
Spring	270	13.93	14.76	−0.82	−0.519	0.604
Ditch	270	0.73	0.09	0.64	1.396	0.163
Field puddle	270	1.04	1.22	−0.18	−0.286	0.774
Cereals						
Rice	270	75.88	76.47	−0.59	−0.807	0.420
Flour	270	1.98	1.24	0.74	2.308	0.021
Maize	270	6.43	7.16	0.73	−1.498	0.134
Chinese sorghum	270	0.49	0.31	0.18	1.744	0.081
Potatoes	270	12.15	12.13	0.02	0.049	0.961

Table 2. Relative risk of certain factors for NPC

	NPC		Controls		χ^2	Odds ratio	AF
	Exposed	Unexposed	Exposed	Unexposed			
Drinking water other than well water	107	163	101	169	0.281	1.098	0.035
House without chimney	219	51	196	74	5.506	1.621	0.311
Fuel with smoke	209	61	186	84	4.988	1.547	0.274
Firewood	207	63	174	96	9.707	1.813	0.344

Table 3. 3,4-Benzpyrene in smoke samples collected from high- and low-risk areass of NPC

	High-risk areas	Low-risk areas	P
No. of samples	27	30	<0.02
3,4-BP (μg/g) $\bar{x} \pm SE$	16.83 ± 2.36	10.29 ± 0.66	

Table 4. 3,4-Benzpyrene in smoke samples collected from houses of NPC patients and non-NPC inhabitants

	NPC house	Non-NPC house	P
No. of samples	5	22	>0.05
3,4-BP (μg/g) $\bar{x} \pm SE$	13.17 ± 0.82	15.59 ± 0.69	

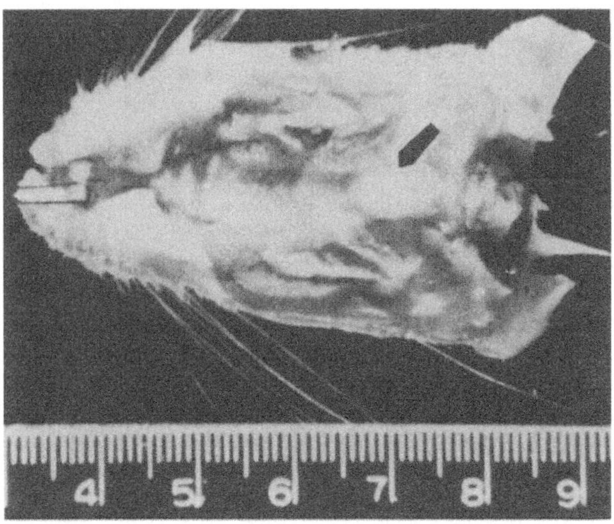

Fig. 2. Nasopharyngeal carcinoma in rats induced by *N*-dinitrosopiperazine. Autopsy No. 1130. *Arrow* shows the tumor mass in the nasopharynx

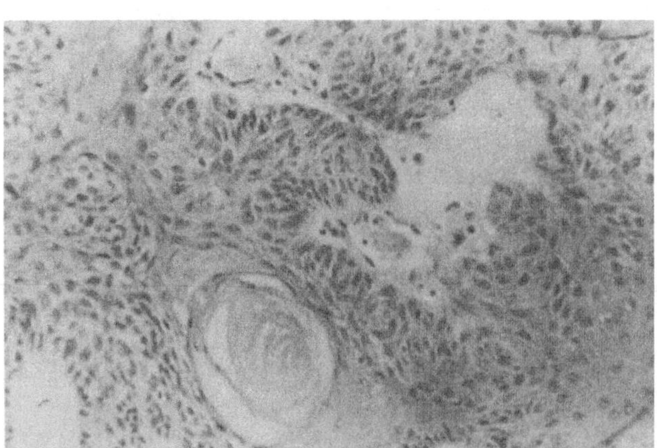

Fig. 3. Histology of the tumor in Fig. 2, showing that the tumor induced is a well-differentiated squamous cell carcinoma (H & E ×450)

Table 5. Consumption of meat, fish and vegetables

Factor	NPC		Controls		Odds ratio	χ^2	AF
	Yes	No	Yes	No			
Smoked meat	211	46	212	45	0.974	0.013	–
Smoked fish	89	168	98	159	0.860	0.681	–
Salted meat	62	195	49	208	1.350	1.942	0.036
Salted fish	79	178	58	199	1.523	4.389	0.064
Salted vegetables	131	126	133	128	1.001	0.000	–
Pickles	134	121	137	118	0.954	0.070	–
Vegetables pickled in soya sauce	87	169	107	150	0.722	3.165	–
Fresh vegetables	244	0	244	0	–	–	–

be the case in Hunan, especially in the west of Hunan. This was demonstrated by a case-control study concerned with the consumption of meat, fish, and vegetables (Table 5).

Promoters in Relation to NPC Carcinogenesis

Because EB virus was originally found in lymphoblasts cultured from tumor biopsies of patients with Burkitt's lymphoma, a number of studies on the interaction of EB virus and B cells were carried out. Several reports indicated that EB virus could be induced and activated from EBV genome-carrying human lymphoblastoid cells by treatment with chemicals, among which TPA and other related chemicals [18] attracted investigators' attention. Zeng et al. [17] tested 495 kinds of Chinese medicinal herbs and found that 15 of them were capable of activating latent EBV. Water extracts from the same herbs also showed an inducing activity. Whether or not the EBV-inducing activities of these Chinese medicinal herbs can be attributed to TPA-like principles, such as is the case in *Croton tiglium,* needs to be further studied. It is very interesting, as Ito et al. [6] pointed out, that the geographical distribution of the provinces where *Croton tiglium* grows and the area where a clustering of NPC occurs show a close similarity. Of course, TPA and related substances in the environment not only act as EBV-inducing chemicals, but also as tumor promoters to the initiated nasopharyngeal epithelial cells. In addition, some trace elements are also considered important for the development of NPC.

Recent studies [7] demonstrated that the contents of nickel and iron, acidity, and total hardness are higher in the drinking water of high-risk areas than those in low-risk areas (Table 6). The results concerning nickel confirmed the study in Guangdong province. Nickel might be a tumor promoter as suggested by some authors [10].

Table 6. Comparison of 12 chemical element contents in drinking water between high-risk and low-risk areas to the west of Hunan Province

	Units	High-risk areas $\bar{x} \pm SE$ (n=45)	Low-risk areas $\bar{x} \pm SE$ (n=30)	P
Acidity	pH	7.29 ±0.10	6.78 ± 0.11	<0.05
Total hardness	$CaCO_3$ mg/liter	105.79 ±9.80	32.53 ± 8.29	<0.05
Nitrogen in nitrates	mg/liter	0.55 ±0.09	1.13 ± 0.57	>0.05
Nitrogen in nitrites	mg/liter	0.009±0.001	0.012± 0.002	>0.05
FE	mg/liter	1.147±0.262	0.368± 0.072	<0.05
Ni	μg/liter	1.69 ±0.20	0.27 ± 0.07	<0.05
Zn	μg/liter	15.6 ±1.7	10.2 ± 1.7	>0.05
Cd	μg/liter	0.44 ±0.05	0.24 ± 0.12	>0.05
Cr	μg/liter	5.6 ±1.6	6.7 ± 2.4	>0.05
Mn	μg/liter	16.8 ±3.4	37.4 ±21.3	>0.05
Pb	μg/liter	6.9 ±0.9	4.0 ± 1.0	>0.05
Cu	μg/liter	2.8 ±0.4	5.0 ± 1.7	>0.05

Genetic Components of Tumor Promotion in NPC

The action of tumor promoters was generally considered reversible. Actually, later stages of tumor promotion are irreversible, and tumor promoters may act on preneoplastic cells to produce stable switches in gene expression that lead to malignancy. Colburn et al. [2] demonstrated, by DNA-mediated gene transfer, the existence of DNA sequence conferring anchorage-independet growth on clonal JB6 cells in response to TPA. Two responsible genes were cloned and designated as Pro_1 and Pro_2 with a size of approximately 3 kb and 12 kb, respectively [8]. In order to obtain a well-defined hybridization probe, Pro_2 recombinants were partially digested and fragments of DNA were inserted into the *EcoR*1 site of plasmid pBR322. Finally, a 3.2-kb fragment *(p32)* containing no repetitive DNA was obtained and used as a probe. Hybridization experiments using genomic DNA of NPC epithelial cells (CNE_1 and CNE_2 cell lines) indicated the presence of Pro_2 homology sequences in genomic DNA of NPC cells. Negative results were encountered in molecular hybridization experiments using genomic DNA extracted from Hela cells, five gynecological tumor cell lines (cervical carcinoma, choriocarcinoma, and endometrial adenocarcinoma), and various leukemia cell lines.

DNA from CNE cells, just like DNA from TPA-sensitive JB6 cells (P^+ cells), can transfer promotion sensitivity when transfected into TPA-resitant JB6 cells (P^- cells). Besides, positive signals were encountered in screening a genomic library of CNE DNA by plaque in situ hybridization with labeled P32 [16].

More experiments should be carried out to identify whether or not the homology sequence to *Pro* genes is present in human NPC and other malignant tumor biopsies.

Acknowledgments. We thank Prof. Zhu Tie-Rong for his helpful suggestion during the preparation of the manuscript and Mr. Deng Xi-Yun for typing it.

References

1. Cancer Research Group of Hunan Medical College: Induction of nasopharyngeal carcinoma in rats by nitroso compounds. Kexue Tongbao 23 (1978) 756-760
2. Colburn NH, Talmadge CB, Ginhart TD: Transfer of sensitivity to tumor promoters by transfection of DNA from sensitive into insensitive mouse JB6 epidermal cells. Mol. cell. Biol. 3 (1983) 1182-1186
3. Fong YY, Walsh EO: Carcinogenic nitrosamines in Cantonese salt-dried fish. Lancet 1971, II: 1032
4. Ho HC: Epidemiology of nasopharyngeal carcinoma. J. roy. Coll. Surg. 20 (1975) 223-235
5. Huang DP, Ho JHC, Saw D et al.: Carcinoma of the nasal and paranasal regions in rats fed Cantonese salted marine fish. In de-Thé G, Ito Y (Eds): Nasopharyngeal Carcinoma: Etiology and Control, pp. 315-328. Lyon: IARC 1978. (IARC Sci. Publ., No. 20)
6. Ito Y, Kishishita M, Morigaki T et al.: Induction and intervention of Epstein-Barr virus expression in human lymphoblastoid cell lines: A simulation model for study of cause and prevention of nasopharyngeal carcinoma and Burkitt's lymphoma. In Grundmann E, Krueger GRF, Ablashi DV (Eds): Nasopharyngeal Carcinoma, pp. 255-262. Stuttgart: Fischer 1981. (Cancer Campaign, Vol. 5)
7. Jiang JW et al.: Preliminary study on the relation of 12 chemical element contents in drinking water to NPC. (In press)
8. Lerman MI, Glenn AH, Colburn NH: Molecular cloning of a new transforming gene induced by tumor promoting 12-O-tetradecanoylphorbol-13-acetate (TPA) in mouse epidermal preneoplastic cells. In Genes and Cancer, No. 191, 1984, pp. 76 ff.
9. Li GY, Luo MJ, Yao KT: Determination of 3,4-benzo(a)pyrene in house-smoke sample collected from high-risk and low-risk area of NPC in Hunan Province. (In press)
10. Ou BX et al.: The promotion action of trace element nickel in the induction of NPC in rats. Guangdong Med. 1 (1980) 32
11. Slaga TJ: Overview of tumor promotion in animals. Environm. Hlth Persp. 50 (1983) 3-14
12. Wu PN, Lin XS, Xiao BS et al.: Second retrospective survey for NPC mortality at 27 counties in the western and southern parts of Hunan Province. (In press)
13. Wu PN, Lin XS, Xiao BS et al.: Field case-control studies on the causative factors of NPC. (In press)
14. Yao KT: Epidemiological characteristics and presumed carcinogenesis of nasopharyngeal carcinoma in Hunan Province based on 1973-1975 cancer mortality survey. Bull. Hunan med. Coll. 7 (1982) 10-17
15. Yao KT, Pan SC, Huang JL et al.: Further investigation of experimental induction of nasopharyngeal carcinoma in rats by dinitrosopiperazine. Bull. Hunan med. Coll. 6 (1981) 1-6
16. Yao KT, Lerman MI, Colburn NH: Unpublished results, 1984
17. Zeng Y, Zhong JM, Mo YK et al.: Epstein-Barr virus early antigen induction in Raji cells by Chinese medicinal herbs. Intervirology 19 (1983) 201-204
18. Zur Hausen H, O'Neill FJ, Freese UK: Persisting oncogenic herpesvirus induced by the tumor promoter TPA. Nature 272 (1978) 373-375

Clinical Course and Therapy of Nasopharyngeal Carcinoma

K.-H. Vosteen and J. Ebbers

Introduction

In 1921, Schmincke and Régaud described, independently of each other, malignant neoplasms arising from the tonsillar tissue of the nasopharynx [31, 29]. Consisting of an intimate mixture of lymphatic and carcinomatous tissue components, they were given the name of "lymphoepitheliomas." Later, a "Schmincke" type with its dominating lymphatic component and fading epithelial strains was discerned from the "Régaud" type, showing only poor lymphatic admixture and rather resembling an anaplastic carcinoma.

The pathohistological classification, however, is difficult, as intermediate forms are observed. In 1978, a standardized nomenclature of nasopharyngeal tumors was established by the WHO, based on Shanmugaratnam's suggestions [34].

A most fascinating trait of certain forms of the nasopharyngeal carcinoma (NPC) is its Epstein-Barr virus (EBV) association. Since 1966, when Old et al. reported on precipitating antibodies against EBV antigens in the sera of NPC patients, we have known that nonkeratinizing, lymphoepithelial, and anaplastic nasopharyngeal carcinomas usually contain EBV genomes [27, 48]. These can be localized in the nuclei of carcinoma cells. The mode of infection, however, is still unclear, as only some B-lymphocytes of man and some primates possess a virus receptor [44, 21]. Although many problems of EBV association remain unsolved at the level of molecular biology, the monitoring of immunoglobulins directed against EBV-encoded antigens in the patients' sera has proved its usefulness for follow-up and even for screening of high-risk populations [43, 45].

Another characteristic of NPC is its peculiar epidemiological distribution: in central Europe and most other countries of the world, it amounts to only about 0.2% of all malignancies [41]. On the other hand, there are regions with a 100-fold and higher incidence, e.g., the province of Canton (south China) [14].

Its age distribution, however, seems to be similar all over the world: the curve shows a peak for the 5th and 6th decades, shifting slightly toward the 4th and 5th decade in high-risk regions. Here, an additional peak at the end of the 2nd decade can be noted [18]. An unusually high incidence in childhood has been reported for Uganda [30]. The reasons for these epidemiological data are unclear. Genetic factors and environmental influences, e.g., the use of popular drugs, have been discussed [35, 46].

Cancer of the Liver, Esophagus, and Nasopharynx
Edited by G. Wagner and Zhang You-Hui

Characteristics of Tumor Spread

Nasopharyngeal carcinoma may arise anywhere in the postnasal space. It is, however, observed most frequently in the pharyngeal roof and the fossa of Rosenmüller [23] (Fig. 1). Submucosal tumor spread is characteristic. The epithelium stays undamaged for a long time. Ulceration and/or exophytic growth are predominantly observed in advanced stages.

Tumor growth may take any direction. Carcinomas arising in the pharyngeal roof tend to invade the nasal cavity and the dorsal cells of the ethmoid. By a more dorsal guide rail, the tumor may infiltrate the prevertebral space. If cranial growth occurs, the sphenoidal sinus will be involved and, after the destruction of its osseous walls, the hypophyseal gland as well as the apex orbitae may be occupied.

Bulb protrusion and impairment of sight are the clinical consequences, as already described by Régaud. A more laterocranial growth leads to an infiltration of the foramen lacerum and the oculomotor, trochlear, and trigeminal nerves. Further dorsolateral spread causes an impairment of the glossopharyngeal, hypoglossal, and accessory nerves. The internal carotid might be affected in this region as well. Sudden hemorrhage from this vessel can terminate the patient's life quickly. Once the osseous skull base has been eroded, a progressive meningoencephalitis will follow. For the topography of the skull base see Fig. 2.

The numerous lymph vessels of the postnasal space are the reason for frequent and early lymph node metastases in NPC. The first filter station is formed by the retropharyngeal lymph nodes. These are found either medially or laterally in the submucosal tissue of the mesopharynx. From here, lymph vessels lead toward the subdigastric lymph nodes and, further, to the cervical chain of lymph nodes along the jugular vein. Most characteristic for NPC, however, is another pattern of lymph node metastasis: the nodes just below the mastoid process and at the dorsal triangle of the neck are attacked [22] (Fig. 3).

Hematogenous metastasis normally occurs at advanced stages of NPC. Compared with other head and neck carcinomas, however, it is frequently observed. Especially infant patients suffer from it most often. The skeleton, the lungs, and the liver are favorite sites of distant metastases [20].

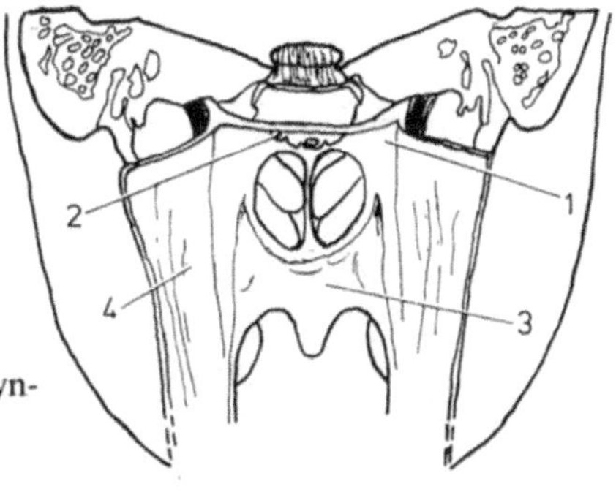

Fig. 1. Topography of the postnasal space as seen from behind. *1*, fossa of Rosenmüller; *2*, nasopharyngeal roof; *3*, back side of the soft palate; *4*, lateral and posterior wall, opened

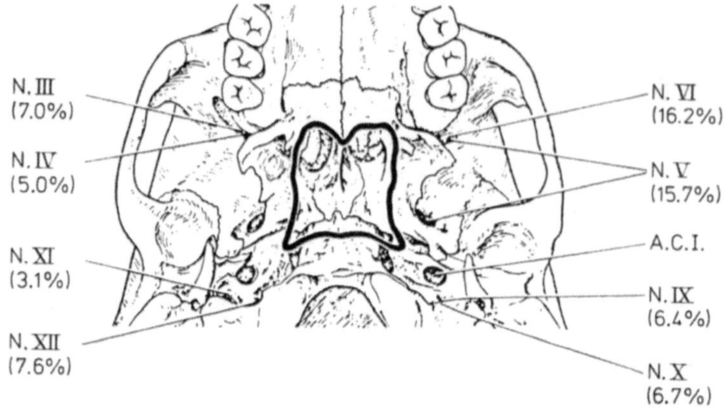

Fig. 2. Topography of the postnasal space as projected to the osseous skull base. The *dark line* shows the margins of the nasopharynx and their relationship to the cranial nerves and the carotid artery *(A. c. i.)*. The *percentages in parentheses* show the relative frequency of involvement in NPC

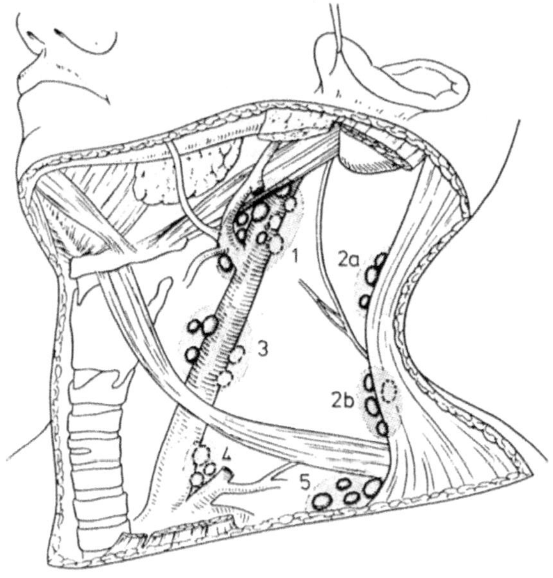

Fig. 3. Possible routes of lymph node metastasis in NPC: *1*, subdigastric lymph nodes; *2a*, upper nuchal lymph nodes; *2b*, lower nuchal lymph nodes; *3*, upper cervical lymph nodes; *4*, lower cervical lymph nodes; *5*, supraclavicular lymph nodes

Symptoms and Diagnosis

There are no early symptoms of NPC, as it grows in a hidden anatomical region. Commonly, the intumescence of neck nodes is the first symptom. Local symptoms (feeling of occlusion, unilateral nose bleeding, or secretion) follow, indicating an advanced primary lesion. Otological symptoms can be registered in nearly all cases of advanced disease, but they may also be provoked by very small tumors. The pathophysiological mechanism is based on a compression of the Eustachian tube,

Table 1. Frequency of different clinical symptoms in NPC. (modified from [10])

Symptoms	Non-Chinese (%)	Chinese (%)
Neck mass	40	50
Hearing impairment	31	25
Nasal obstruction	19	15
Bleeding nose	23	27
Diplopia or n. VI	6	1
Pain	19	13
Paraesthesia or n. V	2	2
Hoarseness or n. X	–	1
n. XII	–	1

thus impairing the ventilation of the middle ear. Serous otitis media and a conductional hearing loss are the consequences.

Neurological and ophthalmological problems are final symptoms. A minute neurological examination can provide quite precise information about the tumor growth along the skull base. Paralysis of the abducens and trigeminal nerve are observed most frequently, followed by the oculomotor and trochlear nerve. The disturbance of other cranial nerves depends on the growth direction of the tumor as described above. Table 1 shows different clinical symptoms and their frequency in NPC [10].

The diagnosis of a really small nasopharyngeal cancer, restricted to the primary site, is a rare event in central Europe even today. This may be due to its hidden site and its uncharacteristic symptoms. Another reason might be its rare incidence, which can lead to a wrong diagnosis, even with a typical combination of symptoms. A study carried out on our own patients showed that, on average, 4 months passed between the onset of symptoms and the first medical consultation, normally by a general practitioner. It took another whole month to establish the correct diagnosis and start treatment at a specialized center.

With the exception of screening procedures in high-risk regions, searching for elevated antibody titers against viral proteins in the blood, the postrhinoscopic examination is the most common and, perhaps, most useful diagnostic method for NPC. The technique of using a small mirror is not easy, however, and is impaired by the submucosal growth of the tumor. Endoscopic methods (oral or nasal access) are less troublesome. They can even detect small mucosal alterations as irregular surface structures, small ulcerations, or an increased injection of vessels, all of which may be signs of tumor growth.

Palpation of the neck for enlarged lymph nodes and a careful examination of the cranial nerves in order to exclude extended tumor growth along the skull base are essential parts of the clinical investigation.

X-ray examinations are important for describing the tumor's spread precisely. Conventional a.p. tomography is still a very effective method for showing even small erosions of the osseous skull base. Computed tomography offers considerable advantages for judging the infiltration of soft tissues. Both techniques are complementary and should be applied routinely. Magnetic resonance tomography seems

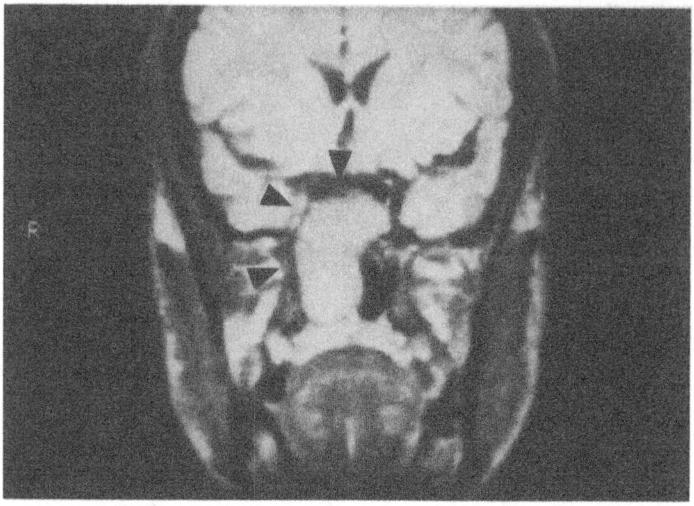

Fig. 4. Magnetic resonance tomography of NPC. The tumor is indicated by *arrows*

to be best suited for demonstrating the exact extension of tumors invading the brain (Fig. 4).

B-scan and Doppler sonography may provide additional information about the consistency of neck nodes and a possible infiltration of major neck vessels.

An early determination of antibody titers against VCA, EA, and EBNA facilitates the diagnosis in unclear cases and represents an important starting value for the patient's follow-up during and after therapy.

A small biopsy from the primary lesion is necessary to confirm the diagnosis histologically. The morphological examination under the light microscope should be supplemented by the immunohistochemical demonstration of the EB nuclear antigen in swab preparations.

Classification

The results of these examinations should lead to a pretherapeutic classification of NPC. This is most important to obtain comparable treatment results. The TNM classification system according to the UICC is internationally accepted today [38].

This system distinguishes the following regions:

1. The roof and the posterior wall, beginning at the boundary between the soft and the hard palate, and ending at the skull base.
2. The lateral wall, including the fossa of Rosenmüller.
3. The anterior wall, formed by the back side of the soft palate. The margins of the choanae are attributed to the nasal cavity.

T1 tumors are restricted to one region. T2 tumors do not occupy more than two regions. T3 tumors have invaded the nasal cavity and/or the oropharynx. T4 tumors have affected the skull base and/or the cranial nerves.

N1 classifies homolateral mobile lymph nodes. N2 means contra- or bilateral mobile lymph nodes. N3 characterizes any fixed lymph node.

Additionally, the TNM system allows for a division into four stages, which is sometimes more versatile, e.g., for statistical evaluations. Stage I corresponds to T1 N0 M0, stage II to T2 N0M0, stage III to T3 N0 M0 or T1-3 N1 M0, and stage IV to T4 N0-1 M0, T1-4 N2-3 M0, or T1-4 N0-3 M1.

Surgery and Radiotherapy

Treatment of NPC is nowadays a domain of radiotherapy. The excellent radiosensitivity of lymphoepitheliomas has already been mentioned by Schmincke himself, and surgical procedures in order to cure the primary tumor are merely of historical interest today [33]. The special anatomical situation of the postnasal space with its intimate neighborhood to the skull base, the cranial nerves, and big vessels offers no prospect of a radical tumor cure by means of surgery.

In selected cases, however, with distinct exophytic tumor growth, a surgical reduction of the tumor masses can be taken into consideration to assist radiotherapy.

There are differing opinions concerning the judgement of surgical treatment of lymph nodes: from a more theoretical point of view, a neck dissection only makes sense if it is possible to remove *en block* the primary tumor together with its complete draining lymph system. The primary lesion and its first filter station, the retropharyngeal lymph nodes, however, escape surgical access. For this reason, most departments avoid primary neck dissection, even if the lymph nodes are palpable. The operation is only used as "salvage surgery" in cases with remaining or recurrent neck masses after radiotherapy.

The chance of survival of the NPC patient also closely depends on the management of the lymph node metastasis. This requires a definite therapeutic strategy. Lymph nodes more than 2-3 cm in diameter cannot be cured regularly by conventional radiotherapy, as tumor cells may become radioresistant due to a radiation-induced hypoxemia of the surrounding tissue [3]. We therefore recommend for some cases primary surgery of neck node metastases for reasons of security.

Unilateral lymph nodes (N1 or N3) are treated by unilateral functional or radical neck dissection, respectively. In cases of bilateral lymph nodes (N2 or N3), a bilateral functional or a unilateral functional and a contralateral radical neck dissection is performed in one operative session. Very few cases with fixed lymph nodes on both sides require a bilateral radical neck dissection. The second neck dissection is performed after the first series of radiotherapy.

Irradiation of the primary tumor and its draining lymph system follows as quickly as possible, normally 10 days after the operation.

If no neck nodes are palpable, we start radiotherapy at once. We also avoid any surgery of patients with palpable lymph nodes but with advanced growth of the primary lesion (T4). In these cases, the prognosis seems too poor to justify the burden of an operation.

Megavoltage radiotherapy offers prospects of a definitive tumor cure, and the former poor results of kilovoltage X-ray therapy have been considerably improved.

The irradiation of NPC requires minute planning due to vulnerable adjacent structures such as eyes, spinal cord, and brain. Computed tomography and a computer-assisted calculation of dosages are useful. Special attention must be paid to a sufficient extension of the fields at the dorsal margins of the tumor along the skull base. Local recurrence in this region is observed occasionally and hardly to be managed. The individual arrangement of the radiation fields depends on the tumor extension.

Normally, the primary lesion and the upper cervical lymph nodes are treated through opposed lateral portals. This therapy is supplemented by an anterior oblique or rotational technique of the primary tumor and anterior tangential irradiation of the upper and lower neck nodes. The total dose normally amounts to 60–70 Gy, divided into an initial series of 40 Gy and – after a 6- to 8-week interval – a second series of 20–30 Gy. The therapy is fractionated to 150–180 cGy/day. It must be given on a megavoltage unit, either a cobalt-60 machine or a linear accelerator.

Interstitial radiotherapy by afterloading techniques can be applied for a local boost or for the management of local recurrent tumors [7].

Neutrons are not as yet routinely applied. They may, however, offer certain advantages, i. e., for the treatment of large neck masses [25].

Cytotoxic Drugs

Children suffering from NPC seem to have an increased risk of hematogenous metastasis [36]. Therefore, radiotherapy should be supplemented by an adjuvant chemotherapy in infant patients, even if there is no evidence of manifest distant disease. General recommendations for defined regimens, however, cannot yet be given. None of the numerous schedules published has proven its statistical value for the survival rate [42]. Schweisguth recommended a combination of vincristine, cyclophosphamide, and Adriamycin [32]. Others see advantages in the use of the ABVD scheme (Table 2) [5].

Cytotoxic drugs are also given to adult patients suffering from hematogenous metastasis. About 30% of all NPC patients develop a distant disease. This is the highest rate of all head and neck carcinomas [26]. Also, for adult NPC patients a defined regimen cannot yet be recommended. The percentage of complete or partial remissions achieved by some schedules is high (67%), but there has been little or no effect on the survival time. Table 3 gives chemotherapeutic results of advanced NPC as reported in the literature. Compared with other head and neck carcinomas, NPC seems to respond better to chemotherapy [8]. Among these, lymphoepithelio-

Table 2. The ABVD-Scheme. [5]

Every 2 weeks	i. v.
Adriamycine	25 mg/m²
Bleomycin	10 mg/m²
Vinblastine	6 mg/m²
Dacarbazine (DTIC)	375 mg/m²

Table 3. Results of Chemotherapy of NPC. Abbreviations: A = adriamycine; B = bleomycin; Bc = BCNU; C = cyclophosphamide; Cc = CNU; D = dacarbazine; F = 5-fluorouracil; M = methotrexate; P = *Cis*-platinum; V = vinblastine; CR = complete remission; PR = partial remission; NC = no change

Authors	Number of cases	Pretreatment	Schedule	CR	PR	NC
Anderson et al. (2)	5	?	M	2	1	2
Brown et al. (6)	8	Various	VBP	1	5	2
Cortes et al. (9)	6	Radiation	BCMF	2	3	1
Galligioni et al. (12)	11	None	ABVD	4	5	2
Goepfert et al. (13)	18	Radiation	BCMF	4	7	7
Huang et al. (19)	7	Surgery/radiation	BMVCc	0	4	3
Lombardi et al. (24)	11 (children)	Radiation	VAC	11	0	0
Presant et al. (28)	5	Radiation	ABcC	1	2	2

mas respond better than squamous cell carcinomas [16]. 5-Fluorouracil, methotrexate, and *cis*-platinum, which in part have shown good effects on other head and neck carcinomas, seem to be less effective in lymphoepitheliomas [4].

Prognosis and Prognostic Factors

Five-year survival rates for all NPC patients differ from 13.8% (in 1959) to 59.0% (in 1976) [1, 17]. Several factors influence the individual prognosis:

Stage of Disease at the Onset of Therapy

Ho reports an approximate 69% 5-year survival rate for T2 tumors versus 36% for T4 tumors [15]. The extent of lymph node metastasis is of importance, as N2 and N3 are associated with distant metastasis in 30% [40].

Histological Type

Lymphoepithelial carcinomas seem to have the best prognosis (66.7% 5-year survival), followed by nonkeratinizing squamous cell carcinomas (20.0%) and undifferentiated carcinomas (12.5%). Keratinizing squamous cell carcinomas, which are not Epstein-Barr virus-associated, exhibit by far the poorest prognosis (4.2%) [47].

Sex

Women show a better prognosis than men for all stages [39].

Age

Most authors agree that in general patients between 20 and 49 years of age have the best survival rates [10].

Outlook for an Improvement of Therapy

Although the prognosis of NPC has been considerably improved during the past 2 decades, there is still a strong need for more effective therapies. At least every second patient will die from his or her disease within 5 years. Only the first out of four prognostically relevant factors listed above should be influenceable to some extent. Especially in high-risk regions, screening programs by serological analysis of EBV-associated antibody titers will be able to increase the relative percentage of early NPC, offering an excellent prognosis after adequate therapy. These promising measures are detailed in Zeng's contribution to his volume.

Screening procedures, however, are useful only in high-risk regions. Thus, further efforts will be necessary to improve actual treatment.

Radiotherapy has demonstrated its primacy, and there is no regimen thinkable today without it. Irradiation itself might be improved by still better planning and optimized combinations of percutaneous and interstitial therapy. A general application of optimally combined photons and neutrons might also contribute to better survival rates.

In addition, there is a need for some sort of "adjuvant therapy." Cytotoxic drugs have been proposed. The presented data, however, have not yet shown a superior effect of any schedule. Further randomized studies, based on large numbers, will be necessary to demonstrate the effects of possible combinations. For statistical reasons they should be performed in high-risk regions.

Much hope has been placed on interferons [37]. Statistically significant data, however, have not yet been presented. Our own data, obtained by the daily application of 10000 IU leukocyte interferon (courtesy of Dr. Cantell) for 2–4 weeks to nude mice bearing NPC xenografts, exhibited no effect on the tumor growth curves. These data provide evidence that a direct effect of leukocyte interferon on NPC does not seem to be very probable. The experiment permits no conclusion about possible indirect effects of leukocyte interferon via activation of NK cells or macrophages, as these are known to be maximally stimulated in nude mice and as human leukocyte interferon only shows slight cross-reactions. The antiviral effects of leukocyte interferon are negligible for NPC as viral replication hardly seems to occur.

Further experimental data on interferons must be obtained before this kind of therapy can be generally recommended.

Another approach can be seen in the development of monoclonal antibodies: compared with other head and neck carcinomas, NPC should offer better prospects of a regular expression of tumor-associated antigenic determinants, due to its monoclonal character [11] and its EBV association. The integrated viral genome is in fact so big that there is a reasonable chance of one or more virus-encoded antigen(s) being expressed in the cellular membrane. The definition of such antigens and the development of monoclonal antibodies suitable for diagnostic and therapeutic approaches to NPC as well is an important task of present and future research.

References

1. Albrecht R: Die Nasenrachentumoren und ihre Behandlung. Arch. Ohr.-, Nas.- u. Kehlk.-Heilk. 175 (1959) 217-221
2. Anderson JM, Fung JHY, Laing D: Arterial infusion chemotherapy for carcinoma of the nasopharynx. Brit. J. clin. Pract. 19 (1965) 565-567
3. Atzinger A, Burger G, Gfirtner H et al.: Aktueller Stand der Bestrahlungsplanung bei malignen Nasopharynxtumoren. Verh. Dtsch. Krebs-Ges. 5 (1984) 305
4. Bodemann HH: Chemotherapie des metastasierenden Nasopharynxkarzinoms. In Wannenmacher M (Hrsg.): Nasopharynx-Tumoren. München: Urban & Schwarzenberg 1984
5. Bonadonna G, Zucali R, Monfardini S et al.: Combination chemotherapy of Hodgkin's disease with Adriamycin, Bleomycin, Vinblastine, and Imidazole Carboxamide versus MOPP. Cancer 36 (1975) 252-259
6. Brown AW, Blom J, Butler WM et al.: Combination chemotherapy with Vinblastine, Bleomycin and *Cis*-Diamminedichloroplatinum (II) in squamous cell carcinoma of the head and neck. Cancer 45 (1980) 2830-2835
7. Busch M, Alberti W: Optimierte Afterloading-Applikation bei Epipharynxtumoren. Strahlentherapie 160 (1984) 77-80
8. Carter SK: The chemotherapy of head and neck cancer. Sem. Oncol. 4 (1977) 413-424
9. Cortes EP, Kalra J, Amin VC et al.: Chemotherapy for head and neck cancer relapsing after radiotherapy. Cancer 47 (1981) 1966-1970
10. Dickson RI: Nasopharyngeal carcinoma: An Evaluation of 209 Patients. Laryngoscope 91 (1981) 333-354
11. Fialkow PJ, Martin GM, Klein G et al.: Evidence for a clonal origin of head and neck tumors. Int. J. Cancer 9 (1972) 133-142
12. Galligioni E, Carbone A, Tirelli U et al.: Combined chemotherapy with Doxorubicin, Bleomycin, Vinblastine, Dacarbazine, and radiotherapy for advanced lymphoepithelioma. Cancer Treatm. Rep. 66 (1982) 1207-1210
13. Goepfert H, Moran ME, Lindberg RD et al.: Chemotherapy of advanced nasopharyngeal carcinoma (NPC). Abstract. Proc. Amer. Soc. clin. Otol. 22 (1981) 427
14. Ho JHC: Nasopharyngeal carcinoma (NPC). Adv. Cancer Res. 15 (1972) 57-92
15. Ho JHC: Nasopharynx. In Halnan KE (Edit.): Treatment of Cancer, pp. 249-267. London: Chapman and Hall 1982
16. Holoye PY, Byers RM, Gard DA et al.: Combination chemotherapy of head and neck cancer. Cancer 42 (1978) 1661-1669
17. Hoppe RT, Goffinet DR, Bagshaw MA: Carcinoma of the nasopharynx. Cancer 37 (1976) 2605-2612
18. Hsu MM, Huang SC, Lynn TC et al.: The survival of patients with nasopharyngeal carcinoma. Otolaryng. Head Neck Surg. 90 (1982) 289-295
19. Huang AT, Lucas VS, Baughn SC et al.: A trial of outpatient chemotherapy for recurrent head and neck tumors. Cancer 45 (1980) 2038-2041
20. Ilberg C von, Kleinmann H, Arnold W: Das Schmincke-Karzinom des Nasopharynx. Laryng. Rhinol. Otol. 55 (1976) 420-428
21. Jondal M, Klein G, Oldstone MBA et al.: Surface markers on human T and B lymphocytes. VIII. Association between complement and Epstein-Barr virus receptors on human lymphoid cells. Scand. J. Immunol. 5 (1976) 401-410
22. Jung H: Intravitale Lymphabflußuntersuchungen vom Nasenrachendach beim Menschen. Laryng. Rhinol. Otol. 53 (1974) 769-773
23. Leipner N, Barwig P, Frommhold H: Karzinome des Nasenrachens. Laryng. Rhinol. Otol. 60 (1981) 321-328
24. Lombardi F, Gasparini M, Gianni C et al.: Nasopharyngeal carcinoma in childhood. Med. pediat. Oncol. 10 (1982) 243-250
25. Maor MH, Hussey DA, Fletcher GH et al.: Fast neutron therapy for locally advanced head and neck tumors. Int. J. Radiat. Oncol. Biol. Phys. 7 (1981) 155-169
26. Merino OR, Lindberg RD, Fletcher GH: An analysis of distant metastasis from squamous cell carcinoma of the upper respiratory and digestive tracts. Cancer 40 (1977) 145-151
27. Old LJ, Boyse EA, Oettgen HF et al.: Precipitating antibody in human serum to an an-

tigen present in cultured Burkitt's lymphoma cells. Proc. nat. Acad. Sci. USA 56 (1966) 1699-1704
28. Presant CA, Ratkin G, Klahr C et al.: Adriamycin, BCNU plus Cyclophosphamide (ABC) in advanced carcinoma of the head and neck. Cancer 44 (1979) 1571-1575
29. Régaud C, Reverchon L: Sur un cas d'épithélioma épidermoide développé dans le massif maxillaire supérieur, étendu aux téguments de la face, aux cavités buccale, nasale et orbitaire, ainsi qu'aux ganglions du cou, guéri par la curiethérapie. Rev. Laryng. 42 (1921) 369-378
30. Schmauz R, Templeton AC: Nasopharyngeal carcinoma in Uganda. Cancer 29 (1972) 610-621
31. Schmincke A: Über lymphoepitheliale Geschwülste. Beitr. path. Anat. 68 (1921) 161-170
32. Schweisguth O: Solide Tumoren im Kindesalter. Stuttgart: Enke 1984
33. Sesterhenn K, Wustrow F, Bertram G: Surgical procedures in diagnosis and treatment of nasopharyngeal carcinoma - a historical review. In Grundmann E, Krueger GRF, Ablashi DV (Eds): Nasopharyngeal Carcinoma, pp. 269-272. Stuttgart: Fischer 1981. (Cancer Campaign, Vol. 5)
34. Shanmugaratnam K, Sobin LH: Histological Typing of Upper Respiratory Tract Tumors. Geneva: WHO 1978. (International Histological Classification of Tumours, No. 19)
35. Simons MJ, Wee GB, Goh EH et al.: Immunogenetic aspects of nasopharyngeal carcinoma. IV. Increased risk in Chinese of nasopharyngeal carcinoma associated with a Chinese-related HLA-profile (A2, Singapore 2). J. nat. Cancer Inst. 57 (1976) 977-980
36. Snow JB: Carcinoma of the nasopharynx in children. Ann. Otol. (St. Louis) 84 (1975) 817-826
37. Treuner J, Niethammer D, Dannecker G et al.: Successful treatment of nasopharyngeal carcinoma with interferon. Lancet 1980, I: 817-818
38. UICC (Hrsg.): TNM-Klassifikation der malignen Tumoren. 3. Aufl. Berlin: Springer 1979
39. Wang CC: Radiation therapy for head and neck neoplasms. Boston: Wright 1983
40. Wannenmacher M: Strahlentherapie der Nasopharynxcarcinome. Verh. Dtsch. Krebs-Ges. 5 (1984) 311
41. Waterhouse J, Muir C, Correa P et al. (Eds): Cancer Incidence in Five Continents. Vol. 3. Lyon: IARC 1976. (IARC Scientific Publications, No. 15)
42. Weidauer H: Chemotherapie der malignen Nasopharynx-Tumoren. Verh. Dtsch. Krebs-Ges. 5 (1984) 333
43. Wilmes E, Wolf H, Deinhardt F et al.: Die Bedeutung von Epstein-Barr Virus-Antikörpern für Diagnose und Verlauf des Nasopharynxkarzinoms. Laryng. Rhinol. Otol. 58 (1979) 911-915
44. Wolf H, zur Hausen H, Becker V: EB viral genomes in epithelial nasopharyngeal carcinoma cells. Nature NB 244 (1973) 245-247
45. Zeng Y, Zhang LG, Li HY et al.: Serological mass survey for early detection of nasopharyngeal carcinoma in Wuzhou City, China. Int. J. Cancer 29 (1982) 139-141
46. Zeng Y, Zhong JM, Mo YK et al.: Epstein-Barr virus early antigen induction in Raji cells by Chinese medicinal herbs. Intervirology 19 (1983) 201-204
47. Ziegler F, Metzger H, Hübener KH: Behandlungsergebnisse beim Nasopharynxkarzinom nach Telekobalttherapie. In Wannenmacher M (Hrsg.): Nasopharynx-Tumoren. München: Urban & Schwarzenberg 1984
48. Zur Hausen H, Schulte-Holthausen H, Klein G et al.: EBV DNA in biopsies of Burkitt tumours and anaplastic carcinomas of the nasopharynx. Nature 228 (1970) 1056-1058

Subject Index

GPSR Compliance

The European Union's (EU) General Product Safety Regulation (GPSR) is a set of rules that requires consumer products to be safe and our obligations to ensure this.

If you have any concerns about our products, you can contact us on ProductSafety@springernature.com

In case Publisher is established outside the EU, the EU authorized representative is:

Springer Nature Customer Service Center GmbH
Europaplatz 3
69115 Heidelberg, Germany

Batch number: 10704763

Printed by Printforce, the Netherlands